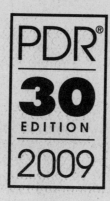

PDR® 30 EDITION 2009

PDR®

for Nonprescription Drugs, Dietary Supplements, and Herbs

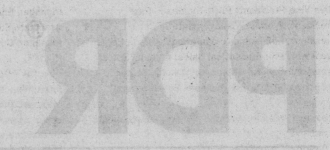

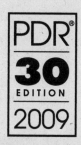

PDR®

for Nonprescription Drugs,
Dietary Supplements, and Herbs

Executive Vice President, PDR: Thomas F. Rice
Vice President, Product Management: Cy Caine
Vice President, Publishing & Operations: Valerie Berger
Vice President, Pharmaceutical Sales: Anthony Sorce
Vice President, Clinical Relations: Mukesh Mehta, RPh
Vice President, Strategy & Business Development:
Ray Zoeller
Vice President, Manufacturing & Vendor Management:
Brian Holland
Senior Director, Copy Sales: Bill Gaffney
Senior Product Manager: Ilyaas Meeran
Solutions Manager: Corey Stone
Director of Sales: Eileen Bruno
Account Manager: Nick W. Clark
Sales Associate: Janet Wallendal

Senior Director, Editorial & Publishing: Bette LaGow
Senior Director, Client Services: Stephanie Struble
Manager, Clinical Services: Nermin Shenouda, PharmD
Drug Information Specialists: Anila Patel, PharmD;
Christine Sunwoo, PharmD; Greg Tallis, RPh

Manager, Editorial Services: Lori Murray
Associate Editors: Sabina Borza, Jennifer Reed
Manager, Customer Service: Todd Taccetta

Director, PDR Production: Jeffrey D. Schaefer
Production Manager, PDR: Steven Maher
Manager, Production Purchasing: Thomas Westburgh
Senior Print Production Manager: Dawn Dubovich
Index Supervisor: Noel Deloughery
Index Editor: Allison O'Hare
Format Editor: Alex Nowalk
Senior Production Coordinator: Yasmin Hernández
Production Coordinators: Eric Udina, Christopher Whalen
Vendor Management Specialist: Gary Lew

Manager, Art Department: Livio Udina
Electronic Publishing Designers: Deana DiVizio,
Carrie Faeth
Digital Imaging Manager: Christopher Husted
Digital Imaging Coordinator: Michael Labruyere

ISBN: 978-1-56363-705-6

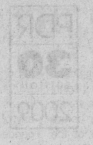

FOREWORD TO THE 30TH EDITION

Physicians' Desk Reference® has been providing unparalleled drug information to doctors and other healthcare professionals for more than 60 years. The variety of *PDR*® reference options is larger than ever before and available in more formats—in print, on CD, on the Internet, and for PDA.

PDR® *for Nonprescription Drugs, Dietary Supplements, and Herbs* features five indices and a full-color Product Identification Guide followed by two distinct sections of product information. The first of these, entitled *Nonprescription Drug Information*, presents manufacturer-supplied labeling of products marketed in compliance with the Code of Federal Regulations labeling requirements for OTC drugs.

The other product section, *Dietary and Herbal Supplement Information*, contains manufacturer-supplied labeling for nutritional supplements and herbal remedies. Please note that these products are marketed under the Dietary Supplement Health and Education Act of 1994 and therefore have not been evaluated by the Food and Drug Administration. Such products are not intended to diagnose, treat, cure, or prevent any disease.

The five indices in the book contain manufacturer contact information, product names, prescribing categories, active ingredients, and a listing of "companion" OTC drugs that may be recommended to relieve symptoms caused by prescription drug therapy.

This book also includes product comparison tables that cover various OTC therapeutic categories—including cough, cold, and flu products—allowing for easy comparison of active ingredients, drug strengths, and dosages.

About This Book

PDR® *for Nonprescription Drugs, Dietary Supplements, and Herbs* is published annually by Thomson Reuters. The book is made possible through the courtesy of the manufacturers whose products appear in it. The information on each product described in the book has been prepared by the manufacturer and edited and approved by the manufacturer's medical department, medical director, or medical counsel. The function of the publisher is the compilation, organization, and distribution of this information. During compilation of this information, the publisher has emphasized the necessity of describing products comprehensively in order to provide all the facts necessary for sound and intelligent decision-making. Descriptions seen here include all information made available by the manufacturer.

In organizing and presenting the material in *PDR*® *for Nonprescription Drugs, Dietary Supplements, and Herbs*, the publisher does not warrant or guarantee any of the products described, or perform any independent analysis in connection with any of the product information contained herein. *Physicians' Desk Reference*® does not assume, and expressly disclaims, any obligation to obtain and include any information other than that provided by the manufacturer. It should be understood that by making this material available the publisher is not advocating the use of any product described herein, nor is the publisher responsible for misuse of a product due to typographical error. Additional information on any product may be obtained from the manufacturer.

Web-Based Clinical Resources

PDR.net, a web portal designed specifically for healthcare professionals, provides a wealth of clinical information, including both full FDA-approved labeling as well as concise drug information, disease monographs, specialty-specific resource centers, patient education, clinical news, and conference information. PDR.net gives prescribers online access to authoritative, evidence-based information they need to support or confirm diagnosis and treatment decisions, including:

- Daily feeds of specialty news, conference coverage, and monthly summaries

- FDA-approved and other manufacturer-provided product labeling for more than 4,000 brand-name drugs

- Full-size product images

- Concise drug information

- Multidrug interaction checker and other tools

- Extensive disease diagnosis and treatment information

- Patient education

- Medical dictionary

- Clinical trial listings

- Professional resources

PDR.net is also home to our **Clinical Resource Centers**, giving you medical news and disease information all in one place. Log on to *www.PDR.net* to learn more about these clinical specialties:

- Allergy and Immunology

- Breast Cancer

- Cardiology
- Dermatology
- Diabetes and Endocrinology
- Nephrology
- Neurology
- Pediatrics
- Psychiatry
- Pulmonology
- Rheumatology
- Urology
- Women's Health
- And more

Online access is **free** for U.S.-based MDs, DOs, dentists, NPs, and PAs in full-time patient practice, as well as for medical students, residents, and other select prescribing allied health professionals. Register today at *www.PDR.net*.

Other Products from PDR

For counseling patients who favor herbal remedies, the newly updated **PDR® for Herbal Medicines Fourth Edition** provides you with evidence-based assessments of more than 700 botanicals. Indexed by scientific and common names (as well as Western, Asian, and homeopathic indications), this volume also includes a Side Effects Index, a Drug/Herb Interactions Guide, an Herb Identification Guide with nearly 400 color photos, and a Safety Guide that lists herbs to be avoided during pregnancy and herbs to be used only under professional supervision. Although botanical products are not officially regulated or monitored in the United States, *PDR for Herbal Medicines* provides you with authoritative information—the findings of the German Regulatory Authority's expert committee on herbal medicines, Commission E.

For more information on these or any other members of the growing family of *PDR* products, please call, toll-free, 800-232-7379 or fax 201-722-2680, or visit *PDRbookstore.com*.

HOW TO USE THIS BOOK

The 2009 edition of *PDR® for Nonprescription Drugs, Dietary Supplements, and Herbs* features a format designed to help you find the information you need as quickly and easily as possible. Now, in addition to consulting the five indices, you can go directly to a specific product comparison table to find the relevant over-the-counter (OTC) products for a particular condition. Details of this organization are outlined below.

FIVE INDICES

- **Manufacturers' Index** lists all pharmaceutical manufacturers that provided OTC drug labeling for this edition. Each entry contains addresses, phone numbers, and emergency contacts, as well as a listing of that manufacturer's products and the corresponding page numbers for labeling information.

- **Product Name Index** provides the page number of each product description in the Nonprescription Drug Information and Dietary and Herbal Supplement Information sections. Listings appear alphabetically by brand name.

- **Product Category Index** lists all fully described products according to therapeutic or pharmaceutical drug category (eg, acetaminophen combinations).

- **Active Ingredients Index** contains product cross-references by generic ingredient.

- **Companion Drug Index** lists OTC products that may be used in conjunction with prescription drug therapy to relieve symptoms of a particular condition or drug-induced side effects.

PRODUCT IDENTIFICATION GUIDE
Organized alphabetically by manufacturer name. This section shows full-color, actual-sized photos of tablets and capsules, plus a variety of other dosage forms and packages.

NONPRESCRIPTION DRUG INFORMATION
Organized alphabetically by manufacturer name. The product labeling in this section includes brand-name OTC drugs and other medical products marketed for home use. **Please keep in mind that the product information included herein is valid as of press time (July 2008).** Additional information, as well as updates to the product labeling, can be obtained from the manufacturer.

DIETARY AND HERBAL SUPPLEMENT INFORMATION
Organized alphabetically by manufacturer name. This section contains product labeling for dietary and herbal supplements marketed under the Dietary Supplement Health and Education Act of 1994. Be aware that these products are not federally regulated and are not intended to diagnose, treat, cure, or prevent any disease.

PRODUCT COMPARISON TABLES
Organized alphabetically by therapeutic category and brand name. These tables provide a quick and easy way to compare the active ingredients and dosages of common brand-name OTC drugs. In all, 24 therapeutic categories are covered, including antacid and heartburn agents; laxatives; and cough, cold, and flu products.

CONTENTS

SECTION 1

MANUFACTURERS' INDEX

This index lists manufacturers that have supplied information for this edition. Each company's entry includes the address, phone, and fax number of its headquarters and regional offices, as well as company contacts for inquiries, orders, and emergency information.

Products with entries in the Nonprescription Drug Information section are listed with their page numbers under the heading "OTC Products Described." Products with entries in the Dietary Supplement Information section are listed with their page numbers under the

heading "Dietary Supplements Described." Other OTC products and dietary supplements available from the manufacturer follow these two sections.

If an entry in the index lists multiple page numbers, the first one shown refers to the photograph of the product, the last one to its prescribing information.

- The ◆ symbol marks drugs shown in the Product Identification Guide.

- *Italic page numbers* signify partial information.

A&Z PHARMACEUTICAL INC.   **624**
180 Oser Avenue, Suite 300
Hauppauge, NY 11788
Direct Inquiries to:
(631) 952-3800

Dietary Supplements Described:
D-Cal Chewable Caplets **624**

AWARENESS   **503, 624**
CORPORATION/dba
AWARENESS LIFE
25 South Arizona Place, Suite 500
Chandler, AZ 85225
Direct Inquiries to:
800-69AWARE
www.awarenesslife.net

Dietary Supplements Described:
Awareness Clear Capsules **624**
◆ Awareness Female Balance **503, 624**
◆ Daily Complete Liquid............ **503, 624**
◆ Experience Capsules **503, 624**
Pure Gardens Cream **624**
◆ PureTrim Mediterranean
    Wellness Shake.............. **503, 624**
◆ SynergyDefense Capsules **503, 625**

BEACH PHARMACEUTICALS   **625**
Division of Beach Products, Inc.
EXECUTIVE OFFICE:
5220 South Manhattan Avenue
Tampa, FL 33611
Direct Inquiries to:
Richard Stephen Jenkins, Executive V.P.:
(813) 839-6565
Clete Harmon, Senior V.P., Regulatory and
Business Affairs:
(864) 277-7282

Manufacturing and Distribution:
1700 Perimeter Road
Greenville, SC 29605
(800) 845-8210

Dietary Supplements Described:
Beelith Tablets......................... **625**

BOEHRINGER   **503, 602**
INGELHEIM
CONSUMER HEALTH
CARE PRODUCTS
Division of Boehringer Ingelheim
Pharmaceuticals, Inc.
900 Ridgebury Road
P.O. Box 368
Ridgefield, CT 06877
Direct Inquiries to:
(888) 285-9159

OTC Products Described:
◆ Dulcolax Stool Softener.......... **503, 602**
◆ Dulcolax Suppositories **503, 602**
◆ Dulcolax Tablets **503, 602**
◆ Zantac 75 Tablets **503, 603**
◆ Maximum Strength Zantac
    150 Tablets................. **503, 603**
◆ Maximum Strength Zantac
    150 Cool Mint Tablets **503, 603**

BOIRON   **503, 604**
6 Campus Blvd.
Newtown Square, PA 19073-3267
Direct Inquiries to:
Boiron Information Center
info@boironusa.com
(800) BOIRON-1 (800-264-7661)
www.boironusa.com

OTC Products Described:
◆ Oscillococcinum **503, 604**

J. R. CARLSON   **625**
LABORATORIES, INC.
15 College Drive
Arlington Heights, IL 60004-1985
Direct Inquiries to:
Customer Service
(888) 234-5656
FAX: (847) 255-1605
www.carlsonlabs.com
For Medical Information Contact:
In Emergencies:
Customer Service
(888) 234-5656
FAX: (847) 255-1605

Dietary Supplements Described:
E-Gems Soft Gels..................... *625*
Med Omega Fish Oil 2800 .... **625**
Norwegian Cod Liver Oil *625*
Super Omega-3 Softgels............... *626*

DOCTOR'S HEALTH   **503, 604**
SUPPLY
2335 Camino Vida Robles
Building B
Carlsbad, CA 92011
Direct Inquiries to:
(760) 431-8047
Fax: (760) 431-0126
www.lifeionizers.com
www.lifedetoxpatch.com

OTC Products Described:
◆ Life Detox Patches............... *503, 604*
◆ Life Ionizer 7500 .... *503, 604*

ENIVA NUTRACEUTICS   503, 626

9702 Ulysses Street NE
Minneapolis, MN 55434
Direct Inquiries to:
(763) 795-8870
FAX: (763) 795-8890
www.eniva.com

Dietary Supplements Described:
◆ Efacor Dietary Supplement **503, 626**
◆ Vibe Liquid Multi-Nutrient
   Supplement **503, 626**

FLEET LABORATORIES   503, 605

Division of C. B. Fleet Company,
Incorporated
Lynchburg, VA 24502
Direct Inquiries to:
Sherrie McNamara, RN, MSN, MBA
Director of Medical Affairs and Product
Safety
(866) 255-6960

OTC Products Described:
◆ Fleet Pedia-Lax Chewable
   Tablets **503, 606**
◆ Fleet Pedia-Lax Enema.......... **503, 606**
◆ Fleet Pedia-Lax Liquid Stool
   Softener...................... **503, 605**
◆ Fleet Pedia-Lax Liquid
   Suppositories................ **504, 605**
◆ Fleet Pedia-Lax Senna Quick
   Dissolve Strips............... **503, 607**
◆ Fleet Pedia-Lax Suppositories ... **504, 605**

4LIFE RESEARCH USA, LLC   628

9850 South 300 West
Sandy, UT 84070
Direct Inquiries to:
(801) 562-3600
FAX: (801) 562-3699
productsupport@4life.com
www.4life.com

Dietary Supplements Described:
4Life Transfer Factor Plus
   Tri-Factor Formula.................. **628**

Other Products Available:
4Life Transfer Factor Belle Vie
4Life Transfer Factor Cardio
4Life Transfer Factor Chewable
4Life Transfer Factor GluCoach
4Life Transfer Factor Immune Spray
4Life Transfer Factor Kids
4Life Transfer Factor MalePro
4Life Transfer Factor ReCall
4Life Transfer Factor RenewAll
4Life Transfer Factor RioVida
4Life Transfer Factor Toothpaste
4Life Transfer Factor Tri-Factor Formula
enummi Face with Transfer Factor E-XF

GREEK ISLAND LABS   628

7620 East McKellips Road
Suite 4 PMB 86
Scottsdale, AZ 85257
Direct Inquiries to:
www.greekislandlabs.com
(888) 841-7363

Dietary Supplements Described:
Natural Joint Capsules **628**
Prostate Complete Dietary
   Supplement....................... *628*

GREEN PHARMACEUTICALS INC.,   607

591 Constitution Ave., #A
Camarillo, CA 93012
**Direct Inquiries and Medical
Emergencies to:**
mail@snorestop.com or
(800) 337-4835

OTC Products Described:
SnoreStop Extinguisher 120 Oral
   Spray **607**
SnoreStop Maximum Strength
   Chewable Tablets.................. **607**

HISAMITSU PHARMACEUTICAL CO., INC.   504, 608

408 Tashiro Daikan-Machi
Tosu Saga 841-0017
Japan
Direct Inquiries to:
+81-3-5293-1720
Fax: +81-3-5293-1724

OTC Products Described:
Salonpas Aqua-Patch.................. **610**
◆ Salonpas Arthritis Pain
   Patches **504, 608**
Salonpas Gel **609**
Salonpas Gel-Patch Hot Soothing **609**
Salonpas-Hot Patch................... **609**
◆ Salonpas Pain Relief Patch...... **504, 608**

HYLAND'S, INC.

(See STANDARD HOMEOPATHIC
COMPANY)

LEGACY FOR LIFE, LLC   629

P.O. Box 410376
Melbourne, FL 32941-0376
Direct Inquiries to:
(800) 557-8477
(321) 951-8815
Technical Inquiries:
(800) 746-0300
info@legacyforlife.net
www.legacyforlife.net

Dietary Supplements Described:
i26 Capsules **629**
i26 Chewable Tablets.................. **629**

MEMORY SECRET   504, 629

1221 Brickell Avenue
Suite 1540
Miami, FL 33131
Direct Inquiries to:
(866) 673-2738
FAX: (305) 675-2279
E-mail: intelectol@memorysecret.net
www.intelectol.com

Dietary Supplements Described:
◆ Intelectol Tablets **504, 629**

MERZ PHARMACEUTICALS   610

Division of Merz, Inc.
4215 Tudor Lane (27410)
P.O Box 18806
Greensboro, NC 27419
Direct Inquiries to:
Medical/Regulatory Affairs
(336) 856-2003
FAX: (336) 217-2439

For Medical Information Contact:
In Emergencies:
Medical/Regulatory Affairs
(336) 856-2003
FAX: (336) 217-2439

OTC Products Described:
Mederma Cream Plus SPF 30 .... **610**

MISSION PHARMACAL COMPANY   610

10999 IH 10 West, Suite 1000
San Antonio, TX 78230-1355
Direct All Inquiries to:
P.O. Box 786099
San Antonio, TX 78278-6099
(800) 292-7364 Customer Service
(M-F 8:30 - 5 C.S.T.)
(210) 696-8400
FAX: (210) 696-6010

OTC Products Described:
Thera-Gesic Creme **610**

Dietary Supplements Described:
Calcet Triple Calcium + Vitamin D
   Tablets............................ **629**

Other Products Available:
Calcet Plus Multivitamin/Mineral Tablets
CitraNatal DHA (Tablets + Capsules)
CitraNatal 90 DHA (Tablets + Capsules)
CitraNatal Rx Tablets
Compete Multivitamin/Mineral Tablets
Fosfree Multivitamin/Mineral Tablets
Iromin-G Multivitamin/Mineral Tablets
Maxilube Personal Lubricant
Mission Prenatal Tablets
Mission Prenatal F.A. Tablets
Mission Prenatal H.P. Tablets
Oncovite Tablets
Thera-Gesic Plus Creme

NOSMO CO., LTD.   630

8414 Dong-Eui Institute of Technology,
San72
Yangjung-Dong, Busanjin-Gu,
Busan
South Korea
Direct Inquiries to:
+82-51-851-7688
www.nosmo.co.kr

Dietary Supplements Described:
NoSmo[King] Stop Smoking Aid **630**

PROCTER & GAMBLE   504, 611

P.O. Box 559
Cincinnati, OH 45201
Direct Inquiries to:
Consumer Relations
(800) 832-3064

Dietary Supplements Described:
Metamucil Capsules................... **611**
Metamucil Powder, Original
   Texture Orange Flavor............. **611**
Metamucil Powder, Original
   Texture Regular Flavor **611**
Metamucil Smooth Texture
   Powder, Orange Flavor............. **611**
◆ Metamucil Smooth Texture
   Powder, Sugar-Free,
   Orange Flavor **504, 611**
Metamucil Smooth Texture
   Powder, Sugar-Free, Regular
   Flavor **611**
Metamucil Wafers, Apple Crisp &
   Cinnamon Spice Flavors........... **611**
◆ Pepto-Bismol Original Liquid,
   Original and Cherry
   Chewable Tablets &
   Caplets **504, 613**

REESE   504, 618
PHARMACEUTICAL
COMPANY

10617 Frank Avenue
Cleveland, OH 44106
Direct Inquiries to:
Voice: (800) 321-7178
FAX: (216) 231-6444
george@reesechemical.com
www.reesepharmaceutical.com

OTC Products Described:
◆ Reese's Pinworm Treatments ...**504, 618**

Other Products Available:
Dentapaine Oral Pain Reliever
Double Tussin DM Intense Strength
    Cough Reliever
Licide Lice-Eliminating Products
ReAzo Urinary Health Products
Refenesen Chest Congestion Relief
    Products

STANDARD HOMEOPATHIC   618
COMPANY

Hyland's
210 West 131st Street
Box 61067
Los Angeles, CA 90061
Direct Inquiries to:
Jay Borneman
(800) 624-9659, Ext. 20

OTC Products Described:
Hyland's BackAche with Arnica
    Caplets **618**
Hyland's Calms Forté Tablets and
    Caplets **618**
Hyland's Calms Forté 4 Kids
    Tablets............................**619**
Hyland's Colic Tablets **619**
Hyland's Cough Syrup with Honey.....**619**
Hyland's Earache Drops..............**619**

STATACOR BIOSCIENCES   632

133 Rollins Avenue
Rockville, MD 20852
Direct Inquiries to:
(888) 782-8226

Dietary Supplements Described:
Omega 3-10 Softgels **632**

TAHITIAN NONI   504, 632
INTERNATIONAL

333 West River Park Drive
Provo, UT 84604
Direct Inquiries to:
(801) 234-1000
www.tahitiannoni.com

Dietary Supplements Described:
◆ Tahitian Noni Leaf Serum
    Soothing Gel **504, 632**
◆ Tahitian Noni Liquid..............**504, 633**
◆ Tahitian Noni Seed Oil **504, 634**

TOPICAL BIOMEDICS,   504, 621
INC.

P.O. Box 494
Rhinebeck, NY 12572-0494
Direct Inquiries to:
Professional Services
(845) 871-4900 ex 1115
FAX: (845) 876-0818
info@topicalbiomedics.com

OTC Products Described:
◆ Topricin Pain Relief and
    Healing Cream **504, 621**

UAS LABORATORIES   634

9953 Valley View Road
Eden Prairie, MN 55344
Direct Inquiries to:
Dr. S.K. Dash
(952) 935-1707
FAX: (952) 935-1650

Dietary Supplements Described:
DDS-Acidophilus Capsules,
    Tablets, and Powder **634**

Other Products Available:
DDS Plus/Multiflora ABF Vegie Capsules
    in 5 Billion Potency
Probioplus DDS Vegie Capsules in 10
    Billion Potency

UPSHER-SMITH   622
LABORATORIES, INC

6701 Evenstad Drive
Maple Grove, MN 55369
Direct Inquiries to:
Medical Information:
(800) 654-2299

OTC Products Described:
Amlactin AP Anti-Itch Moisturizing
    Cream *622*
Amlactin Moisturizing Body Lotion
    and Cream.......................*622*
Amlactin XL Moisturizing Lotion *622*

WELLNESS INTERNATIONAL   634
NETWORK, LTD.

5800 Democracy Drive
Plano, TX 75024
Direct Inquiries to:
Product Inquiries
(972) 312-1100
E-mail: winproducts@winltd.com

Branch Offices:
WIN Worldwide BV
Kruisweg 583-2132 NA
Hoofdoorp, Netherlands

Wellness International Network S.A.
(Pty) Ltd.
Old Mutual Building
1 Nicol Grove
Nicol Grove Office Park
Fourways, Johannesburg, South Africa

WIN Worldwide Mexico, S. de R.L. de C.V.
Av. Lázaro Cárdenas 2321 Pte.
Piso 3-HQ
Residencial San Agustín
San Pedro Garza García
Nuevo Léon, México 66260

Dietary Supplements Described:
Accelerator Tablets **634**
BioLean Free Tablets **635**
BioLean II Tablets.......................**635**
Clarity Capsules **636**
DHEA Plus Tablets **636**
Elasticity Capsules **636**
Elixir Capsules..........................**636**
Essential Capsules **637**
Feminine Capsules **637**
Flexibility Capsules **637**
Food For Thought Dietary
    Supplement........................**637**
LipoTrim Capsules **638**
Lovpil Capsules.........................**638**
Masculine Capsules **638**
Mass Appeal Tablets **638**
Phyto-Vite Tablets......................**639**
Protector Capsules **639**
ProXtreme Protein Supplement........**639**
Relief Capsules.........................**640**
Satieté Tablets.........................**640**
Sleep-Tite Caplets **640**
Sure2Endure Tablets **641**
Tranquility Capsules **641**
WIN CoQ10 Gelcaps **641**
WINOmeg3complex Gelcaps..........**642**
Winrgy Dietary Supplement...........**642**

SECTION 2

PRODUCT NAME INDEX

This index includes all entries in the Product Information sections. Products are listed alphabetically by brand name.

If an entry in the index lists multiple page numbers, the first one shown refers to the photograph of the product, the last one to its prescribing information.

- **Bold page numbers** indicate that the entry contains full product information.

- *Italic page numbers* signify partial information.

SECTION 3

PRODUCT CATEGORY INDEX

This index cross-references each brand by pharmaceutical category. All fully described products in the Product Information sections are included.

If an entry in the index lists multiple page numbers, the first one shown refers to the photograph of the product, the last one to its prescribing information.

The classification of each product is determined by the publisher in cooperation with the product's manufacturer or, when necessary, by the publisher alone.

SECTION 4

ACTIVE INGREDIENTS INDEX

This index cross-references each brand by its generic ingredients. All entries in the Product Information sections are included. Under each generic heading, all fully described products are listed first, followed by those with only partial descriptions.

If an entry in the index lists multiple page numbers, the first one shown refers to the photograph of the product, the last one to its prescribing information.

- **Bold page numbers** indicate full product information.

- *Italic page numbers* signify partial information.

Classification of products under these headings has been determined in cooperation with the products' manufacturers or, if necessary, by the publisher alone.

Italic Page Number **Indicates Brief Listing**

Italic Page Number **Indicates Brief Listing**

SECTION 5

COMPANION DRUG INDEX

This index is a quick-reference guide to OTC products that may be used in conjunction with prescription drug therapy to reverse drug-induced side effects, relieve symptoms of the illness itself, or treat sequelae of the initial disease. All entries are derived from the FDA-approved prescribing information published by *PDR*.

The products listed are generally considered effective for temporary symptomatic relief. They may not, however, be appropriate for sustained therapy, and each case must be approached on an individual basis. Certain common side effects may be harbingers of more serious reactions. When making a recommendation, be sure to adjust for the patient's age, concurrent medical conditions, and complete drug regimen. Consider timing as well, since simul-

taneous ingestion may not be recommended in all instances.

Please note that only products fully described in *Physicians' Desk Reference* and its companion volumes are included in this index. The publisher therefore cannot guarantee that all entries are totally accurate or complete. Keep in mind, too, that although a given OTC product is usually an appropriate companion for an entire class of prescription medications, certain drugs within the class may be exceptions. If you have any doubt about the suitability of a particular OTC product in a given situation, be sure to check the underlying *PDR* prescribing information and the relevant medical literature.

HYPERTHYROIDISM, NUTRIENTS DEFICIENCY SECONDARY TO

Hyperthyroidism may be treated with methimazole or propylthiouracil. The following products may be recommended for relief of nutrients deficiency:

HYPOKALEMIA

May result from the use of corticosteroids, diuretics, thiazides, aldesleukin, amphotericin b, carboplatin, foscarnet sodium, mycophenolate mofetil, pamidronate disodium or tacrolimus. The following products may be recommended:

HYPOMAGNESEMIA

May result from the use of aldesleukin, aminoglycosides, amphotericin b, caroboplatin, cisplatin, cyclosporine, diuretics, foscarnet, pamidronate, sargramostim or tacrolimus. The following products may be recommended:

HYPOPARATHYROIDISM

May be treated with vitamin d sterols. The following products may be recommended for relief of symptoms:

HYPOTHYROIDISM, CONSTIPATION SECONDARY TO

Hypothyroidism may be treated with thyroid hormones. The following products may be recommended for relief of constipation:

INFECTIONS, BACTERIAL, UPPER RESPIRATORY TRACT

May be treated with amoxicillin-clavulanate, cephalosporins, doxycycline, erythromycin, macrolide antibiotics, penicillins or minocycline hydrochloride. The following products may be recommended for relief of symptoms:

IRRITABLE BOWEL SYNDROME

May be treated with 5-ht3 receptor antagonists, anticholinergic and combinations, dicyclomine hydrochloride or hyoscyamine sulfate. The following products may be recommended for relief of symptoms:

NASAL POLYPS, RHINORRHEA SECONDARY TO

Nasal polyps may be treated with nasal steroidal anti-inflammatory agents. The following products may be recommended for relief of rhinorrhea:

OSTEOPOROSIS

May be treated with biphosphonates, calcitonin or estrogens. The following products may be recommended for relief of symptoms:

OSTEOPOROSIS, SECONDARY

May result from the use of chemotherapeutic agents, phenytoin, prolonged glucocorticoid therapy, thyroid hormones, carbamazepine, heparin or methotrexate sodium. The following products may be recommended:

OTITIS MEDIA, ACUTE

May be treated with amoxicillin, amoxicillin-clavulanate, cephalosporins, erythromycin-sulfisoxazole, macrolide antibiotics or sulfamethoxazole-trimethoprim. The following products may be recommended for relief of symptoms:

PANCREATIC INSUFFICIENCY, NUTRIENTS DEFICIENCY SECONDARY TO

Pancreatic insufficiency may be treated with pancrelipase. The following products may be recommended for relief of nutrients deficiency:

PARKINSON'S DISEASE, CONSTIPATION SECONDARY TO

Parkinson's disease may be treated with COMT inhibitors, centrally active anticholinergic agents, dopaminergic agents, selective inhibitor of mao type b, carbidopa or levodopa. The following products may be recommended for relief of constipation:

PEPTIC ULCER DISEASE

May be treated with histamine h2 receptor antagonists, proton pump inhibitors or sucralfate. The following products may be recommended for relief of symptoms:

PHARYNGITIS

May be treated with cephalosporins, macrolide antibiotics or penicillins. The following products may be recommended for relief of symptoms:

RENAL OSTEODYSTROPHY, HYPOCALCEMIA SECONDARY TO

Renal osteodystrophy may be treated with vitamin d sterols. The following products may be recommended for relief of hypocalcemia:

RESPIRATORY TRACT ILLNESS, INFLUENZA A VIRUS-INDUCED

May be treated with amantadine hydrochloride, oseltamivir phosphate or rimantadine hydrochloride. The following products may be recommended for relief of symptoms:

RHEUMATOID ARTHRITIS, KERATOCONJUNCTIVITIS SICCA SECONDARY TO

Rheumatoid arthritis may be treated with biologicals, corticosteroids, nonsteroidal anti-inflammatory drugs or azathioprine. The following products may be recommended for relief of keratoconjunctivitis sicca:

RHINITIS, NONALLERGIC

May be treated with nasal steroids or ipratropium bromide. The following products may be recommended for relief of symptoms:

SINUSITIS

May be treated with amoxicillin, amoxicillin-clavulanate, cefprozil, cefuroxime axetil or clarithromycin. The following products may be recommended for relief of symptoms:

SKIN IRRITATION

May result from the use of transdermal drug delivery systems. The following products may be recommended:

TUBERCULOSIS, NUTRIENTS DEFICIENCY SECONDARY TO

Tuberculosis may be treated with capreomycin sulfate, ethambutol hydrochloride, ethionamide, isoniazid, pyrazinamide, rifampin or streptomycin sulfate. The following products may be recommended for relief of nutrients deficiency:

XERODERMA

May result from the use of aldesleukin, protease inhibitors, retinoids, topical acne preparations, topical corticosteroids, topical retinoids, benzoyl peroxide, clofazimine, interferon alfa-2a, recombinant, interferon alfa-2b, recombinant or pentostatin. The following products may be recommended:

POISON CONTROL CENTERS

The American Association of Poison Control Centers (AAPCC) uses a single, nationwide emergency number to automatically link callers with their regional poison center. This toll-free number, **800-222-1222**, also works for **teletype lines (TTY)** for the hearing-impaired and **telecommunication devices (TTD)** for individuals who are deaf. However, a few local poison centers and the ASPCA/Animal Poison Control Center are not part of this nationwide system and continue to use separate numbers.

Most of the centers listed below are certified by the AAPCC. **Certified centers are marked by an asterisk after the name.**

Each has to meet certain criteria. It must, for example, serve a large geographic area; it must be open 24 hours a day and provide direct-dial or toll-free access; it must be supervised by a medical director; and it must have registered pharmacists or nurses available to answer questions from the public.

Within each state, centers are listed alphabetically by city. Some state poison centers also list their original emergency numbers (including TTY/TDD), which only work within that state. For these listings, callers may use either the state number or the nationwide 800 number.

ALABAMA

BIRMINGHAM
Regional Poison Control Center, The Children's Hospital of Alabama (*)

1600 7th Ave. South
Birmingham, AL 35233-1711
Business: 205-939-9201
Emergency: 800-222-1222
www.chsys.org

TUSCALOOSA
Alabama Poison Center (*)

2503 Phoenix Dr.
Tuscaloosa, AL 35405
Business: 205-345-0600
Emergency: 800-222-1222
800-462-0800 (AL)
www.alapoisoncenter.org

ALASKA

JUNEAU
Alaska Poison Control System

Section of Community
Health and EMS
410 Willoughby Ave.
Room 103
Box 110616
Juneau, AK 99811-0616
Business: 907-465-3027
Emergency: 800-222-1222
www.chems.alaska.gov

(PORTLAND, OR)
**Oregon Poison Center (*)
Oregon Health Sciences University**

3181 SW Sam Jackson Park Rd.
CB550
Portland, OR 97239
Business: 503-494-8968
Emergency: 800-222-1222
www.oregonpoison.com

ARIZONA

PHOENIX
**Banner Poison Control Center (*)
Banner Good Samaritan Medical Center**

901 E. Willetta St.
Room 2701
Phoenix, AZ 85006
Business: 602-495-4884
Emergency: 800-222-1222
www.bannerpoisoncontrol.com

TUCSON
Arizona Poison and Drug Information Center

1295 N. Martin Ave.
Drachman Hall B308
Tucson, AZ 85724
Business: 520-626-7899
Emergency: 800-222-1222

ARKANSAS

LITTLE ROCK
Arkansas Poison and Drug Information Center College of Pharmacy - UAMS

4301 West Markham St.
Mail Slot 522-2
Little Rock, AR 72205-7122
Business: 501-686-6161
Emergency: 800-222-1222
800-376-4766 (AR)
TDD/TTY: 800-641-3805

ASPCA/Animal Poison Control Center

1717 South Philo Rd.
Suite 36
Urbana, IL 61802
Business: 217-337-5030
Emergency: 888-426-4435
800-548-2423
www.napcc.aspca.org

CALIFORNIA

FRESNO/MADERA
**California Poison Control System-Fresno/Madera Div. (*)
Children's Hospital of Central California**

9300 Valley Children's Place
MB 15
Madera, CA 93638-8762
Business: 559-622-2300
Emergency: 800-222-1222
800-876-4766 (CA)
TDD/TTY: 800-972-3323
www.calpoison.org

SACRAMENTO
**California Poison Control System-Sacramento Div.(*)
UC Davis Medical Center**

Room HSF 1024
2315 Stockton Blvd.
Sacramento, CA 95817
Business: 916-227-1400
Emergency: 800-222-1222
800-876-4766 (CA)
TDD/TTY: 800-972-3323
www.calpoison.org

SAN DIEGO
**California Poison Control System-San Diego Div. (*)
UC San Diego Medical Center**

200 West Arbor Dr.
San Diego, CA 92103-8925
Business: 858-715-6300
Emergency: 800-222-1222
800-876-4766 (CA)
TDD/TTY: 800-972-3323
www.calpoison.org

SAN FRANCISCO
**California Poison Control System-San Francisco Div. (*)
San Francisco General Hospital University of California San Francisco**

Box 1369
San Francisco, CA 94143-1369
Business: 415-502-6000
Emergency: 800-222-1222
800-876-4766 (CA)
TDD/TTY: 800-972-3323
www.calpoison.org

COLORADO

DENVER
Rocky Mountain Poison and Drug Center (*)

777 Bannock St.
Mail Code 0180
Denver, CO 80204-4507
Business: 303-739-1100
Emergency: 800-222-1222
TDD/TTY: 303-739-1127 (CO)
www.RMPDC.org

CONNECTICUT

FARMINGTON
**Connecticut Regional Poison Control Center (*)
University of Connecticut Health Center**

263 Farmington Ave.
Farmington, CT 06030-5365
Business: 860-679-4540
Emergency: 800-222-1222
TDD/TTY: 866-218-5372
http://poisoncontrol.uchc.edu

DELAWARE

(PHILADELPHIA, PA)
**The Poison Control Center (*)
Children's Hospital of Philadelphia**

34th St. & Civic Center Blvd.
Philadelphia, PA 19104-4303
Business: 215-590-2003
Emergency: 800-222-1222
TDD/TTY: 215-590-8789
www.poisoncontrol.chop.edu

DISTRICT OF COLUMBIA

WASHINGTON, DC
National Capital Poison Center (*)

3201 New Mexico Ave., NW
Suite 310
Washington, DC 20016
Business: 202-362-3867
Emergency: 800-222-1222
www.poison.org

FLORIDA

JACKSONVILLE

Florida Poison Information
Center-Jacksonville (*)
SHANDS Hospital

655 West 8th St.
Jacksonville, FL 32209
Business: 904-244-4465
Emergency: 800-222-1222
http://fpicjax.org

MIAMI

Florida Poison Information
Center-Miami (*)
University of Miami–
Department of Pediatrics

PO Box 016960 (R-131)
Miami, FL 33101
Business: 305-585-5250
Emergency: 800-222-1222
www.miami.edu/poison-center

TAMPA

Florida Poison
Information Center-Tampa (*)
Tampa General Hospital

PO Box 1289
Tampa, FL 33601-1289
Business: 813-844-7044
Emergency: 800-222-1222
www.poisoncentertampa.org

GEORGIA

ATLANTA

Georgia Poison Center (*)
Hughes Spalding Children's
Hospital, Grady Health System

80 Jesse Hill Jr. Dr., SE
PO Box 26066
Atlanta, GA 30303-3050
Business: 404-616-9237
Emergency: 800-222-1222
                404-616-9000
                (Atlanta)
TDD: 404-616-9287
www.georgiapoisoncenter.org

HAWAII

(DENVER, CO)

Rocky Mountain Poison
and Drug Center (*)

777 Bannock St.
Mail Code 0180
Denver, CO 80204-4507
Business: 303-739-1100
Emergency: 800-222-1222
www.RMPDC.org

IDAHO

(DENVER, CO)

Rocky Mountain Poison
and Drug Center (*)

777 Bannock St.
Mail Code 0180
Denver, CO 80204-4507
Business: 303-739-1100
Emergency: 800-222-1222
www.RMPDC.org

ILLINOIS

CHICAGO

Illinois Poison Center (*)

222 South Riverside Plaza
Suite 1900
Chicago, IL 60606
Business: 312-906-6136
Emergency: 800-222-1222
TDD/TTY: 312-906-6185
www.illinoispoisoncenter.org

INDIANA

INDIANAPOLIS

Indiana Poison Control Center (*)
Clarian Health Partners
Methodist Hospital

I-65 at 21st St.
Indianapolis, IN 46206-1367
Business: 317-962-2335
Emergency: 800-222-1222
                800-382-9097
                317-962-2323
                (Indianapolis)
TTY: 317-962-2336
www.clarian.org/poisoncontrol

IOWA

SIOUX CITY

Iowa Statewide Poison
Control Center
Iowa Health System and the
University of Iowa Hospitals and
Clinics

401 Douglas St.
Suite 402
Sioux City, IA 51101
Business: 712-279-3710
Emergency: 800-222-1222
                712-277-2222 (IA)
www.iowapoison.org

KANSAS

KANSAS CITY

University of Kansas
Poison Control Medical Center

3901 Rainbow Blvd.
Room B-400
Kansas City, KS 66160-7231
Business   913-588-6638
Emergency: 800-222-1222
                800-332-6633 (KS)
TDD: 913-588-6639
www.kumc.com/bodyside.cmf?2144

KENTUCKY

LOUISVILLE

Kentucky Regional
Poison Center (*)

PO Box 35070
Louisville, KY 40232-5070
Business: 502-629-7264
Emergency: 800-222-1222
www.krpc.com

LOUISIANA

MONROE

Louisiana Drug and Poison
Information Center (*)
University of Louisiana at
Monroe

700 University Ave.
Monroe, LA 71209-6430
Business: 318-342-3648
Emergency: 800-222-1222
                800-256-9822
                (LA only)
www.lapcc.org

MAINE

PORTLAND

Northern New England
Poison Center

Maine Medical Center
22 Bramhall St.
Portland, ME 04102
Business: 207-662-0111
Emergency: 800-222-1222
                207-871-2879 (ME)
TDD/TTY: 207-662-4900 (ME)
www.nnepc.org

MARYLAND

BALTIMORE

Maryland Poison Center (*)
University of Maryland at
Baltimore
School of Pharmacy

220 Arch St.
Office Level 1
Baltimore, MD 21201
Business: 410-706-7604
Emergency: 800-222-1222
TDD: 410-706-1858
www.mdpoison.com

(WASHINGTON, DC)

National Capital
Poison Center (*)

3201 New Mexico Ave., NW
Suite 310
Washington DC 20016
Business: 202-362-3867
Emergency: 800-222-1222
TDD/TTY: 202-362-8563 (MD)
www.poison.org

MASSACHUSETTS

BOSTON

Regional Center for Poison
Control and Prevention (*)
(Serving Massachusetts and
Rhode Island)

300 Longwood Ave.
Boston, MA 02115
Business: 617-355-6609
Emergency: 800-222-1222
TDD/TTY: 888-244-5313
www.maripoisoncenter.com

MICHIGAN

DETROIT

Regional Poison
Control Center (*)
Children's Hospital of Michigan

4160 John R. Harper
    Professional Office Bldg.
Suite 616
Detroit, MI 48201
Business: 313-745-5335
Emergency: 800-222-1222
TDD/TTY: 800-356-3232
www.mitoxic.org/pcc

GRAND RAPIDS

DeVos Children's Hospital
Regional Poison Center (*)

100 Michigan St., NE
Grand Rapids, MI 49503
Business: 616-391-3690
Emergency: 800-222-1222
http://poisoncenter.
    devoschildrens.org

MINNESOTA

MINNEAPOLIS

Minnesota Poison Control
System (*) Hennepin County
Medical Center

701 Park Ave.
Mail Code RL
Minneapolis, MN 55415
Business: 612-873-3144
Emergency: 800-222-1222
www.mnpoison.org

MISSISSIPPI

JACKSON

Mississippi Regional Poison
Control Center, University of
Mississippi Medical Center

2500 North State St.
Jackson, MS 39216
Business: 601-984-1680
Emergency: 800-222-1222

MISSOURI

ST. LOUIS

Missouri Regional
Poison Center (*)
Cardinal Glennon
Children's Hospital

7980 Clayton Rd.
Suite 200
St. Louis, MO 63117
Business: 314-772-5200
Emergency: 800-222-1222
TDD/TTY: 314-612-5705
www.cardinalglennon.com

MONTANA

(DENVER, CO)
Rocky Mountain Poison and Drug Center (*)

777 Bannock St.
Mail Code 0180
Denver, CO 80204-4507
Business: 303-739-1100
Emergency: 800-222-1222
TDD/TTY: 303-739-1127
www.RMPDC.org

NEBRASKA

OMAHA
The Poison Center (*)
Children's Hospital

8401 W. Dodge St.
Suite 115
Omaha, NE 68114
Business: 402-955-5555
Emergency: 800-222-1222
www.nebraskapoison.com

NEVADA

(DENVER, CO)
Rocky Mountain Poison and Drug Center (*)

777 Bannock St.
Mail Code 0180
Denver, CO 80204-4507
Business: 303-739-1100
Emergency: 800-222-1222
www.RMPDC.org

(PORTLAND, OR)
Oregon Poison Center (*)
Oregon Health Sciences University

3181 SW Sam Jackson Park Rd.
Portland, OR 97201
Business: 503-494-8600
Emergency: 800-222-1222
www.oregonpoison.com

NEW HAMPSHIRE

(PORTLAND, ME)
Northern New England Poison Center

Maine Medical Center
22 Bramhall St.
Portland, ME 04102
Business: 207-662-0111
Emergency: 800-222-1222
www.nnepc.org

NEW JERSEY

NEWARK
New Jersey Poison Information and Education System (*)
UMDNJ

65 Bergen St.
Newark, NJ 07101
Business: 973-972-9280
Emergency: 800-222-1222
TDD/TTY: 973-926-8008
www.njpies.org

NEW MEXICO

ALBUQUERQUE
New Mexico Poison and Drug Information Center (*)

MSC09-5080
1 University of New Mexico
Albuquerque, NM 87131-0001
Business: 505-272-4261
Emergency: 800-222-1222
http://HSC.UNM.edu/pharmacy/poison

NEW YORK

BUFFALO
Western New York Regional Poison Control Center (*)
Children's Hospital of Buffalo

219 Bryant St.
Buffalo, NY 14222
Business: 716-878-7654
Emergency: 800-222-1222
www.fingerlakespoison.org

MINEOLA
Long Island Regional Poison and Drug Information Center (*)
Winthrop University Hospital

259 First St.
Mineola, NY 11501
Business: 516-663-2650
Emergency: 800-222-1222
TDD: 516-747-3323
(Nassau)
631-924-8811
(Suffolk)
www.lirpdic.org

NEW YORK CITY
New York City Poison Control Center (*)
NYC Dept. of Health

455 First Ave.
Room 123
New York, NY 10016
Business: 212-447-8152
Emergency: 800-222-1222
(English) 212-340-4494
212-POISONS
(212-764-7667)

Emergency: 212-venenos
(Spanish) (212-836-3667)
TDD: 212-689-9014

ROCHESTER
Finger Lakes Regional Poison and Drug Information Center(*)
University of Rochester Medical Center

601 Elmwood Ave.
Box 321
Rochester, NY 14642
Business: 585-273-4155
Emergency: 800-222-1222
TTY: 585-273-3854

SYRACUSE
Central New York Poison Center (*)
SUNY Upstate Medical University

750 East Adams St.
Syracuse, NY 13210
Business: 315-464-7078
Emergency: 800-222-1222
www.cnypoison.org

NORTH CAROLINA

CHARLOTTE
Carolinas Poison Center (*)
Carolinas Medical Center

PO Box 32861
Charlotte, NC 28232
Business: 704-512-3795
Emergency: 800-222-1222
www.ncpoisoncenter.org

NORTH DAKOTA

BISMARK
ND Department of Health Injury Prevention Program

600 E. Boulevard Ave.
Bismark, ND 58505
Business: 612-873-3144
Emergency: 800-222-1222
www.ndpoison.org

OHIO

CINCINNATI
Cincinnati Drug and Poison Information Center (*)
Regional Poison Control System

3333 Burnet Ave.
Vernon Place, 3rd Floor
Cincinnati, OH 45229
513-636-5063
Emergency: 800-222-1222
TDD/TTY: 800-253-7955
www.cincinnatichildrens.org/dpic

CLEVELAND
Greater Cleveland Poison Control Center

11100 Euclid Ave.
MP 6007
Cleveland, OH 44106-6007
Business: 216-844-1573
Emergency: 800-222-1222
216-231-4455
(OH)

COLUMBUS
Central Ohio Poison Center (*)

700 Children's Dr.
Room L032
Columbus, OH 43205-2696
Business: 614-722-2635
Emergency: 800-222-1222
TTY: 614-228-2272
www.bepoisonsmart.com

OKLAHOMA

OKLAHOMA CITY
Oklahoma Poison Control Center (*)
Children's Hospital at OU Medical Center

940 Northeast 13th St.
Room 3510
Oklahoma City, OK 73104
Business: 405-271-5062
Emergency: 800-222-1222
www.oklahomapoison.org

OREGON

PORTLAND
Oregon Poison Center (*)
Oregon Health Sciences University

3181 S.W. Sam Jackson Park Rd.,
CB550
Portland, OR 97239
Business: 503-494-8968
Emergency: 800-222-1222
www.ohsu.edu/poison

PENNSYLVANIA

PHILADELPHIA
The Poison Control Center (*)
Children's Hospital of Philadelphia

34th Street & Civic Center Blvd.
Philadelphia, PA 19104-4399
Business: 215-590-2003
Emergency: 800-222-1222
215-386-2100 (PA)
TDD/TTY: 215-590-8789
www.poisoncontrol.chop.edu

PITTSBURGH
Pittsburgh Poison Center (*)
Children's Hospital of Pittsburgh

3705 Fifth Ave.
Pittsburgh, PA 15213
Business: 412-390-3300
Emergency: 800-222-1222
412-681-6669
www.chp.edu/clinical/03a_poison.php

RHODE ISLAND

(BOSTON, MA)
Regional Center for Poison Control and Prevention (*)

(Serving Massachusetts and Rhode Island)

300 Longwood Ave.
Boston, MA 02115
Business: 617-355-6609
Emergency: 800-222-1222
TDD/TTY: 888-244-5313
www.maripoisoncenter.com

SOUTH DAKOTA

(MINNEAPOLIS, MN)
Hennepin Regional Poison Center (*) Hennepin County Medical Center

701 Park Ave.
Minneapolis, MN 55415
Business: 612-873-3144
Emergency: 800-222-1222
www.mnpoison.org

SIOUX FALLS
Provides education only—Does not manage exposure cases.

Sioux Valley Poison Control Center (*)

1305 W. 18th St.
Box 5039
Sioux Falls, SD 57117-5039
Business: 605-328-6670
www.sdpoison.org

TENNESSEE

NASHVILLE
Tennessee Poison Center (*)

1161 21st Ave. South
501 Oxford House
Nashville, TN 37232-4632
Business: 615-936-0760
Emergency: 800-222-1222
www.poisonlifeline.org

TEXAS

AMARILLO
Texas Panhandle Poison Center (*) Northwest Texas Hospital

1501 S. Coulter Dr.
Amarillo, TX 79106
Business: 806-354-1630
Emergency: 800-222-1222
www.poisoncontrol.org

DALLAS
North Texas Poison Center (*) Texas Poison Center Network Parkland Health and Hospital System

5201 Harry Hines Blvd.
Dallas, TX 75235
Business: 214-589-0911
Emergency: 800-222-1222
www.poisoncontrol.org

EL PASO
West Texas Regional Poison Center (*) Thomason Hospital

4815 Alameda Ave.
El Paso, TX 79905
Business 915-534-3800
Emergency: 800-222-1222
www.poisoncontrol.org

GALVESTON
Southeast Texas Poison Center (*) The University of Texas Medical Branch

3.112 Trauma Bldg.
301 University Blvd.
Galveston, TX 77555-1175
Business: 409-772-9142
Emergency: 800-222-1222
www.poisoncontrol.org

SAN ANTONIO
South Texas Poison Center (*) The University of Texas Health Science Center–San Antonio

7703 Floyd Curl Dr., MSC 7849
San Antonio, TX 78229-3900
Business: 210-567-5762
Emergency: 800-222-1222
www.poisoncontrol.org

TEMPLE
Central Texas Poison Center (*) Scott & White Memorial Hospital

2401 South 31st St.
Temple, TX 76508
Business: 254-724-7401
Emergency: 800-222-1222
www.poisoncontrol.org

UTAH

SALT LAKE CITY
Utah Poison Control Center (*)

585 Komas Dr.
Suite 200
Salt Lake City, UT 84108
Business: 801-587-0600
Emergency: 800-222-1222
http://uuhsc.utah.edu/poison

VERMONT

(PORTLAND, ME)
Northern New England Poison Center

Maine Medical Center
22 Bramhall St.
Portland, ME 04102
Business: 207-662-7220
Emergency: 800-222-1222
www.nnepc.org

VIRGINIA

CHARLOTTESVILLE
Blue Ridge Poison Center (*) University of Virginia Health System

PO Box 800774
Charlottesville, VA 22908-0774
Business: 434-924-0347
Emergency: 800-222-1222
www.healthsystem.virginia.edu.brpc

RICHMOND
Virginia Poison Center (*) Virginia Commonwealth University

PO Box 980522
Richmond, VA 23298-0522
Business: 804-828-4780
Emergency: 800-222-1222
804-828-9123
www.vcu.edu/mcved/vpc

WASHINGTON

SEATTLE
Washington Poison Center (*)

155 NE 100th St.
Suite 400
Seattle, WA 98125-8011
Business: 206-517-2359
Emergency: 800-222-1222
www.wapc.org

WEST VIRGINIA

CHARLESTON
West Virginia Poison Center (*)

3110 MacCorkle Ave. SE
Charleston, WV 25304
Business: 304-347-1212
Emergency: 800-222-1222
www.wvpoisoncenter.org

WISCONSIN

MILWAUKEE
Wisconsin Poison Center

Suite CC 660
PO Box 1997
Milwaukee, WI 53201
Business: 414-266-2952
Emergency: 800-222-1222
TDD/TTY: 414-266-2542
www.wisconsinpoison.org

WYOMING

(OMAHA, NE)
The Poison Center (*) Nebraska Regional Poison Center

8401 W. Dodge St.
Suite 115
Omaha, NE 68114
Business: 402-955-5555
Emergency: 800-222-1222
www.nebraskapoison.com

PRODUCT IDENTIFICATION GUIDE

For quick identification, this section provides full-color reproductions of product packaging, as well as some actual-sized photographs of tablets and capsules.

Products in this section are arranged alphabetically by manufacturer. In some instances, not all dosage forms and sizes are pictured. For more information on any of the products in this section, please turn to the page indicated above the product's photo or check directly with the product's manufacturer.

While every effort has been made to guarantee faithful reproduction of the photos in this section, changes in size, color, and design are always a possibility. Be sure to confirm a product's identity with the manufacturer or your pharmacist.

MANUFACTURER'S INDEX

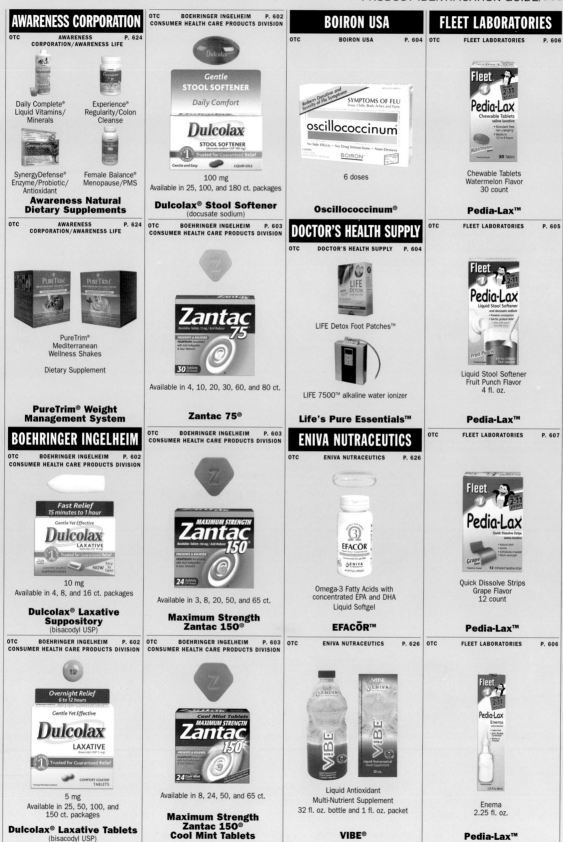

AWARENESS CORPORATION

OTC   AWARENESS   P. 624
CORPORATION/AWARENESS LIFE

Daily Complete®
Liquid Vitamins/
Minerals

Experience®
Regularity/Colon
Cleanse

SynergyDefense®
Enzyme/Probiotic/
Antioxidant

Female Balance®
Menopause/PMS

**Awareness Natural
Dietary Supplements**

OTC   AWARENESS   P. 624
CORPORATION/AWARENESS LIFE

PureTrim®
Mediterranean
Wellness Shakes

Dietary Supplement

**PureTrim® Weight
Management System**

BOEHRINGER INGELHEIM

OTC   BOEHRINGER INGELHEIM   P. 602
CONSUMER HEALTH CARE PRODUCTS DIVISION

Fast Relief
15 minutes to 1 hour

Gentle Yet Effective

Dulcolax
LAXATIVE

10 mg
Available in 4, 8, and 16 ct. packages

**Dulcolax® Laxative
Suppository**
(bisacodyl USP)

OTC   BOEHRINGER INGELHEIM   P. 602
CONSUMER HEALTH CARE PRODUCTS DIVISION

Overnight Relief
6 to 12 hours

Gentle Yet Effective

Dulcolax
LAXATIVE

5 mg
Available in 25, 50, 100, and
150 ct. packages

Dulcolax® Laxative Tablets
(bisacodyl USP)

OTC   BOEHRINGER INGELHEIM   P. 602
CONSUMER HEALTH CARE PRODUCTS DIVISION

Gentle
STOOL SOFTENER

Daily Comfort

Dulcolax
STOOL SOFTENER

100 mg
Available in 25, 100, and 180 ct. packages

Dulcolax® Stool Softener
(docusate sodium)

OTC   BOEHRINGER INGELHEIM   P. 603
CONSUMER HEALTH CARE PRODUCTS DIVISION

Zantac
75

Available in 4, 10, 20, 30, 60, and 80 ct.

Zantac 75®

OTC   BOEHRINGER INGELHEIM   P. 603
CONSUMER HEALTH CARE PRODUCTS DIVISION

MAXIMUM STRENGTH
Zantac
150

Available in 3, 8, 20, 50, and 65 ct.

**Maximum Strength
Zantac 150®**

OTC   BOEHRINGER INGELHEIM   P. 603
CONSUMER HEALTH CARE PRODUCTS DIVISION

Cool Mint Tablets
MAXIMUM STRENGTH
Zantac
150

Available in 8, 24, 50, and 65 ct.

**Maximum Strength
Zantac 150®
Cool Mint Tablets**

BOIRON USA

OTC   BOIRON USA   P. 604

SYMPTOMS OF FLU
Fever, Chills, Body Aches and Pains

oscillococcinum

BOIRON

6 doses

Oscillococcinum®

DOCTOR'S HEALTH SUPPLY

OTC   DOCTOR'S HEALTH SUPPLY   P. 604

LIFE Detox Foot Patches™

LIFE 7500™ alkaline water ionizer

Life's Pure Essentials™

ENIVA NUTRACEUTICS

OTC   ENIVA NUTRACEUTICS   P. 626

EFACOR

Omega-3 Fatty Acids with
concentrated EPA and DHA
Liquid Softgel

EFACŌR™

OTC   ENIVA NUTRACEUTICS   P. 626

VIBE

Liquid Antioxidant
Multi-Nutrient Supplement
32 fl. oz. bottle and 1 fl. oz. packet

VIBE®

FLEET LABORATORIES

OTC   FLEET LABORATORIES   P. 606

Fleet
Pedia-Lax
Chewable Tablets
saline laxative

Chewable Tablets
Watermelon Flavor
30 count

Pedia-Lax™

OTC   FLEET LABORATORIES   P. 605

Fleet
Pedia-Lax
Liquid Stool Softener
oral docusate sodium

Liquid Stool Softener
Fruit Punch Flavor
4 fl. oz.

Pedia-Lax™

OTC   FLEET LABORATORIES   P. 607

Fleet
Pedia-Lax
Quick Dissolve Strips
senna laxative

Quick Dissolve Strips
Grape Flavor
12 count

Pedia-Lax™

OTC   FLEET LABORATORIES   P. 606

Fleet
Pedia-Lax
Enema

Enema
2.25 fl. oz.

Pedia-Lax™

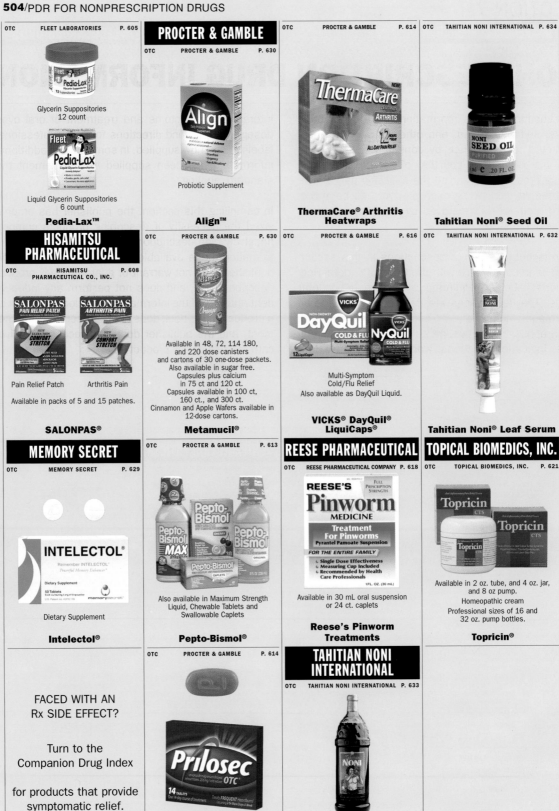

OTC   FLEET LABORATORIES   P. 605

Glycerin Suppositories
12 count

Liquid Glycerin Suppositories
6 count

Pedia-Lax™

HISAMITSU PHARMACEUTICAL

OTC   HISAMITSU   P. 608
PHARMACEUTICAL CO., INC.

Pain Relief Patch   Arthritis Pain

Available in packs of 5 and 15 patches.

SALONPAS®

MEMORY SECRET

OTC   MEMORY SECRET   P. 629

INTELECTOL®

Dietary Supplement

Intelectol®

FACED WITH AN
Rx SIDE EFFECT?

Turn to the
Companion Drug Index

for products that provide
symptomatic relief.

PROCTER & GAMBLE

OTC   PROCTER & GAMBLE   P. 630

Probiotic Supplement

Align™

OTC   PROCTER & GAMBLE   P. 630

Available in 48, 72, 114 180,
and 220 dose canisters
and cartons of 30 one-dose packets.
Also available in sugar free.
Capsules plus calcium
in 75 ct and 120 ct.
Capsules available in 100 ct,
160 ct., and 300 ct.
Cinnamon and Apple Wafers available in
12-dose cartons.

Metamucil®

OTC   PROCTER & GAMBLE   P. 613

Also available in Maximum Strength
Liquid, Chewable Tablets and
Swallowable Caplets

Pepto-Bismol®

OTC   PROCTER & GAMBLE   P. 614

20 mg

Prilosec OTC®

OTC   PROCTER & GAMBLE   P. 614

**ThermaCare® Arthritis
Heatwraps**

OTC   PROCTER & GAMBLE   P. 616

Multi-Symptom
Cold/Flu Relief
Also available as DayQuil Liquid.

**VICKS® DayQuil®
LiquiCaps®**

REESE PHARMACEUTICAL

OTC   REESE PHARMACEUTICAL COMPANY   P. 618

**REESE'S
Pinworm
MEDICINE**

Treatment
For Pinworms
Pyrantel Pamoate Suspension

FOR THE ENTIRE FAMILY
- Single Dose Effectiveness
- Measuring Cup Included
- Recommended by Health
  Care Professionals

Available in 30 mL oral suspension
or 24 ct. caplets

**Reese's Pinworm
Treatments**

TAHITIAN NONI INTERNATIONAL

OTC   TAHITIAN NONI INTERNATIONAL   P. 633

Dietary Supplement

Tahitian Noni® Juice

OTC   TAHITIAN NONI INTERNATIONAL   P. 634

Tahitian Noni® Seed Oil

OTC   TAHITIAN NONI INTERNATIONAL   P. 632

Tahitian Noni® Leaf Serum

TOPICAL BIOMEDICS, INC.

OTC   TOPICAL BIOMEDICS, INC.   P. 621

Available in 2 oz. tube, and 4 oz. jar,
and 8 oz pump.
Homeopathic cream
Professional sizes of 16 and
32 oz. pump bottles.

Topricin®

NONPRESCRIPTION DRUG INFORMATION

This section presents information on nonprescription drugs, self-testing kits, and other medical products marketed for home use by consumers. It is made possible through the courtesy of the manufacturers whose products appear on the following pages. The information concerning each product has been prepared, edited, and approved by the manufacturer's professional staff.

Pharmaceutical product descriptions in this section must be in compliance with the Code of Federal Regulations' labeling requirements for over-the-counter drugs. The descriptions are designed to provide all information necessary for informed use, including, when applicable, active ingredients, inactive ingredients, indications, actions, warnings, cautions, drug interactions, symptoms and treatment of oral overdosage, dosage and directions for use, professional labeling, and how supplied. In some cases, additional information has been supplied to complement the standard labeling.

In compiling this section, the publisher has emphasized the necessity of describing products comprehensively. The descriptions seen here include all information made available by the manufacturer. The publisher does not warrant or guarantee any product described here, and does not perform any independent analysis of the information provided. Inclusion of a product in this book does not represent an endorsement, and the publisher does not necessarily advocate the use of any product listed.

Boehringer Ingelheim Consumer Health Care Products

DIVISION OF BOEHRINGER INGELHEIM PHARMACEUTICALS, INC.
900 RIDGEBURY ROAD
P.O. BOX 368
RIDGEFIELD, CT 06877

Direct Inquiries to:
(888) 285-9159

DULCOLAX®
LAXATIVE TABLETS
[dul cō-lax]
brand of bisacodyl USP
Tablets of 5 mg laxative

Drug Facts

Active ingredient (in each tablet):	Purpose
Bisacodyl USP, 5 mg	Stimulant laxative

Use
• for temporary relief of occasional constipation and irregularity
• this product generally produces bowel movement in 6 to 12 hours

Warnings
Do not use if you cannot swallow without chewing
Ask a doctor before use if you have
• stomach pain, nausea or vomiting
• a sudden change in bowel habits that lasts more than 2 weeks
When using this product
• do not chew or crush tablet(s)
• do not use within 1 hour after taking an antacid or milk
• it may cause stomach discomfort, faintness and cramps
Stop use and ask a doctor if
• you have rectal bleeding or no bowel movement after using this product. These could be signs of a serious condition.
• you need to use a laxative for more than 1 week
If pregnant or breast-feeding, ask a health professional before use.
Keep out of reach of children. In case of overdose, get medical help or contact a Poison Control Center right away.

Directions   take with a glass of water

adults and children 12 years of age and over	1 to 3 tablets in a single daily dose
children 6 to under 12 years of age	1 tablet in a single daily dose
children under 6 years of age	ask a doctor

Other information
• store at 20-25°C (68-77°F)
• protect from excessive humidity
• questions about DULCOLAX? 1-888-285-9159 (English/Spanish)
• www.Dulcolax.com

• blister packaged for your protection. do not use if individual seals are broken.

Inactive ingredients   acacia, acetylated monoglyceride, carnauba wax, cellulose acetate phthalate, corn starch, dibutyl phthalate, docusate sodium, gelatin, glycerin, iron oxides, kaolin, lactose, magnesium stearate, methylparaben, pharmaceutical glaze, polyethylene glycol, povidone, propylparaben, Red No. 30 lake, sodium benzoate, sorbitan monooleate, sucrose, talc, titanium dioxide, white wax, Yellow No. 10 lake.

How supplied: Boxes of 25, 50, 100 and 150 comfort coated tablets

Boehringer Ingelheim Consumer Health Care Products

Division of Boehringer Ingelheim Pharmaceuticals, Inc., Ridgefield, CT 06877

Made in Mexico

Copyright © 2008, Boehringer Ingelheim Pharmaceuticals, Inc. All rights reserved.

Shown in Product Identification Guide, page 503

DULCOLAX® LAXATIVE SUPPOSITORIES
[dul cō-lax]
brand of bisacodyl USP
Suppositories of 10 mg laxative

Drug Facts

Active ingredient (in each suppository)	Purpose
Bisacodyl USP, 10 mg	Stimulant laxative

Use
• for temporary relief of occasional constipation and irregularity
• this product generally produces bowel movement in 15 minutes to 1 hour

Warnings

For rectal use only

Ask a doctor before use if you have
• stomach pain, nausea or vomiting
• a sudden change in bowel habits that lasts more than 2 weeks

When using this product it may cause stomach discomfort, faintness, rectal burning and mild cramps

Stop use and ask a doctor if
• you have rectal bleeding or no bowel movement after using this product. These could be signs of a serious condition.
• you need to use a laxative for more than 1 week

If pregnant or breast-feeding, ask a health professional before use.

Keep out of reach of children. If swallowed, get medical help or contact a Poison Control Center right away.

Directions

adults and children 12 years of age and over	1 suppository in a single daily dose. Peel open plastic. Insert suppository well into rectum, pointed end first. Retain about 15 to 20 minutes.
children 6 to under 12 years of age	½ suppository in a single daily dose
children under 6 years of age	ask a doctor

Other information
• do not store above 30ºC (86ºF)
• questions about DULCOLAX? 1-888-285-9159 (English/Spanish)
• www.Dulcolax.com
• do not use this product if the individual seal is broken

Inactive ingredient   hydrogenated vegetable oil

How supplied: Boxes of 4, 8 and 16 comfort shaped suppositories

Boehringer Ingelheim Consumer Health Care Products
Division of Boehringer Ingelheim Pharmaceuticals, Inc., Ridgefield, CT 06877
Made in Italy
Copyright © 2008, Boehringer Ingelheim Pharmaceuticals, Inc. All rights reserved.

Shown in Product Identification Guide, page 503

DULCOLAX® STOOL SOFTENER
[dul cō-lax]
brand of docusate sodium USP
Liquid gel of 100 mg stool softener

Drug Facts

Active ingredient (in each liquid gel)	Purpose
Docusate sodium, 100 mg	Stool softener laxative

Use
• for temporary relief of occasional constipation and irregularity
• this product generally produces bowel movement in 12 to 72 hours

Warnings
Ask a doctor before use if you have
• stomach pain, nausea or vomiting
• a sudden change in bowel habits that lasts more than 2 weeks
Ask a doctor or pharmacist before use if you are presently taking mineral oil
Stop use and ask a doctor if
• you have rectal bleeding or no bowel movement after using this product. These could be signs of a serious condition
• you need to use a laxative for more than 1 week
If pregnant or breast-feeding, ask a health professional before use
Keep out of reach of children. In case of overdose, get medical help or contact a Poison Control Center right away

Directions	take with a glass of water
adults and children 12 years of age and over	1 to 3 liquid gels daily. This dose may be taken as a single daily dose or in divided doses
children 2 to under 12 years of age	1 liquid gel daily
children under 2 years of age	ask a doctor

Other information:
- store at 15-30°C (59-86°F)
- protect from excessive humidity
- questions about DULCOLAX? 1-888-285-9159 (English/Spanish)
- www.Dulcolax.com
- do not use this product if the safety seal under the cap is torn or missing

Inactive ingredients FD&C Red #40, FD&C Yellow #6, gelatin, glycerin, hypromellose, polyethylene glycol, propylene glycol, purified water, sorbitol special, titanium dioxide.

How supplied: Bottles of 25, 100 and 180 Liquid Gels

Boehringer Ingelheim Consumer Health Care Products
Division of Boehringer Ingelheim Pharmaceuticals, Inc., Ridgefield, CT 06877
Copyright © 2008, Boehringer Ingelheim Pharmaceuticals, Inc. All rights reserved.

Shown in Product Identification Guide, page 503

ZANTAC 75®
brand of ranitidine USP
Tablet of 75 mg acid reducer

Drug Facts
Active Ingredient
(in each tablet) **Purpose**
Ranitidine 75 mg (as ranitidine hydrochloride 84 mg) .... Acid reducer

Uses
- relieves heartburn associated with acid indigestion and sour stomach
- prevents heartburn associated with acid indigestion and sour stomach brought on by certain foods and beverages

Warnings
Allergy alert: Do not use if you are allergic to ranitidine or other acid reducers
Do not use
- if you have trouble or pain swallowing food, vomiting with blood, or bloody or black stools. These may be signs of a serious condition. See your doctor.
- with other acid reducers
Ask a doctor before use if you have
- frequent **chest pain**
- frequent wheezing, particularly with heartburn
- unexplained weight loss
- nausea or vomiting
- stomach pain
- had heartburn over 3 months. This may be a sign of a more serious condition

- heartburn with **lightheadedness, sweating or dizziness**
- chest pain or shoulder pain with shortness of breath; sweating; pain spreading to arms, neck or shoulders; or lightheadedness
Stop use and ask a doctor if
- your heartburn continues or worsens
- you need to take this product for more than 14 days
If pregnant or breast-feeding, ask a health professional before use.
Keep out of reach of children. In case of overdose, get medical help or contact a Poison Control Center right away.

Directions
- adults and children 12 years and over:
  - to **relieve** symptoms, swallow 1 tablet with a glass of water
  - to **prevent** symptoms, swallow 1 tablet with a glass of water **30 to 60 minutes before** eating food or drinking beverages that cause heartburn
  - can be used up to twice daily (do not take more than 2 tablets in 24 hours)
- children under 12 years: ask a doctor

Other information
- do not use if printed foil under bottle cap is open or torn
- store at 20°–25°C (68°–77°F)
- avoid excessive heat or humidity
- this product is sodium and sugar free

Inactive ingredients
Hypromellose, magnesium stearate, microcrystalline cellulose, synthetic red iron oxide, titanium dioxide, triacetin
Questions?
Call **1-888-285-9159**
Or visit **www.zantacotc.com**
Shown in Product Identification Guide, page 503

MAXIMUM STRENGTH ZANTAC 150®
brand of ranitidine USP
Tablet of 150 mg acid reducer

Drug Facts
Active ingredient
(in each tablet) **Purpose**
Ranitidine 150 mg (as ranitidine hydrochloride 168 mg) ...... Acid reducer

Uses
- relieves heartburn associated with acid indigestion and sour stomach
- prevents heartburn associated with acid indigestion and sour stomach brought on by certain foods and beverages

Warnings
Allergy alert: Do not use if you are allergic to ranitidine or other acid reducers
Do not use
- if you have trouble or pain swallowing food, vomiting with blood, or bloody or black stools. These may be signs of a serious condition. See your doctor.
- with other acid reducers
- if you have kidney disease, except under the advice and supervision of a doctor
Ask a doctor before use if you have
- frequent **chest pain**
- frequent wheezing, particularly with heartburn

- unexplained weight loss
- nausea or vomiting
- stomach pain
- had heartburn over 3 months. This may be a sign of a more serious condition.
- heartburn with **lightheadedness, sweating or dizziness**
- chest pain or shoulder pain with shortness of breath; sweating; pain spreading to arms, neck or shoulders; or lightheadedness
Stop use and ask a doctor if
- your heartburn continues or worsens
- you need to take this product for more than 14 days
If pregnant or breast-feeding, ask a health professional before use.
Keep out of reach of children. In case of overdose, get medical help or contact a Poison Control Center right away.

Directions
- adults and children 12 years and over:
  - to **relieve** symptoms, swallow 1 tablet with a glass of water
  - to **prevent** symptoms, swallow 1 tablet with a glass of water **30 to 60 minutes before** eating food or drinking beverages that cause heartburn
  - can be used up to twice daily (do not take more than 2 tablets in 24 hours)
- children under 12 years: ask a doctor
Other information
- do not use if printed foil under bottle cap is open or torn
- store at 20°–25°C (68°–77°F)
- avoid excessive heat or humidity
- this product is sodium and sugar free
Inactive ingredients
Hypromellose, magnesium stearate, microcrystalline cellulose, synthetic red iron oxide, titanium dioxide, triacetin
Questions?
Call **1-888-285-9159**
Or visit **www.zantacotc.com**
Shown in Product Identification Guide, page 503

MAXIMUM STRENGTH ZANTAC 150®
COOL MINT TABLETS
brand of ranitidine USP
Cool Mint Tablet of 150 mg acid reducer

Drug Facts
Active Ingredient **Purpose**
(in each tablet)
Ranitidine 150 mg (as ranitidine hydrochloride 168 mg) ...... Acid reducer
Uses
- relieves heartburn associated with acid indigestion and sour stomach
- prevents heartburn associated with acid indigestion and sour stomach brought on by eating or drinking certain foods and beverages
Warnings
Allergy alert: Do not use if you are allergic to ranitidine or other acid reducers
Do not use
- with other acid reducers
- if you have kidney disease, except under the advice and supervision of a doctor

Continued on next page

Zantac 150 Cool Mint—Cont.

- if you have trouble or pain swallowing food, vomiting with blood, or bloody or black stools. These may be signs of a serious condition. See your doctor.

Ask a doctor before use if you have
- nausea or vomiting
- stomach pain
- unexplained weight loss
- frequent **chest pain**
- frequent wheezing, particularly with heartburn
- had heartburn over 3 months. This may be a sign of a more serious condition.
- heartburn with **lightheadedness, sweating or dizziness**
- chest pain or shoulder pain with shortness of breath; sweating; pain spreading to arms, neck or shoulders; or lightheadedness

Stop use and ask a doctor if
- your heartburn continues or worsens
- you need to take this product for more than 14 days

If pregnant or breast-feeding, ask a health professional before use.

Keep out of reach of children. In case of overdose, get medical help or contact a Poison Control Center right away.

Directions
- adults and children 12 years and over:
  - to **relieve** symptoms, swallow 1 tablet with a glass of water
  - to **prevent** symptoms, swallow 1 tablet with a glass of water **30 to 60 minutes before** eating food or drinking beverages that cause heartburn
  - can be used up to twice daily (up to 2 tablets in 24 hours)
  - do not chew tablet
- children under 12 years: ask a doctor

Other information
- do not use if individual unit is open or torn
- store at 20°–25°C (68°–77°F)
- avoid excessive heat or humidity
- this product is sodium and sugar free

Inactive ingredients
Hypromellose, magnesium stearate, microcrystalline cellulose, synthetic red iron oxide, titanium dioxide, triacetin
Questions?
Call **1-888-285-9159**
Or visit **www.zantacotc.com**
Shown in Product Identification Guide, page 503

UNKNOWN DRUG?
Consult the
Product Identification Guide
(Gray Pages)
for full-color photos of
leading over-the-counter
medications

Boiron
**6 CAMPUS BOULEVARD
NEWTOWN SQUARE, PA
19073-3267**

Direct inquires to:
Boiron Information Center
info@boironusa.com
1-800-BOIRON-1 (1-800-264-7661)
www.boironusa.com

OSCILLOCOCCINUM®   **OTC**
No Side Effects • No Drug
Interactions • Non-Drowsy

Drug Facts
Active ingredient   **Purpose**
Anas barbariae hepatis et ..... To reduce cordis extractum   the duration
200CK HPUS   and severity of flu symptoms
The letters HPUS indicate that this ingredient is officially included in the Homeopathic Pharmacopoeia of the United States.

Uses:
Temporarily relieves symptoms of flu such as fever, chills, body aches and pains.

Warnings:
Do not use if glued carton end flaps are open or if the tray seal is broken.
Ask a doctor before use in children under 2 years of age.
Stop use and ask a doctor if symptoms persist for more than 3 days or worsen.
If pregnant or breast-feeding, ask a health professional before use. **Keep out of reach of children.**

Directions

Age	Dose
Adults and children 2 years of age and older	Dissolve entire contents of one tube in the mouth every 6 hours, up to 3 times a day.
Children under 2 years of age	Ask a doctor.

Other Information
- store at 68-77°F (20-25°C)
- contains 1g of sugar per dose
Inactive ingredients
sucrose, lactose

How Supplied: **3 DOSES, 6 DOSES**
0.04 oz. each
HOMEOPATHIC MEDICINE
Questions, Comments?
www.boironusa.com
info@boironusa.com
1-800-BOIRON-1 (1-800-264-7661)
Boiron Information Center
6 Campus Boulevard
Newtown Square, PA 19073-3267
Shown in Product Identification Guide, page 503

Doctor's Health Supply
**2335 CAMINO VIDA ROBLES
BUILDING B
CARLSBAD, CA 92011**

Phone: 760-431-8047
Fax: 760-431-0126
www.lifeionizers.com
www.lifedetoxpatch.com

LIFE DETOX PATCHES

Key Facts: LIFE Detox Patches are a unique and innovative way to rid the body of accumulated toxins. The technique is both simple and noninvasive. LIFE Detox Foot Patches use all natural ingredients(Zeolite and Tourmaline) and negative ions that have been shown to help rid your body of harmful toxins safely and effectively. Using LIFE Detox Foot Patches™ is a natural way to help your body remove heavy metals, metabolic waste, microscopic organisms, chemical residue, and all kinds of natural and artificial toxins!
These statements have not been evaluated by the Food & Drug Administration. This product is not intended to diagnose, treat, cure or prevent any disease.
Shown in Product Identification Guide, page 503

LIFE IONIZER 7500
Counter and under-counter models

Key Facts: Revolutionary New Alkaline Water Ionizer with new SMPS Power System. Same power system that runs High Definition Televisions. Life 7500 - Artificial intelligence function for customer convenience & ionizer protection.
New LIFE 7500 MESH Technology System -
1. Seven (7) platinum coated titanium plates
2. Dual Filter System with nine (9) stages + Free Pre-filter & housing
3. 8 modes - four levels of alkaline, two acidic and one purify mode
4. 4 Amperage settings to adjust for water conditions
5. Flow rate indicator and heat sensor to prevent excessive usage
6. SMPS- Power source that replaces old fashioned transformer. Same system that powers High Definition Television.
7. Automatic cleaning
5 year warranty: LIFE Ionizers latest high technology systems are so well-built that we confidently offer a five year warranty - 3 years parts & labor and 2 years additional labor.
- pH production are dependent upon water source.
These statements have not been evaluated by the Food & Drug Administra-

tion. **This product is not intended to diagnose, treat, cure or prevent any disease.**
Shown in Product Identification Guide, page 503　.

Fleet Laboratories
Division of C.B. Fleet Company, Incorporated
LYNCHBURG, VA 24502

Direct Inquiries to:
Sherrie McNamara, RN, MSN, MBA
Director of Medical Affairs and Product Safety
1-866-255-6960

FLEET® PEDIA-LAX®　　　　　OTC
DOCUSATE SODIUM LIQUID STOOL SOFTENER
Stool softener laxative

Drug Facts
Active ingredient	Purpose
(in each tablespoon – 15 mL)	
Docusate sodium 50 mg	Stool softener

Uses:
• to help prevent dry, hard stools
• to relieve occasional constipation

Description:
Docusate sodium is a stool softener laxative, given orally, which usually produces a bowel movement within 12 to 72 hours. Stool softener laxatives penetrate and soften the stool, thereby promoting bowel movement.

INFORMATION FOR PATIENT
DRUG INTERACTION PRECAUTION: Do not give this product to child if child is presently taking mineral oil, unless directed by a doctor.

WARNINGS:
Ask a doctor before using any laxative if your child has
• abdominal pain, nausea or vomiting
• a sudden change in bowel habits lasting more than 2 weeks
• already used a laxative for more than 1 week
Stop using this product and consult a doctor if your child has
• rectal bleeding
• no bowel movement after 72 hours of taking this product
These symptoms may be signs of a serious condition.
Keep this and all drugs out of the reach of children. In case of overdose, get medical help or contact a Poison Control Center right away.

Directions: Doses may be taken as a single daily dose or in divided doses.
Doses must be given in a 6-8 ounce glass of milk or juice, to prevent throat irritation.

Each tablespoon (15 mL) contains 13 mg sodium.

Dosing Chart

Age	Starting Dose	Maximum Dose per Day
Children 2 to 11 years	1–3 tablespoons	3 tablespoons
Children under 2	Ask a doctor	Ask a doctor

Inactive ingredients: citric acid, edetate disodium, FD&C Red #3, flavor, methylparaben, polyethylene glycol, povidone, propylene glycol, propylparaben, sodium citrate, sorbitol, sucralose, water, zanthan gum, xylitol.

How Supplied: 4 fl.oz. (118 mL) bottles with child-resistant cap. Fruit punch flavor.
Is this product OTC?
Yes.
QUESTIONS? Call 1-866-255-6960 or visit www.Pedia-Lax.com
Shown in Product Identification Guide, page 503

FLEET® PEDIA-LAX®　　　　　OTC
GLYCERIN LAXATIVES: SUPPOSITORIES AND LIQUID GLYCERIN SUPPOSITORIES
Hyperosmotic laxative

Drug Facts
Active ingredient	Purpose
(in each 2.7 mL delivered dose)	
Glycerin 2.8 g	Hyperosmotic laxative

Drug Facts
Active ingredient	Purpose
(in each suppository)	
Glycerin 1 g	Hyperosmotic laxative

Use:
• to relieve occasional constipation

Description:
Glycerin is a hyperosmotic laxative, given rectally, which usually produces a bowel movement within 15 minutes to 1 hour. Hyperosmotic laxatives encourage bowel movements by drawing water into the bowel from surrounding tissues. This produces a softer stool mass and increased bowel action. These products are used for fast, predictable relief of occasional constipation. However, rectal irritation may occur with its use.

INFORMATION FOR PATIENT
WARNINGS
This product may cause rectal discomfort or a burning sensation.
General Laxative Warnings:
Ask a doctor before using any laxative if your child has
• abdominal pain, nausea or vomiting
• a sudden change in bowel habits lasting more than 2 weeks
• already used a laxative for more than 1 week

Stop using this product and consult a doctor if your child has
• rectal bleeding
• no bowel movement after 1 hour of taking this product
These symptoms may be signs of a serious condition.
Keep this and all drugs out of the reach of children. In case of accidental overdose or ingestion, seek professional assistance or contact a Poison Control Center right away.

Directions:
FLEET® Pedia-Lax® Liquid Glycerin Suppositories

Dosing Chart

Age	Single daily dosage
children 2 to 5 years	1 suppository or as directed by a doctor
children under 2	ask a doctor

Preferred position: Place child on left side with knees bent and arms resting comfortably, or have child kneel, then lower head and chest forward until left side of face is resting on surface with left arm folded comfortably.
CAUTION: REMOVE ORANGE PROTECTIVE SHIELD FROM TIP BEFORE INSERTING. Hold the unit upright, grasping the bulb with fingers. Grasp the orange protective shield with the other hand; pull gently to remove. With steady pressure, gently insert the tip into the rectum with a slight side-to-side movement, with the tip pointing towards navel. **DISCONTINUE USE IF RESISTANCE IS ENCOUNTERED. FORCING THE TIP CAN RESULT IN INJURY.** Insertion may be easier if child receiving the liquid suppository bears down as if having a bowel movement. This helps relax the muscles around the anus. Squeeze the bulb until nearly all liquid has been expelled. While continuing to squeeze the bulb, remove the tip from the rectum and discard the unit. It is not necessary to empty the unit completely. The unit contains more than the amount of liquid needed for effective use. A small amount of liquid will remain in the unit after squeezing.
FLEET®　　Pedia-Lax®　　Glycerin Suppositories

Dosing Chart

Age	Single daily dosage
children 2 to 5 years	1 suppository or as directed by a doctor
children under 2	ask a doctor

Insert suppository fully into the rectum. The suppository need not melt completely to produce laxative action. Store the container tightly closed and keep away from excessive heat.

Continued on next page

Fleet Pedia-Lax Laxatives—Cont.

How Supplied: FLEET® Pedia-Lax® Liquid Glycerin Suppositories Each box contains 6 child rectal applicators (4 mL each).
FLEET® Pedia-Lax® Glycerin Suppositories Available in jars of 12.
IS THIS PRODUCT OTC? Yes.
QUESTIONS?
Call 1-866-255-6960 or visit www.Pedia-Lax.com

Shown in Product Identification Guide, page 504

FLEET® PEDIA-LAX® ENEMA OTC
Saline laxative

Drug Facts

Active ingredient (in each 59-mL delivered dose)	Purpose
Monobasic sodium phosphate 9.5 g	Saline laxative/ bowel cleanser
Dibasic sodium phosphate 3.5 g	Saline laxative/ bowel cleanser

Uses:
• to relieve occasional constipation
• bowel cleansing before rectal exam

Description:
Each **latex-free** FLEET® PEDIA-LAX® ENEMA unit, with a 2 inch, pre-lubricated Comfortip®, contains 2.25 fl. oz. (66 mL) of enema solution in a ready-to-use squeeze bottle.
FLEET® PEDIA-LAX® ENEMAS are designed for quick, convenient administration by nurse or parent according to instructions. Each is disposable after a single use.
ELEMENTAL AND ELECTROLYTIC CONTENT

mEq Phosphate (PO_4) per mL	4.15
mEq Sodium (Na) per mL	1.61
mg Sodium (Na) per mL	37
mmole Phosphorus (P) per mL	1.38

Each FLEET® PEDIA-LAX® ENEMA 59 mL delivered dose contains 2.2 grams sodium.
When used as directed, FLEET® PEDIA-LAX® ENEMAS provide thorough yet safe cleansing action and induce complete emptying of the left colon, usually within 1 to 5 minutes, without pain or spasm.
INFORMATION FOR PATIENT

WARNINGS:
Using more than one enema in 24 hours can be harmful.
Ask a doctor before using this product if the child is on a sodium-restricted diet or has a kidney disease.
IF, AFTER THE ENEMA SOLUTION IS ADMINISTERED THERE IS NO RETURN OF LIQUID, CONTACT A PHYSICIAN IMMEDIATELY, AS ELECTROLYTE DISTURBANCES AND CONSEQUENT SERIOUS SIDE EFFECTS COULD OCCUR.
DO NOT USE ANY FLEET® ENEMA IN CHILDREN UNDER 2 YEARS OF AGE.
DO NOT ADMINISTER A FULL 2.25 FL. OZ. FLEET® PEDIA-LAX® ENEMA TO CHILDREN UNDER 5 YEARS OF AGE.
FOR CHILDREN 2 TO UNDER 5 YEARS, USE ONE-HALF BOTTLE OF 2.25 FL. OZ. FLEET® PEDIA-LAX® ENEMA.
IMPORTANT: FLEET® PEDIA-LAX® ENEMAS ARE NOT INTENDED FOR ORAL CONSUMPTION in any dosage size.
General Laxative Warnings:
Ask a doctor before using any laxative if your child has
• abdominal pain, nausea or vomiting
• a sudden change in bowel habits lasting more than 2 weeks
• already used a laxative for more than 1 week
Stop using this product and consult a doctor if your child has
• rectal bleeding
• no bowel movement after 30 minutes of taking this product
These symptoms may be signs of a serious condition.
Keep this and all drugs out of the reach of children. In case of accidental overdose or ingestion, seek professional assistance or contact a Poison Control Center right away.
Use ONLY the Fleet® Pedia-Lax® enema in children.

Drug Interactions: Do not give child other sodium phosphates products such as Fleet® Phospho-soda® oral solution or sodium phosphates tablets while child is taking this product.

Hydration: Additional liquids by mouth are recommended.

Directions:
Do not use more unless directed by a doctor. See Warnings.

Dosing Chart

Age	Single daily dosage
children 5 to 11 years	one bottle or as directed by a doctor
children 2 to under 5 years	one-half bottle (see below) or as directed by a doctor
children under 2 years	DO NOT USE

One-half bottle preparation: Unscrew cap and remove 2 Tablespoons of liquid with a measuring spoon. Replace cap and follow DIRECTIONS on back of carton.
REMOVE ORANGE PROTECTIVE SHIELD FROM TIP BEFORE INSERTING.
Preferred position: Place child on left side with knees bent and arms resting comfortably, or have child kneel, then lower head and chest forward until left side of face is resting on surface with left arm folded comfortably.
The diaphragm at base of tube prevents reflux and assures controlled flow of the enema solution. FLEET® PEDIA-LAX® ENEMA should be used at room temperature.

How Supplied: FLEET® PEDIA-LAX® ENEMA is supplied in a 2.25 fl. oz. (66 mL) ready-to-use squeeze bottle.
QUESTIONS? Call 1-866-255-6960 or visit www.Pedia-Lax.com.

Shown in Product Identification Guide, page 503

FLEET® PEDIA-LAX®   OTC
MAGNESIUM HYDROXIDE
CHEWABLE TABLETS
Saline laxative

Drug Facts

Active ingredient (in each tablet):	Purpose
Magnesium hydroxide 400 mg	Saline laxative

Use:
• to relieve occasional constipation

Description:
Magnesium hydroxide is a saline laxative, given orally, which usually produces a bowel movement within 30 minutes to 6 hours. Saline laxatives increase water in the intestine thereby promoting bowel movement.

INFORMATION FOR PATIENT
WARNINGS:
Ask a physician before using this product if child has a magnesium-restricted diet or a kidney disease.
Ask a doctor before using any laxative if your child has
• abdominal pain, nausea or vomiting
• a sudden change in bowel habits lasting more than 2 weeks
• already used a laxative for more than 1 week
Stop using this product and consult a doctor if your child has
• rectal bleeding
• no bowel movement after 6 hours of taking this product
These symptoms may be signs of a serious condition.
Keep this and all drugs out of the reach of children. In case of overdose, get medical help or contact a Poison Control Center right away.

Directions: Doses may be taken as a single daily dose or in divided doses. **Have child drink a full glass (8 fluid ounces) of liquid with each tablet.**
Each tablet contains 170 mg magnesium.

Dosing Chart

Age	Starting Dose	Maximum Dose per Day
Children 6 to 11 years	3–6 tablets	6 tablets

Children 2 to 5 years	1–3 tablets	3 tablets
Children under 2	Ask a doctor	Ask a doctor

Inactive ingredients: colloidal silicon dioxide, FD&C Red #40 aluminum lake, flavor, magnesium stearate, maltodextrin, mannitol, sorbitol, stearic acid, sucralose

How Supplied: 30 Pedia-Lax Chewable Tablets per bottle with child-resistant cap. Watermelon flavor.

Is this product OTC?

Yes.

QUESTIONS?

Call 1-866-255-6960 or visit www.Pedia-Lax.com

Shown in Product Identification Guide, page 503

FLEET® PEDIA-LAX® SENNA OTC QUICK DISSOLVE STRIPS

Stimulant laxative

Drug Facts

Active ingredient (in each strip)	**Purpose**
Standardized Sennosides 8.6 mg	Stimulant laxative

Use:
• to relieve occasional constipation

Description:

Senna is a stimulant laxative, given orally, which usually produces a bowel movement within 6 to 12 hours. Stimulant laxatives promote bowel movement by one or more direct actions on the intestine.

INFORMATION FOR PATIENT

WARNINGS:

Ask a physician before using this product if child is taking non-steroidal anti-inflammatory drugs (NSAIDs).

Ask a doctor before using any laxative if your child has
• abdominal pain, nausea, or vomiting
• a sudden change in bowel habits lasting more than 2 weeks
• already used a laxative for more than 1 week

Stop using this product and consult a doctor if your child has
• rectal bleeding
• no bowel movement after 12 hours of taking this product

These symptoms may be signs of a serious condition.

Keep this and all drugs out of the reach of children. In case of overdose, get medical help or contact a Poison Control Center right away.

Directions:

Dosing Chart

Age	Starting Dose	Maximum Dose per Day
Children 6 to 11 years	2 strips	Do not exceed 4 strips in 24 hours
Children 2 to 5 years	1 strip	Do not exceed 2 strips in 24 hours
Children under 2	Ask a doctor	Ask a doctor

Place quick dissolve strip on child's tongue or have child place on the tongue. Allow strip to dissolve. Encourage child to drink plenty of liquids.

Inactive ingredients: butylated hydroxytoluene, FD&C Red #40, flavor, hydroxypropyl methylcellulose, malic acid, methylparaben, polydextrose, polyethylene oxide, simethicone, sodium bicarbonate, sucralose, white ink.

How Supplied: 12 Pedia-Lax Quick-Dissolve Strips per carton. Grape flavor.

Other Information: Color of strips may vary. Store at controlled room temperature 59°–86°F (15°–30°C).

Is this product OTC?

Yes.

QUESTIONS?

Call 1-866-255-6960 or visit www.Pedia-Lax.com

Shown in Product Identification Guide, page 503

Green Pharmaceuticals® Inc.,

591 CONSTITUTION AVE, #A CAMARILLO, CA 93012

Direct Inquiries and Medical Emergencies:

mail@snorestop.com or (800) 337-4835

SNORESTOP®　　　　OTC EXTINGUISHER™ 120 ORAL SPRAYS HOMEOPATHIC ANTI-SNORING MEDICINE

Description: Uniquely formulated (U.S. Patent No. 6,491,954) to temporarily relieve the symptoms commonly associated with non-apneic snoring. No known side effects or drug interactions.

Important Information: This product contains no ephedrine, no pseudoephedrine, no tropane or indole alkaloids. Each substance has been highly diluted according to the *Homeopathic Pharmacopoeia of the United*

States: 4X is equal to one-part-per-ten thousand, 6X is equal to one-part-per-million, and 12 X is equal to one-part-per-trillion.

Mode of Action: Decongestive, anti-inflammatory, anti-histaminic and mucolytic.

Active Ingredients (HPUS): Nux vomica 4X, 6X, Belladonna 6X, Ephedra vulgaris 6X, Hydrastis canadensis 6X, Kali bichromicum 6X, Teucrium marum 6X, Histaminum hydrochloricum 12 X.

Directions: Children over 5 years of age and Adults. Shake before each use. Spray once under the tongue and once in the back of throat at bedtime. When improvement is noticed, you may use *every other night.*

Warnings: Do not use if seal around the bottle is broken. Do not use on children under 5 years of age. This product does not treat sleep apnea. For sleep apnea, consult with a specialist. If symptoms worsen, discontinue use and consult with a licensed health care professional. **If pregnant or breast-feeding,** ask a health care professional before use. Keep this and all medications out of the reach of children. This product is non-addictive and may be used up to 4 times a day.

Inactive Ingredients: Purified water 75%, USP Alcohol 15%, Glycerin 9.9%, Potassium sorbate 0.1%.

How Supplied: 0.4 fl oz bottle delivering 120 metered sprays (NDC 61152-196-12). 0.3 fl.oz bottle delivering 60 metered sprays (NDC 61152-196-09)

SNORESTOP®　　　　OTC MAXIMUM STRENGTH CHEWABLE TABLETS HOMEOPATHIC ANTI-SNORING MEDICINE

Description: Uniquely formulated* to temporarily relieve the symptoms of non-apneic snoring. No known side effects or drug interactions. Non-habit forming. *This formula has been the subject of a peer-reviewed, randomized, double blind, placebo controlled independent clinical study whose positive results have been published in the medical journal *Sleep and Breathing.* Vol.3. No.2. 1999.

Important Information: This product contains no ephedrine, no pseudoephedrine, no tropane or indole alkaloids. Each substance has been highly diluted according to the *Homeopathic Pharmacopoeia of the United States:* 4X is equal to one-part-per-ten thousand, 6X is equal to one-part-per-million, and 12 X is equal to one-part-per-trillion.

Mode of Action: Decongestive, anti-inflammatory, anti-histaminic and mucolytic.

Continued on next page

SnoreStop Tablets—Cont.

Active Ingredients (HPUS): Nux vomica 4X, 6X, Belladonna 6X, Ephedra vulgaris 6X, Hydrastis canadensis 6X, Kali bichromicum 6X, Teucrium marum 6X, Histaminum hydrochloricum 12 X.

Directions: Children over 5 years of age and Adults. Chew or suck one tablet when lying in bed. When improvement is noticed, you may start using *every other night* until no longer needed.

Warnings: Do not use if blister seal around the tablet is broken. Do not use on children under 5 years of age. This product does not treat sleep apnea. For sleep apnea, consult with a specialist. If symptoms worsen, discontinue use and consult with a licensed health care professional. **If you are pregnant or breastfeeding,** ask a health care professional before use. Keep this and all medications out of the reach of children.

Inactive Ingredients: Lactose 297 mg, magnesium stearate 3 mg.

How Supplied: Boxes of 10 tablets (NDC 61152-195-10), 20 tablets (NDC 61152-195-20), 60 tablets (NDC 61152-195-60).

Hisamitsu Pharmaceutical Co., Inc.

**408 TASHIRO DAIKAN-MACHI
TOSU SAGA 841-0017
JAPAN**

Direct Inquiries to:
Tel: +81-3-5293-1720
Fax: +81-3-5293-1724

SALONPAS®   OTC
ARTHRITIS PAIN
Pain Relieving Patch

Drug Facts:
Active ingredients:
(in each patch)   **Purpose:**
Menthol 3%   Topical analgesic
Methyl Salicylate
    10% (NSAID*)   Topical analgesic
*nonsteroidal anti-inflammatory drug

Uses:
Temporarily relieves mild to moderate aches & pains of muscles & joints associated with:
• arthritis • sprains • strains • bruises
• simple backache

Warnings:
For external use only
Stomach bleeding warning
This product contains an NSAID, which may cause stomach bleeding. The chance is small but higher if you:
• are age 60 or older
• have had stomach ulcers or bleeding problems

• take a blood thinning (anticoagulant) or steroid drug
• take other drugs containing an NSAID [aspirin, ibuprofen, naproxen, or others]
• have 3 or more alcoholic drinks every day while using this product
• take more or for a longer time than directed

Do not use
• on the face or rashes
• on wounds or damaged skin
• if allergic to aspirin or other NSAIDs
• with a heating pad
• when sweating (such as from exercise or heat)
• any patch from a pouch that has been open for 14 or more days
• right before or after heart surgery

Ask a doctor before use if
• you are allergic to topical products
• the stomach bleeding warning applies to you
• you have high blood pressure, heart disease, or kidney disease
• you are taking a diuretic

When using this product
• wash hands after applying or removing patch. Avoid contact with eyes. If eye contact occurs, rinse thoroughly with water.
• the risk of heart attack or stroke may increase if you use more than directed or for longer than directed

Stop use and ask a doctor if
• you feel faint, vomit blood, or have bloody or black stools. These are signs of stomach bleeding.
• rash, itching or skin irritation develops
• condition worsens
• symptoms last for more than 3 days
• symptoms clear up and occur again within a few days
• stomach pain or upset gets worse or lasts

If pregnant or breast-feeding, ask a doctor before use during the first 6 months of pregnancy. Do not use during the last 3 months of pregnancy because it may cause problems in the unborn child or complications during delivery.

Keep out of reach of children.
If put in mouth, get medical help or contact a Poison Control Center right away. Package not child resistant.

Directions:
Adults 18 years and older:
• clean and dry affected area
• remove patch from backing film and apply to skin
• apply one patch to the affected area and leave in place for up to 8 to 12 hours
• if pain lasts after using the first patch, a second patch may be applied for up to another 8 to 12 hours
• only use one patch at a time
• do not use more than 2 patches per day
• do not use for more than 3 days in a row

Children under 18 years of age:
• do not use

Other Information:
• some individuals may not experience pain relief until several hours after applying the patch
• avoid storing product in direct sunlight
• protect product from excessive moisture
• store at 20-25°C (68-77°F)

Inactive ingredients: alicyclic saturated hydrocarbon resin, backing cloth, film, mineral oil, polyisobutylene, polyisobutylene 1,200,000, styrene-isoprene-styrene block copolymer, synthetic aluminum silicate

Questions or comments?
Toll free 1-87-SALONPAS
MON-FRI 9AM to 5PM (PST)

How Supplied: Available in 3 patches, 5 patches & 15 patches 2 3/4 × 3 15/16 inch (7cm ×10cm)
Shown in Product Identification Guide, page 504

SALONPAS® PAIN RELIEF   OTC
PATCH
Pain Relieving Patch

Drug Facts:
Active ingredients: **Purpose:**
(in each patch).
Menthol 3%   Topical analgesic
Methyl salicylate
    10% (NSAID*)   Topical analgesic
*nonsteroidal anti-inflammatory drug

Uses:
Temporarily relieves mild to moderate aches & pains of muscles & joints associated with:
• strains • sprains • simple backache
• arthritis • bruises

Warnings:
For external use only
Stomach bleeding warning:
This product contains an NSAID, which may cause stomach bleeding. The chance is small but higher if you:
• are age 60 or older
• have had stomach ulcers or bleeding problems
• take a blood thinning (anticoagulant) or steroid drug
• take other drugs containing an NSAID [aspirin, ibuprofen, naproxen, or others]
• have 3 or more alcoholic drinks every day while using this product
• take more or for a longer time than directed

Do not use
• on the face or rashes
• on wounds or damaged skin
• if allergic to aspirin or other NSAIDs
• with a heating pad
• when sweating (such as from exercise or heat)
• any patch from a pouch that has been open for 14 or more days
• right before or after heart surgery

Ask a doctor before use if
• you are allergic to topical products
• the stomach bleeding warning applies to you
• you have high blood pressure, heart disease, or kidney disease
• you are taking a diuretic

When using this product
• wash hands after applying or removing patch. Avoid contact with eyes. If eye contact occurs, rinse thoroughly with water.
• the risk of heart attack or stroke may increase if you use more than directed or for longer than directed

Stop use and ask a doctor if
- you feel faint, vomit blood, or have bloody or black stools. These are signs of stomach bleeding.
- rash, itching or skin irritation develops
- condition worsens
- symptoms last for more than 3 days
- symptoms clear up and occur again within a few days
- stomach pain or upset gets worse or lasts

If pregnant or breast-feeding, ask a doctor before use during the first 6 months of pregnancy. Do not use during the last 3 months of pregnancy because it may cause problems in the unborn child or complications during delivery.

Keep out of reach of children
If put in mouth, get medical help or contact a Poison Control Center right away. Package not child resistant.

Directions:
Adults 18 years and older:
- clean and dry affected area
- remove patch from backing film and apply to skin
- apply one patch to the affected area and leave in place for up to 8 to 12 hours
- if pain lasts after using the first patch, a second patch may be applied for up to another 8 to 12 hours
- only use one patch at a time
- do not use more than 2 patches per day
- do not use for more than 3 days in a row

Children under 18 years of age:
- do not use

Other information:
- some individuals may not experience pain relief until several hours after applying the patch
- avoid storing product in direct sunlight
- protect product from excessive moisture
- store at 20-25°C (68-77°F)

Inactive ingredients: alicyclic saturated hydrocarbon resin, backing cloth, film, mineral oil, polyisobutylene, polyisobutylene 1,200,000, styrene-isoprene-styrene block copolymer, synthetic aluminum silicate

Questions or comments?
Toll free 1-87-SALONPAS
MON-FRI 9AM to 5PM (PST)

How Supplied: Available in 3 patches, 5 patches & 15 patches 2 3/4 × 3 15/16 inch (7cm ×10cm)

Shown in Product Identification Guide, page 504

SALONPAS® GEL   OTC

Drug Facts:

Active Ingredients:	Purpose:
Menthol 7%	Topical analgesic
Methyl Salicylate 15%	Topical analgesic

Uses:
For temporary relief of minor aches & pains of muscles & joints associated with:

- simple backache • arthritis • strains
- bruises • sprains

Warnings:
For external use only
Do not use
- on wounds or damaged skin.
- if you are allergic to aspirin or salicylates.
- with a heating pad.
- with, or at the same times as, other external analgesic products.

Ask a doctor before use, if you are allergic to any ingredients of this product.
When using this product
- **do not use otherwise than as directed.**
- avoid contact with the eyes, mucous membranes or rashes.
- do not bandage tightly.

Stop use and ask a doctor if
- **rash, itching or excessive skin irritation develops.**
- conditions worsen.
- symptoms persist for more than 7 days.
- symptoms clear up and occur again within a few days.

Keep out of reach of children. If swallowed, get medical help or contact a Poison Control Center right away.

Directions:
Adults and children 2 years of age and over:
- Clean and dry affected area.
- Apply to affected area not more than 3 to 4 times daily for 7 days.

Children under 2 years of age:
- Consult a doctor.

Other Information:
- Avoid storing product in direct sunlight.
- Protect product from excessive moisture.

Inactive ingredients:
carbomer, denatured alcohol, hydroxypropyl cellulose, perfume, polyoxyethylene oleylamine, propylene glycol, water

How Supplied: Available in 40g

SALONPAS® GEL-PATCH   OTC
HOT SOOTHING

Drug Facts:

Active Ingredients:		Purpose:
Capsicum extract	0.025% as Capsaicin	Topical analgesic
Menthol	1.25%	Topical analgesic

Uses:
For temporary relief of minor aches & pains of muscles & joints associated with:

- simple backache • arthritis • strains
- bruises • sprains

Warnings: For external use only
Discontinue use at least 1 hour before a bath or shower and do not use immediately after a bath or shower.
Do not use
- on wounds or damaged skin.
- with a heating pad.
- with, or at the same time as, other external analgesic products.

Ask a doctor before use, if you are allergic to any ingredients of this product.
When using this product
- **do not use otherwise than as directed.**
- avoid contact with the eyes, mucous membranes or rashes.

Stop use and ask a doctor if
- **rash, itching or excessive skin irritation develops.**
- conditions worsen.
- symptoms persist for more than 7 days.
- symptoms clear up and occur again within a few days.

Keep out of reach of children. If swallowed, get medical help or contact a Poison Control Center right away.

Directions:
Adults and children 12 years of age and over:
- Clean and dry affected area.
- Remove patch from film.
- Apply to affected area not more than 3 to 4 times daily for 7 days.
- Remove patch from the skin after at most 8 hour's application.

Children under 12 years of age:
- Consult a doctor.

Other Information:
- Store at 15-30°C (59-86°F)
- Avoid storing product in direct sunlight.
- Protect product from excessive moisture.
- The active ingredients of this product increase blood circulation.

This may cause redness on the application site. Upon removal of the patch, the redness should disappear after a few hours. If redness persists, stop using the product and consult a doctor.

Inactive ingredients: aluminum silicate, edetate disodium, gelatin, glycerin, magnesium aluminometasilicate, oleyl alcohol, polyacrylic acid, polyethylene glycol, polyvinyl alcohol, sodium polyacrylate, sorbitan monooleate, tartaric acid, titanium dioxide, water

How Supplied: Available in 6 patch 5.51 IN x 3.94 IN (14cm x 10cm)

SALONPAS®-HOT   OTC
Capsicum Patch

Drug Facts:

Active Ingredient:		Purpose:
Capsicum extract	0.025% as Capsaicin	Topical analgesic

Uses:
For temporary relief of minor aches & pains of muscles & joints associated with:

- simple backache • arthritis • strains
- bruises • sprains

Warnings:
For external use only
Discontinue use at least 1 hour before a bath or shower and do not use immediately after a bath or shower.

Continued on next page

Salonpas-Hot Patch—Cont.

Do not use
- on wounds or damaged skin.
- with a heating pad.
- with, or at the same time as, other external analgesic products.
- if you are allergic to any ingredients of this product.

When using this product
- do not use otherwise than as directed.
- avoid contact with the eyes, mucous membranes or rashes.

Stop use and ask a doctor if
- rash, itching or excessive skin irritation develops.
- conditions worsen.
- symptoms persist for more than 7 days.
- symptoms clear up and occur again within a few days.

Keep out of reach of children. If swallowed, get medical help or contact a Poison Control Center right away.

Directions:
Adults and children 12 years of age and over:
- Clean and dry affected area.
- Remove patch from film.
- Apply to affected area not more than 3 to 4 times daily for 7 days.
- Remove patch from the skin after at most 8 hour's application.

Children under 12 years of age:
- Consult a doctor.

Other Information:
- Avoid storing product in direct sunlight.
- Protect product from excessive moisture.

Inactive ingredients: butylated hydroxytoluene, hydrogenated rosin glycerol ester, maleated rosin glycerin ester, natural rubber, polybutene, polyisobutylene, silicon dioxide, titanium dioxide, zinc oxide

How Supplied: Available in 1 patch 5.12 IN × 7.09 IN

SALONSIP® AQUA-PATCH®   OTC
Pain Relieving Cooling Patch

Drug Facts:
Active Ingredient: **Purpose:**
Menthol 1.25%   Topical analgesic

Uses:
For temporary relief of minor aches & pains of muscles & joints associated with:
- simple backache • arthritis • strains
- bruises • sprains

Warnings: For external use only
Do not use
- if you are allergic to any ingredients of this product.
- on wounds or damaged skin.
- with a heating pad.
- with, or at the same time as, other external analgesic products.

When using this product
- do not use otherwise than as directed.
- avoid contact with the eyes, mucous membranes or rashes.

Stop use and ask a doctor if
- rash, itching or excessive skin irritation develops.
- conditions worsen.
- symptoms persist for more than 7 days.
- symptoms clear up and occur again within a few days.

Keep out of reach of children. If swallowed, get medical help or contact a Poison Control Center right away.

Directions:
Adults and children 12 years of age and over:
- Clean and dry affected area.
- Remove patch from film.
- Apply to affected area not more than 3 to 4 times daily for 7 days.
- Remove patch from the skin after at most 8 hour's application.

Children under 12 years of age:
- Consult a doctor.

Other Information:
- Avoid storing product in direct sunlight.
- Protect product from excessive moisture.

Inactive ingredients: agar, aluminum silicate, edetate disodium, glycerin, isopropyl myristate, magnesium aluminometasilicate, polyethylene glycol monostearate, polyacrylic acid, polyvinyl alcohol, sodium polyacrylate, tartaric acid, titanium dioxide, water

How Supplied:
Available in 5 patch 5.51 IN × 3.94 IN 14cm × 10cm

Merz Pharmaceuticals
DIVISION OF MERZ, INC.
4215 TUDOR LANE (27410)
P.O. BOX 18806
GREENSBORO, NC 27419

Direct Inquiries to:
Medical/Regulatory Affairs
(336) 856-2003
FAX: (336) 217-2439
For Medical Information Contact:
In Emergencies:
Medical/Regulatory Affairs
(336) 856-2003
FAX: (336) 217-2439

MEDERMA® CREAM   OTC
PLUS SPF 30
[ma-der-mă]

Description: Mederma® Cream helps old and new scars appear softer, smoother and less noticeable. Mederma® Cream offers the added protection of SPF 30 in a cream formulation to help protect scars from the sun's UV rays. Mederma® Cream is a greaseless, topical cream that is safe for use on all skin types.

Active Ingredients: Avobenzone 3%, Octocrylene 10%, Oxybenzone 6%

Inactive Ingredients: Water, Allium Cepa (Onion) Bulb Extract, C12-15 Alkyl Benzoate, Dicaprylyl Carbonate, Hydrogenated Lecithin, Caprylic/Capric Triglyceride, Panthenol, Pentylene Glycol, Phenoxyethanol, Butyrospermum Parkii (Shea Butter), Glycerin, Ammonium Acryloyl – Dimethyltaurate/VP Copolymer, Fragrance, Squalane, Methylparaben, Xanthan Gum, Disodium EDTA, Ceramide 3, Sodium Hyaluronate, Butylparaben, Ethylparaben, Propylparaben, Isobutylparaben.

Dosage And Administration Evenly apply a small amount of Mederma® Cream and gently massage into the scar 3 times daily and as needed before sun exposure. Mederma® Cream should be used for 8 weeks on new scars and 3-6 months on existing scars. Children under 6 months of age: ask a doctor.

Warnings: For external use only. When using this product keep out of eyes. Rinse with water to remove. Stop use and ask doctor if rash or irritation develops and lasts. Do not use on open wounds. Keep out of reach of children. If swallowed, get medical help or contact a Poison Control Center right away.

Storage Store at room temperature

How Supplied: Mederma® Cream is available in:
- 20g tube (a three-month supply for scars up to three inches long)
- 50g tube (a three-month supply for scars eight to ten inches long)

Manufactured for:
Merz Pharmaceuticals, Greensboro, NC 27410
5011234   Rev. 09/07

Mission Pharmacal Company
10999 IH 10 WEST, SUITE 1000
SAN ANTONIO, TX 78230-1355

Direct Inquiries to:
P.O. Box 786099
San Antonio, TX 78278-6099
(800) 292-7364; (210) 696-8400

THERA-GESIC® Maximum Strength
Analgesic Pain Relieving Creme

Drug Facts
Active Ingredients: **Purpose:**
Menthol 1% .... Analgesic
Methyl Salicylate 15% . Counterirritant

Use:
temporary relief of minor aches and pains of muscles and joints associated with:
- arthritis • simple backaches • strains
- bruises • sprains

Warnings:
For external use only. Use only as directed. Avoid contact with eyes or mucous membranes.

Do not bandage tightly, wrap or cover until after washing the areas where THERA-GESIC® has been applied.

Do not use
- immediately after shower or bath
- if skin is sensitive to oil of wintergreen (methyl salicylate)
- on wounds or damaged skin

Ask a doctor before use
- for children under 2 and to 12 years of age
- if prone or sensitive to allergic reactions from aspirin or salicylate

When using this product
- discontinue use if skin irritation develops, or redness is present
- do not swallow
- do not use a heating pad after application of THERA-GESIC®

Stop use and ask a doctor if condition worsens, or if symptoms persist for more than 7 days or clear up and occur again within a few days.

If pregnant or breast-feeding, ask a health professional before use.

Keep out of reach of children to avoid accidental poisoning. If swallowed, get medical help or contact a Poison Control Center right away.

Directions:
Adults and children 12 or more years of age: Apply thin layers of creme into and around the sore or painful area, not more than 3 to 4 times daily. The number of thin layers controls the intensity of the action of THERA-GESIC®. One thin layer provides a mild effect, two thin layers provide a strong effect and three thin layers provide a very strong effect. SEE WARNINGS. Wash hands thoroughly after application.

Other Information:
Once THERA-GESIC® has penetrated the skin, the area may be washed, leaving it dry, clean and fragrance-free without decreasing the effectiveness of the product. Avoid contact with clothing or other surfaces. Store at 20–25°C (68–77°F).

Inactive Ingredients:
Carbomer 934, Dimethicone, Glycerine, Methylparaben, Propylparaben, Sodium Lauryl Sulfate, Trolamine, Water.

Questions?
(210) 696-8400 (M-F 8:30-5:00 CST)

How Supplied: Net wt. 3 oz., NDC 0178-0320-03; Net wt. 5 oz., NDC 0178-0320-05.

Procter & Gamble
P.O. BOX 559
CINCINNATI, OH 45201

Direct Inquiries to:
Consumer Relations
(800) 832-3064

METAMUCIL® FIBER LAXATIVE
[met uh-mü sil]
(psyllium husk)

*Also see **Metamucil Dietary Fiber Supplement** in PDR for Nonprescription Drugs*

Description: Metamucil contains psyllium husk (from the plant *Plantago ovata*), a bulk forming, natural therapeutic fiber for restoring and maintaining regularity when recommended by a physician. Metamucil contains no chemical stimulants and does not disrupt normal bowel function. Each dose of Metamucil powder and Metamucil Fiber Wafers contains approximately 3.4 grams of psyllium husk (or 2.4 grams of soluble fiber). Each dose of Metamucil capsules fiber laxative (5 capsules) contains approximately 2.6 grams of psyllium husk (or 2.0 grams of soluble fiber). Inactive ingredients, sodium, calcium, potassium, calories, carbohydrate, dietary fiber, and phenylalanine content are shown in the following table for all versions and flavors. Metamucil Smooth Texture Sugar-Free Unflavored and Metamucil capsules contains no sugar and no artificial sweeteners; Metamucil Smooth Texture Sugar-Free Orange Flavor contains aspartame (phenylalanine content per dose is 25 mg). Metamucil powdered products and Metamucil capsules are gluten-free. Metamucil Fiber Wafers contain gluten: Apple contains 0.7g/dose, Cinnamon contains 0.5g/dose. Each two-wafer dose contains 5 grams of fat.

Actions: The active ingredient in Metamucil is psyllium husk, a natural fiber which promotes elimination due to its bulking effect in the colon. This bulking effect is due to both the water-holding capacity of undigested fiber and the increased bacterial mass following partial fiber digestion. These actions result in enlargement of the lumen of the colon, and softer stool, thereby decreasing intraluminal pressure and straining, and speeding colonic transit in constipated patients.

Indications: Metamucil is indicated for the treatment of occasional constipation, and when recommended by a physician, for chronic constipation and constipation associated with irritable bowel syndrome, diverticulosis, hemorrhoids, convalescence, senility and pregnancy. Pregnancy: Category B. If considering use of Metamucil as part of a cholesterol-lowering program, see **Metamucil Dietary Fiber Supplement** in Dietary Supplement Section.

Drug Facts

Active Ingredient: (in each DOSE)	Purpose:
Psyllium husk approximately 3.4 g	Fiber therapy for regularity

For Metamucil capsules each dose of 5 capsules contains approximately 2.6 gm of psyllium husk.

Uses:
- effective in treating occasional constipation and restoring regularity

Warnings:
Choking: Taking this product without adequate fluid may cause it to swell and block your throat or esophagus and may cause choking. Do not take this product if you have difficulty in swallowing. If you experience chest pain, vomiting, or difficulty in swallowing or breathing after taking this product, seek immediate medical attention.

Allergy alert: This product may cause allergic reaction in people sensitive to inhaled or ingested psyllium.

Ask a doctor before use if you have:
- a sudden change in bowel habits persisting for 2 weeks
- abdominal pain, nausea or vomiting

Stop use and ask a doctor if:
- constipation lasts more than 7 days
- rectal bleeding occurs

These may be signs of a serious condition.

Keep out of reach of children. In case of overdose, get medical help or contact a Poison Control Center right away.

Directions: For Powders: Put one dose into an empty glass. Fill glass with at least 8 oz of water or your favorite beverage. Stir briskly and drink promptly. If mixture thickens, add more liquid and stir. Mix this product (child or adult dose) with at least 8 ounces (a full glass) of water or other fluid. **For Capsules:** Take product with 8 oz of liquid (swallow 1 capsule at a time) up to 3 times daily. Take this product with at least 8 oz (a full glass) of liquid. **For Wafers:** Take this product (child or adult dose) with at least 8 ounces (a full glass) of liquid. Taking these products without enough liquid may cause choking. See choking warning.

Adults 12 yrs. & older	Powders: 1 dose in 8 oz of liquid. Capsules: 5 capsules with 8 oz of liquid (swallow one capsule at a time). Wafers: 1 dose with 8 oz of liquid. Take at the first sign of irregularity; can be taken up to 3 times daily. Generally produces effect in 12 – 72 hours.
6 – 11 yrs.	Powders: ½ adult dose in 8 oz of liquid. Wafers: 1 wafer with 8 oz of liquid. Can be taken up to 3 times daily. Capsules: consider use of powder or wafer products
Under 6 yrs.	consult a doctor

Continued on next page

Metamucil Fiber Laxative/Dietary Fiber Supplement

Versions/Flavors	Ingredients (alphabetical order)	Sodium mg/ dose	Calcium mg/ dose	Potassium mg/ dose	Calories kcal/ dose	Total Carbohydrate g/dose	Dietary Fiber/ (Soluble) g/dose	Dosage (Weight in gms)	How Supplied
Smooth Texture Orange Flavor Metamucil Powder	Citric Acid, FD&C Yellow #6, Natural and Artificial Flavor, Psyllium Husk, Sucrose	5	7	30	45	12	3 (2.4)	1 rounded tablespoon ~12g	Canisters: Doses: 48, 72, 114, 188; Cartons: 30 single-dose packets.
Smooth Texture Sugar-Free Orange Flavor Metamucil Powder	Aspartame, Citric Acid, FD&C Yellow #6, Maltodextrin, Natural and Artificial Flavor, Psyllium Husk	5	7	30	20	5	3 (2.4)	1 rounded teaspoon ~5.8g	Canisters: Doses: 30, 48, 72, 114, 180, 220; Cartons: 30 single-dose packets.
Smooth Texture Sugar-Free Unflavored Metamucil Powder	Citric Acid, Maltodextrin, Psyllium Husk	4	7	30	20	5	3 (2.4)	1 rounded teaspoon ~5.4g	Canisters: Doses: 48, 72 114.
Coarse Milled Unflavored Metamucil Powder	Psyllium Husk, Sucrose	3	6	30	25	7	3 (2.4)	1 rounded teaspoon ~7g	Canisters: Doses: 48, 72 114.
Coarse Milled Orange Flavor Metamucil Powder	Citric Acid, FD&C Yellow #6, Natural and Artificial Flavor, Psyllium Husk, Sucrose	5	6	30	40	11	3 (2.4)	1 rounded tablespoon ~11g	Canisters: Doses: 48,72 114.
Metamucil Capsules	Caramel color, FD&C Blue No. 1 Aluminum Lake, FD&C Red No. 40 Aluminum Lake, FD&C Yellow No. 6 Aluminum Lake, gelatin, polysorbate 80, psyllium husk	0	5	30	10	3	3 (2.4)	6 capsules 3.2g	Bottles: 100 ct, 160 ct, 300 ct
Fiber Laxative Wafers **Apple** Metamucil Wafers	(1)	20	14	60	120	17	6	2 wafers 24 g	Cartons: 12 doses
Cinnamon Metamucil Wafers	(2)	20	14	60	120	17	6	2 wafers 24 g	Cartons: 12 doses

(1) ascorbic acid, brown sugar, cinnamon, corn oil, corn starch, fructose, lecithin, molasses, natural and artificial flavors, oat hull fiber, psyllium husk, sodium bicarbonate, sucrose, water, wheat flour
(2) ascorbic acid, cinnamon, corn oil, corn starch, fructose, lecithin, molasses, natural and artificial flavors, nutmeg, oat hull fiber, oats, psyllium husk, sodium bicarbonate, sucrose, water, wheat flour

---

Metamucil—Cont.

Laxatives, including bulk fibers, may affect how well other medicines work. If you are taking a prescription medicine by mouth, take this product at least 2 hours before or 2 hours after the prescribed medicine. As your body adjusts to increased fiber intake, you may experience changes in bowel habits or minor bloating. **New Users:** Start with 1 dose per day; gradually increase to 3 doses per day as necessary.

Other Information:
- **Each product contains:** Potassium; sodium (See table for amount/dose)
- **PHENYLKETONURICS:** Smooth Texture Sugar Free Orange product contains phenylalanine 25 mg per dose
- Each product contains a 100% natural, therapeutic fiber

[See table above]

Inactive Ingredients: See table Notice to Health Care Professionals:

To minimize the potential for allergic reaction, health care professionals who frequently dispense powdered psyllium products should avoid inhaling airborne dust while dispensing these products. Handling and Dispensing: To minimize generating airborne dust, spoon product from the canister into a glass according to label directions.

How Supplied: Powder: canisters and cartons of single-dose packets. Capsules: 100, 160 and 300 count bottles. Wafers: cartons of single dose packets. (See table)

***Questions?* 1-800-983-4237**

Shown in Product Identification Guide, page 504

PEPTO-BISMOL®
ORIGINAL LIQUID,
MAXIMUM STRENGTH LIQUID,
ORIGINAL AND CHERRY FLAVOR
CHEWABLE TABLETS
AND EASY-TO-SWALLOW CAPLETS
For upset stomach, indigestion, heartburn, nausea and diarrhea.

Multi-symptom Pepto-Bismol® contains bismuth subsalicylate and is the only leading OTC stomach remedy clinically proven effective for both upper and lower GI symptoms. It has been clinically proven in double-blind placebo-controlled trials for relief of upset stomach symptoms and diarrhea.

Active Ingredient:
(per tablespoon/per tablet/per caplet)
Original Liquid/Tablets/Caplets
Bismuth subsalicylate 262 mg
Maximum Strength Liquid
Bismuth subsalicylate 525 mg

Inactive Ingredients:
[Original Liquid] benzoic acid, flavor, magnesium aluminum silicate, methylcellulose, red 22, red 28, saccharin sodium, salicylic acid, sodium salicylate, sorbic acid, water
[Cherry Liquid] benzoic acid, flavor, magnesium aluminum silicate, methylcellulose, red 22, red 28, saccharin sodium, salicylic acid, sodium salicylate, sorbic acid, sucralose, water
[Maximum Strength Liquid] benzoic acid, flavor, magnesium aluminum silicate, methylcellulose, red 22, red 28, saccharin sodium, salicylic acid, sodium salicylate, sorbic acid, water
[Original Tablets] calcium carbonate, flavor, magnesium stearate, mannitol, povidone, red 27 aluminum lake, saccharin sodium, talc
[Cherry Tablets] adipic acid, calcium carbonate, flavor, magnesium stearate, mannitol, povidone, red 27 aluminum lake, red 40 aluminum lake, saccharin sodium, talc
[Caplets] calcium carbonate, magnesium stearate, mannitol, microcrystalline cellulose, polysorbate 80, povidone, red 27 aluminum lake, silicon dioxide, sodium starch glycolate.

Other Information:
Sodium Content
Original Liquid—each Tbsp contains: sodium 6 mg • low sodium
Cherry Liquid—each Tbsp contains: sodium 6 mg • low sodium
Maximum Strength Liquid—each Tbsp contains: sodium 6 mg • low sodium
Chewable Tablets—each Original or Cherry Flavor Tablet contains: calcium 140 mg, sodium less than 1 mg • very low sodium
Caplets—each Caplet contains: calcium 27 mg, sodium 3 mg • low sodium
Salicylate Content
Original Liquid—each Tbsp contains: salicylate 130 mg
Cherry Liquid—each Tbsp contains: salicylate 118 mg
Maximum Strength Liquid—each Tbsp contains: salicylate 236 mg

Chewable Tablets—each tablet contains:
[original] salicylate 102 mg
[cherry] salicylate 99 mg
Caplets—each caplet contains: salicylate 99 mg
All Forms are sugar free.

Indications:
• relieves upset stomach symptoms (i.e., indigestion, heartburn, nausea and fullness caused by over-indulgence in food and drink) without constipating; and,
• controls diarrhea.

Actions: For upset stomach symptoms, the active ingredient is believed to work via a topical effect on the stomach mucosa. For diarrhea, it is believed to work by several mechanisms in the gastrointestinal tract, including: 1) normalizing fluid movement via an antisecretory mechanism, 2) binding bacterial toxins and 3) antimicrobial activity.

Warnings:
Reye's syndrome: Children and teenagers who have or are recovering from chicken pox or flu-like symptoms should not use this product. When using this product, if changes in behavior with nausea and vomiting occur, consult a doctor because these symptoms could be an early sign of Reye's syndrome, a rare but serious illness.
Allergy alert: Contains salicylate.
Do not take if you are
• allergic to salicylates (including aspirin)
• taking other salicylate products
Do not use if you have
• an ulcer
• a bleeding problem
• bloody or black stool
Ask a doctor before use if you have
• fever
• mucus in the stool
Ask a doctor or pharmacist before use if you are taking any drug for
• anticoagulation (thinning the blood)
• diabetes
• gout
• arthritis
When using this product a temporary, but harmless, darkening of the stool and/or tongue may occur
Stop use and ask a doctor if
• symptoms get worse
• ringing in the ears or loss of hearing occurs
• diarrhea lasts more than 2 days
If pregnant or breast feeding, ask a health professional before use.
Keep out of reach of children. In case of overdose, get medical help or contact a Poison Control Center right away.
Notes: May cause a temporary and harmless darkening of the tongue or stool. Stool darkening should not be confused with melena.
While no lead is intentionally added to Pepto-Bismol, this product contains certain ingredients that are mined from the ground and thus contain small amounts of naturally occurring lead. For example, bismuth, contained in the active ingredient of Pepto-Bismol, is mined and therefore contains some naturally occurring lead. The small amounts of naturally oc-

curring lead in Pepto-Bismol are low in comparison to average daily lead exposure; this is for the information of healthcare professionals. Pepto-Bismol is indicated for treatment of acute upset stomach symptoms and diarrhea. It is not intended for chronic use.

Overdosage: In case of overdose, patients are advised to contact a physician or Poison Control Center. Emesis induced by ipecac syrup is indicated in large ingestions provided ipecac can be administered within one hour of ingestion. Activated charcoal should be administered after gastric emptying. Patients should be evaluated for signs and symptoms of salicylate toxicity.

Directions:
Pepto-Bismol® Original Liquid, Original & Cherry Flavor Chewable Tablets, and Caplets
[Original Liquid]
• shake well before using
• for accurate dosing, use dose cup
[Original Tablet, Cherry Tablets]
• chew or dissolve in mouth
[Caplets]
• swallow with water, do not chew
• adults and children 12 years and over: 1 dose (2 Tbsp or 30 ml; 2 tablets or 2 caplets) every 1/2 to 1 hour as needed
• do not exceed 8 doses (16 Tbsp or 240 ml); 16 tablets or capsules in 24 hours
• use until diarrhea stops but not more than 2 days
• children under 12 years: ask a doctor
• drink plenty of clear fluids to help prevent dehydration caused by diarrhea
Pepto-Bismol® Maximum Strength Liquid
• shake well before use
• for accurate dosing, use dose cup
• adults and children 12 years and over: 1 dose (2 Tbsp 30 ml) every 1 hour as needed
• do not exceed 4 doses (8 Tbsp or 120 ml) in 24 hours
• use until diarrhea stops but not more than 2 days
• children under 12 years: ask a doctor
• drink plenty of clear fluids to help prevent dehydration caused by diarrhea

How Supplied: Pepto-Bismol® Original, Cherry, and Maximum Strength Liquids are pink. Pepto-Bismol® Original and Cherry Liquids are available in: 4, 8, 12 and 16 fl oz bottles. Pepto-Bismol® Maximum Strength Liquid is available in: 4, 8 and 12 fl oz bottles. Pepto-Bismol® Original and Cherry Flavor Tablets are pink, round, chewable tablets imprinted with a debossed triangle and "Pepto-Bismol" on one side. Tablets are available in: boxes of 30 and 48. Pepto-Bismol® Caplets are pink and imprinted with "Pepto-Bismol" on one side. Caplets are available in bottles of 24 and 40.
• avoid excessive heat (over 104°F or 40°C)
• protect liquids from freezing
Questions: 1-800-717-3786
www.pepto-bismol.com
Shown in Product Identification Guide, page 504

Continued on next page

PRILOSEC OTC® TABLETS
[prī-lō-sĕk]

Drug Facts

Active Ingredient: **Purpose:**
(in each tablet)
Omeprazole magnesium
    delayed-release tablet
    20.6 mg (equivalent to 20 mg
    omeprazole) .... Acid reducer

Use:
* treats frequent heartburn (occurs 2 or more days a week)
* not intended for immediate relief of heartburn; this drug may take 1 to 4 days for full effect

Warnings:

Allergy alert: Do not use if you are allergic to omeprazole

Do not use if you have trouble or pain swallowing food, vomiting with blood, or bloody or black stools.
These may be signs of a serious condition. See your doctor.

Ask a doctor before use if you have
* had heartburn over 3 months. This may be a sign of a more serious condition.
* heartburn with **lightheadedness, sweating or dizziness**
* chest pain or shoulder pain with shortness of breath; sweating; pain spreading to arms, neck or shoulders; or lightheadedness
* frequent **chest pain**
* frequent wheezing, particularly with heartburn
* unexplained weight loss
* nausea or vomiting
* stomach pain

Ask a doctor or pharmacist before use if you are taking
* warfarin (blood-thinning medicine)
* prescription antifungal or anti-yeast medicines
* diazepam (anxiety medicine)
* digoxin (heart medicine)
* tacrolimus (immune system medicine)
* atazanavir (medicine for HIV infection)

Stop use and ask a doctor if
* your heartburn continues or worsens
* you need to take this product for more than 14 days
* you need to take more than 1 course of treatment every 4 months

If pregnant or breast-feeding, ask a health professional before use.

Keep out of reach of children. In case of overdose, get medical help or contact a Poison Control Center right away.

Directions:
* adults 18 years of age and older
* this product is to be used once a day (every 24 hours), every day for 14 days
* it may take 1 to 4 days for full effect, although some people get complete relief of symptoms within 24 hours

14-Day Course of Treatment
* swallow 1 tablet with a glass of water before eating in the morning
* take every day for 14 days
* do not take more than 1 tablet a day
* do not chew or crush the tablets
* do not crush tablets in food
* do not use for more than 14 days unless directed by your doctor

Repeated 14-Day Courses (if needed)
* you may repeat a 14-day course every 4 months

* **do not take for more than 14 days or more often than every 4 months unless directed by a doctor**
* children under 18 years of age: ask a doctor

Other Information:
* read the directions, warnings and package insert before use
* keep the carton and package insert. They contain important information.
* store at 20–25°C (68–77°F)
* keep product out of high heat and humidity
* protect product from moisture

How Prilosec OTC Works For Your Frequent Heartburn
Prilosec OTC works differently from other OTC heartburn products, such as antacids and other acid reducers. Prilosec OTC stops acid production at the source – the **acid pump** that produces stomach acid. Prilosec OTC is to be used once a day (every 24 hours), every day for 14 days.

What to Expect When Using Prilosec OTC
Prilosec OTC is a different type of medicine from antacids and other acid reducers. Prilosec OTC may take 1 to 4 days for full effect, although some people get complete relief of symptoms within 24 hours. Make sure you take the entire 14 days of dosing to treat your frequent heartburn.

Safety Record
For years, doctors have prescribed Prilosec to treat acid-related conditions in millions of people safely.

Who Should Take Prilosec OTC
This product is for adults (18 years and older) with **frequent heartburn**-when you have heartburn 2 or more days a week.
* Prilosec OTC is **not** intended for those who have heartburn infrequently, one episode of heartburn a week or less, or for those who want immediate relief of heartburn.

Tips for Managing Heartburn
* Do not lie flat or bend over soon after eating.
* Do not eat late at night or just before bedtime.
* Certain foods or drinks are more likely to cause heartburn, such as rich, spicy, fatty and fried foods, chocolate, caffeine, alcohol and even some fruits and vegetables.
* Eat slowly and do not eat big meals.
* If you are overweight, lose weight.
* If you smoke, quit smoking.
* Raise the head of your bed.
* Wear loose-fitting clothing around your stomach.

Inactive Ingredients:
glyceryl monostearate, hydroxypropyl cellulose, hypromellose, iron oxide, magnesium stearate, methacrylic acid copolymer, microcrystalline cellulose, paraffin, polyethylene glycol 6000, polysorbate 80, polyvinylpyrrolidone, sodium stearyl fumarate, starch, sucrose, talc, titanium dioxide, triethyl citrate

How Supplied:
Prilosec OTC is available in 14 tablet, 28 tablet and 42 tablet sizes. These sizes contain one, two and three 14-day courses of treatment, respectively. Do not use for more than 14 days in a row unless directed by your doctor. For the 28 count (two 14-day courses) and the 42 count (three 14-day courses), you may repeat a 14-day course every 4 months.

Questions? 1-800-289-9181

Shown in Product Identification Guide, page 504

THERMACARE®
Therapeutic Heat Wraps
Arthritis

Arthritis Hand/Wrist

PLEASE READ ALL INSTRUCTIONS AND WARNINGS BEFORE USE. ADDITIONAL WARNINGS ARE INCLUDED IN THE PACKAGE INSERT. TO REDUCE THE RISK OF BURNS, FIRE, AND PERSONAL INJURY, THIS PRODUCT MUST BE USED IN ACCORDANCE WITH THE USE INSTRUCTIONS AND WARNINGS.

Uses: Provides temporary relief of minor muscular and joint aches and pains associated with overexertion, strains, sprains, and arthritis.

Directions: Tear open pouch when ready to use. It may take up to 30 minutes for ThermaCare to reach its therapeutic temperature. Do not place the heat cells on the palm of the hand. Place on pain area on back of hand with thumb through slit and darker discs toward skin. Wrap straps under palm of hand and fasten. Overtightening may cause discomfort. Adjust as needed. Be careful when applying to the hand and wrist – do not overlap the heat cells. For maximum effectiveness, we recommend you wear ThermaCare for 12 hours. Do not wear for more than 12 hours in any 24-hour period. Please keep in mind as you use this product, that due to differences in body temperature not everyone senses heat on the hand/wrist the same. Therefore, the product may not feel as warm as you might expect.

WARNING: THIS PRODUCT CAN CAUSE BURNS. CHECK SKIN FREQUENTLY DURING USE. IF YOU FIND IRRITATION OR A BURN, REMOVE PRODUCT IMMEDIATELY.

55 OR OLDER: YOUR RISK OF BURNING INCREASES AS YOU AGE. IF YOU ARE 55 YEARS OF AGE OR OLDER, DO NOT USE DURING SLEEP.

ADDITIONAL WARNINGS: Each heat disc contains iron (~2 grams), which can be harmful if ingested. If ingested, rinse mouth with water and call a Poison Control Center immediately. If heat disc contents come in contact with your skin or eyes, rinse right away with water. Never heat product in a microwave or attempt to reheat, as wrap could catch fire. Keep out of reach of children and pets.

DO NOT MICROWAVE

ASK A DOCTOR BEFORE USE if you have
- DIABETES
- poor circulation or heart disease
- rheumatoid arthritis
- or are pregnant

WHEN USING THIS PRODUCT check skin frequently for signs of burns or blisters – if found, stop use
- if product feels too hot – stop use or wear over clothing
- do not place extra pressure over the product
- do not use for more than 12 hours in a 24-hour period

DO NOT USE with pain rubs, medicated lotions, creams or ointments
- on unhealthy, damaged or broken skin
- on areas of bruising or swelling that have occurred within 48 hours
- on people unable to follow all use instructions
- on areas of the body where you can't feel heat
- with other forms of heat
- on people unable to remove the product, including children, infants, and some elderly

STOP USE AND ASK A DOCTOR if you experience any discomfort, burning, swelling, rash or other changes in your skin that persist where the wrap is worn
- if after 7 days your pain gets worse or remains unchanged, as this may be a sign of a more serious condition

Arthritis Neck/Shoulder/Wrist
PLEASE READ ALL INSTRUCTIONS AND WARNINGS BEFORE USE. ADDITIONAL WARNINGS ARE INCLUDED IN THE PACKAGE INSERT. TO REDUCE THE RISK OF BURNS, FIRE, AND PERSONAL INJURY, THIS PRODUCT MUST BE USED IN ACCORDANCE WITH THE USE INSTRUCTIONS AND WARNINGS.

Uses: Provides temporary relief of minor muscular and joint aches and pains associated with overexertion, strains, sprains, and arthritis.

Directions: Tear open pouch when ready to use. It may take up to 30 minutes for ThermaCare to reach its therapeutic temperature. Peel away paper to reveal adhesive side. Place on pain area with adhesive against the skin. Attach firmly. Be careful when applying to the wrist – do not overlap the heat cells. For maximum effectiveness, we recommend you wear ThermaCare for 12 hours. Do not wear for more than 12 hours in any 24-hour period.

WARNING: **THIS PRODUCT CAN CAUSE BURNS. CHECK SKIN FREQUENTLY DURING USE. IF YOU FIND IRRITATION OR A BURN, REMOVE PRODUCT IMMEDIATELY.**
55 OR OLDER: **YOUR RISK OF BURNING INCREASES AS YOU AGE. IF YOU ARE 55 YEARS OF AGE OR OLDER, DO NOT USE DURING SLEEP.**
ADDITIONAL WARNINGS: Each heat disc contains iron (~2 grams), which can be harmful if ingested. If ingested, rinse mouth with water and call a Poison Control Center immediately. If heat disc contents come in contact with your skin or

eyes, rinse right away with water. Never heat product in a microwave or attempt to reheat, as wrap could catch fire. Keep out of reach of children and pets.
DO NOT MICROWAVE

ASK A DOCTOR BEFORE USE if you have
- DIABETES
- poor circulation or heart disease
- rheumatoid arthritis
- or are pregnant

WHEN USING THIS PRODUCT check skin frequently for signs of burns or blisters – if found, stop use
- if product feels too hot – stop use or wear over clothing
- do not place extra pressure over the product
- do not use for more than 12 hours in a 24-hour period

DO NOT USE with pain rubs, medicated lotions, creams or ointments
- on unhealthy, damaged or broken skin
- on areas of bruising or swelling that have occurred within 48 hours
- on people unable to follow all use instructions
- on areas of the body where you can't feel heat
- with other forms of heat
- on people unable to remove the product, including children, infants, and some elderly

STOP USE AND ASK A DOCTOR if you experience any discomfort, burning, swelling, rash or other changes in your skin that persist where the wrap is worn
- if after 7 days your pain gets worse or remains unchanged, as this may be a sign of a more serious condition

Arthritis Knee/Elbow
PLEASE READ ALL INSTRUCTIONS AND WARNINGS BEFORE USE. ADDITIONAL WARNINGS ARE INCLUDED IN THE PACKAGE INSERT. TO REDUCE THE RISK OF BURNS, FIRE, AND PERSONAL INJURY, THIS PRODUCT MUST BE USED IN ACCORDANCE WITH THE USE INSTRUCTIONS AND WARNINGS.

Uses: Provides temporary relief of minor muscular and joint aches and pains associated with overexertion, strains, sprains, and arthritis.

Directions: Tear open pouch when ready to use. It may take up to 30 minutes for ThermaCare to reach its therapeutic temperature. Peel away paper to reveal adhesive tabs. Using adhesive is optional if you have sensitive skin or have body hair around the knee or elbow area.

Knee: Do not place heat cells on the back of the knee. Bend knee slightly and place opening over kneecap. Secure tabs to skin (optional). Wrap straps around knee and fasten. Over-tightening may cause discomfort. Adjust as needed.

Elbow: Do not place heat cells on the inside of the bend of the arm. Bend elbow slightly and place opening over elbow. Secure tabs to skin (optional). Wrap straps around elbow and fasten. Over-tightening may cause discomfort. Adjust as needed.

For maximum effectiveness, we recommend you wear ThermaCare for 12 hours. Do not wear for more than 12 hours in any 24-hour period.

WARNING: **THIS PRODUCT CAN CAUSE BURNS. CHECK SKIN FREQUENTLY DURING USE. IF YOU FIND IRRITATION OR A BURN, REMOVE PRODUCT IMMEDIATELY.**
55 OR OLDER: **YOUR RISK OF BURNING INCREASES AS YOU AGE. IF YOU ARE 55 YEARS OF AGE OR OLDER, WEAR THERMACARE OVER A TOWEL OR CLOTH SUCH AS A WASHCLOTH, NOT DIRECTLY AGAINST YOUR SKIN, AND DO NOT WEAR WHILE SLEEPING.**
ADDITIONAL WARNINGS: Each heat disc contains iron (~2 grams), which can be harmful if ingested. If ingested, rinse mouth with water and call a Poison Control Center immediately. If heat disc contents come in contact with your skin or eyes, rinse right away with water. Never heat product in a microwave or attempt to reheat, as wrap could catch fire. Keep out of reach of children and pets.
DO NOT MICROWAVE

ASK A DOCTOR BEFORE USE if you have
- DIABETES
- poor circulation or heart disease
- rheumatoid arthritis
- or are pregnant

WHEN USING THIS PRODUCT check skin frequently for signs of burns or blisters – if found, stop use
- if product feels too hot – stop use or wear over clothing
- do not place extra pressure or tight clothing over the product
- do not use for more than 12 hours in a 24-hour period

DO NOT USE with pain rubs, medicated lotions, creams or ointments
- on unhealthy, damaged or broken skin
- on areas of bruising or swelling that have occurred within 48 hours
- on people unable to follow all use instructions
- on areas of the body where you can't feel heat
- with other forms of heat
- on people unable to remove the product, including children, infants, and some elderly

STOP USE AND ASK A DOCTOR if you experience any discomfort, burning, swelling, rash or other changes in your skin that persist where the wrap is worn
- if after 7 days your pain gets worse or remains unchanged, as this may be a sign of a more serious Condition

QUESTIONS?
1-800-323-3383 or visit
www.thermacare.com

How Supplied:
Available in boxes of 2 (Hand/Wrist & Knee/Elbow) or 3 (Neck/Shoulder/Wrist) or in single use pouches.

Shown in Product Identification Guide, page 504

Continued on next page

VICKS® DAYQUIL® LIQUID
VICKS® DAYQUIL® LIQUICAPS®
VICKS® DAYQUIL® COLD & FLU MULTI-SYMPTOM RELIEF
Acetaminophen [-] [for] aches/fever
Dextromethorphan [-] [for] cough
Phenylephrine [-] [for] nasal congestion
Non-drowsy

Drug Facts
Active Ingredients:
(in each 15 ml tablespoon)   Purpose:
Acetaminophen
    325 mg .... Pain reliever/fever reducer
Dextromethorphan HBr
    10 mg .... Cough suppressant
Phenylephrine HCl
    5 mg .... Nasal decongestant

Uses: temporarily relieves common cold/flu symptoms:
- nasal congestion
- cough due to minor throat and bronchial irritation
- sore throat
- headache
- minor aches and pains
- fever

Warnings:
Liver warning: This product contains acetaminophen. Severe liver damage may occur if:
- adult takes more than 6 doses in 24 hours
- child takes more than 5 doses in 24 hours
- taken with other drugs containing acetaminophen
- adult has 3 or more alcoholic drinks every day while using this product

Sore throat warning: If sore throat is severe, persists for more than two days, is accompanied or followed by a fever, headache, rash, nausea, or vomiting, consult a doctor promptly.

Do not use
- with any other drug containing acetaminophen (prescription or nonprescription). Ask a doctor or pharmacist before using with other drugs if you are not sure.
- if you are now taking a prescription monoamine oxidase inhibitor (MAOI) (certain drugs for depression, psychiatric or emotional conditions, or Parkinson's disease), or for 2 weeks after stopping the MAOI drug. If you do not know if your prescription drug contains an MAOI, ask a doctor or pharmacist before taking this product.

Ask a doctor before use if you have
- liver disease
- heart disease
- thyroid disease
- diabetes
- high blood pressure
- trouble urinating due to enlarged prostate gland
- cough that occurs with too much phlegm (mucus)
- persistent or chronic cough as occurs with smoking, asthma, or emphysema
- a sodium-restricted diet

When using this product, do not use more than directed

Stop use and ask a doctor if
- you get nervous, dizzy or sleepless
- symptoms get worse or last more than 5 days (children) or 7 days (adults)
- fever gets worse or lasts more than 3 days
- redness or swelling is present
- new symptoms occur
- cough comes back, or occurs with rash or headache that lasts.

These could be signs of a serious condition.

If pregnant or breast-feeding, ask a health professional before use.

Keep out of reach of children.

Overdose warning: Taking more than the recommended dose can cause serious health problems. In case of overdose, get medical help or contact a Poison Control Center right away. Quick medical attention is critical for adults as well as for children even if you do not notice any signs or symptoms.

Directions:
- take only as recommended — see Overdose warning
- use dose cup or tablespoon (TBSP)
- do not exceed 5 doses (children) or 6 doses (adults) per 24 hours

adults and children 12 years and over	30 ml (2 TBSP) every 4 hours
children 6 to under 12 years	15 ml (1 TBSP) every 4 hours
children 2 to under 6 years	ask a doctor
children under 2 years	do not use

- **when using other DayQuil or NyQuil products, carefully read each label to insure correct dosing**

Other Information:
- **each tablespoon contains** sodium 50 mg
- store at room temperature

Inactive Ingredients: carboxymethylcellulose sodium, citric acid, disodium EDTA, FD&C Yellow No. 6, flavor, glycerin, propylene glycol, purified water, saccharin sodium, sodium benzoate, sodium chloride, sodium citrate, sorbitol sucraoofe

Questions? 1-800-251-3374

How Supplied: Available in 6, 10, and 12 OZ, twin pack and quad pack.

Drug Facts
Active Ingredients
(in each LiquiCap)   Purpose:
Acetaminophen
    325 mg .... Pain reliever/fever reducer
Dextromethorphan HBr
    10 mg .... Cough suppressant
Phenylephrine HCl
    5 mg .... Nasal decongestant

Uses:
temporarily relieves common cold/flu symptoms:
- nasal congestion
- cough due to minor throat and bronchial irritation
- sore throat
- headache
- minor aches and pains
- fever

Warnings:
Liver warning: This product contains acetaminophen. Severe liver damage may occur if you take:
- more than 6 doses in 24 hours
- with other drugs containing acetaminophen
- 3 or more alcoholic drinks every day while using this product

Sore throat warning: If sore throat is severe, persists for more than two days, is accompanied or followed by a fever, headache, rash, nausea, or vomiting, consult a doctor promptly.

Do not use
- with any other drug containing acetaminophen (prescription or nonprescription). Ask a doctor or pharmacist before using with other drugs if you are not sure.
- if you are now taking a prescription monoamine oxidase inhibitor (MAOI) (certain drugs for depression, psychiatric or emotional conditions, or Parkinson's disease), or for 2 weeks after stopping the MAOI drug. If you do not know if your prescription drug contains an MAOI, ask a doctor or pharmacist before taking this product.

Ask a doctor before use if you have
- liver disease
- heart disease
- thyroid disease
- diabetes
- high blood pressure
- trouble urinating due to enlarged prostate gland
- cough that occurs with too much phlegm (mucus)
- persistent or chronic cough as occurs with smoking, asthma, or emphysema

When using this product, do not use more than directed

Stop use and ask a doctor if
- you get nervous, dizzy or sleepless
- symptoms get worse or last more than 5 days (children) or 7 days (adults)
- fever gets worse or lasts more than 3 days
- redness or swelling is present
- new symptoms occur
- cough comes back, or occurs with rash or headache that lasts.

These could be signs of a serious condition.

If pregnant or breast-feeding, ask a health professional before use.

Keep out of reach of children.

Overdose warning: Taking more than the recommended dose can cause serious health problems. In case of overdose, get medical help or contact a Poison Control Center right away. Quick medical attention is critical for adults as well as for children even if you do not notice any signs or symptoms.

Directions:
- take only as recommended — see Overdose warning
- do not exceed 6 doses per 24 hours

adults and children 12 years and over	2 LiquiCaps with water every 4 hours
children 2 to under 12 years	ask a doctor
children under 2 years	do not use

- when using other DayQuil or NyQuil products, carefully read each label to insure correct dosing

Other Information:
- store at room temperature

Inactive Ingredients: FD&C Red No. 40, FD&C Yellow No. 6, gelatin, glycerin, polyethylene glycol, povidone, propylene glycol, purified water, sorbitol special, titanium dioxide

Questions? 1-800-251-3374

How Supplied: Available in boxes of 2, 12, 20, 24, 40, and 60.

Shown in Product Identification Guide, page 504

VICKS® NYQUIL® LIQUICAPS®
VICKS® NYQUIL® LIQUID
VICKS® NYQUIL® COLD & FLU MULTI-SYMPTOM RELIEF
Acetaminophen [-] pain reliever/fever reducer
Dextromethorphan [-] cough suppressant
Doxylamine [-] antihistamine

Drug Facts:
Active ingredients:
(in each LiquiCap) **Purpose:**
Acetaminophen
325 mg .... Pain reliever/fever reducer
Dextromethorphan HBr
15 mg .... Cough suppressant
Doxylamine succinate
6.25 mg .... Antihistamine

Uses: temporarily relieves common cold/flu symptoms:
- cough due to minor throat and bronchial irritation
- sore throat
- headache
- minor aches and pains
- fever
- runny nose and sneezing

Warnings:
Liver warning: This product contains acetaminophen. Severe liver damage may occur if you take:
- more than 4 doses in 24 hours
- with other drugs containing acetaminophen
- 3 or more alcoholic drinks every day while using this product

Sore throat warning: If sore throat is severe, persists for more than two days, is accompanied or followed by fever, headache, rash, nausea, or vomiting, consult a doctor promptly.

Do not use
- with any other drug containing acetaminophen (prescription or nonprescription). Ask a doctor or pharmacist before using with other drugs if you are not sure.
- if you are now taking a prescription monoamine oxidase inhibitor (MAOI) (certain drugs for depression, psychiatric or emotional conditions, or Parkinson's disease), or for 2 weeks after stopping the MAOI drug. If you do not know if your prescription drug contains an MAOI, ask a doctor or pharmacist before taking this product.
- to make a child sleep

Ask a doctor before use if you have
- liver disease
- glaucoma
- cough that occurs with too much phelgm (mucus)
- a breathing problem or chronic cough that lasts or as occurs with smoking, asthma, chronic bronchitis or emphysema
- trouble urinating due to enlarged prostate gland

Ask a doctor or pharmacist before use if you are taking sedatives or tranquilizers.

When using this product
- **do not use more than directed**
- excitability may occur, especially in children
- marked drowsiness may occur
- avoid alcoholic drinks
- be careful when driving a motor vehicle or operating machinery
- alcohol, sedatives, and tranquilizers may increase drowsiness

Stop use and ask a doctor if
- pain or cough gets worse or lasts more than 7 days
- fever gets worse or lasts more than 3 days
- redness or swelling is present
- new symptoms occur
- cough comes back or occurs with rash or headache that lasts.

These could be signs of a serious condition.

If pregnant or breast-feeding, ask a health professional before use.

Keep out of reach of children.

Overdose warning: Taking more than the recommended dose can cause serious health problems. In case of overdose, get medical help or contact a Poison Control Center right away. Quick medical attention is critical for adults as well as for children even if you do not notice any signs or symptoms.

Directions:
- take only as recommended - see Overdose warning
- do not exceed 4 doses per 24 hours

adults and children 12 years and over	2 LiquiCaps with water every 6 hours
children 2 to under 12 yrs	ask a doctor
children under 2 yrs	do not use

- when using other DayQuil or NyQuil products, carefully read each label to insure correct dosing

Other Information:
- store at room temperature

Inactive Ingredients: D&C Yellow No. 10, FD&C Blue No. 1, gelatin, glycerin, polyethylene glycol, povidone, propylene glycol, purified water, sorbitol special, titanium dioxide

Questions? 1-800-362-1683

How Supplied:
Available in boxes of 2, 12, 20, 24, 40 and 60.

Drug Facts
Active ingredients:
(in each 15 ml tablespoon) **Purpose:**
Acetaminophen
500 mg .... Pain reliever/fever reducer
Dextromethorphan HBr
15 mg .... Cough suppressant
Doxylamine succinate
6.25 mg .... Antihistamine

Uses: temporarily relieves common cold/ flu symptoms:
- cough due to minor throat and bronchial irritation
- sore throat
- headache
- minor aches and pains
- fever
- runny nose and sneezing

Warnings:
Liver warning: This product contains acetaminophen. Severe liver damage may occur if you take:
- more than 4 doses in 24 hours.
- with other drugs containing acetaminophen
- 3 or more alcoholic drinks every day while using this product

Sore throat warning: If sore throat is severe, persists for more than two days, is accompanied or followed by fever, headache, rash, nausea, or vomiting, consult a doctor promptly.

Do not use
- with any other drug containing acetaminophen (prescription or nonprescription). Ask a doctor or pharmacist before using with other drugs if you are not sure.
- if you are now taking a prescription monoamine oxidase inhibitor (MAOI) (certain drugs for depression, or emotional conditions, or Parkinson's disease), or for 2 weeks after stopping the MAOI drug. If you do not know if your prescription drug contains an MAOI, ask a doctor or pharmacist before taking this product.
- to make a child sleep

Ask a doctor before use if you have
- liver disease
- glaucoma
- cough that occurs with too much phelgm (mucus)
- a breathing problem or chronic cough that lasts or as occurs with smoking, asthma, chronic bronchitis or emphysema
- trouble urinating due to enlarged prostate gland
- a sodium-restricted diet

Ask a doctor or pharmacist before use if you are taking sedatives or tranquilizers.

When using this product
- **do not use more than directed**
- excitability may occur, especially in children
- marked drowsiness may occur
- avoid alcoholic drinks
- be careful when driving a motor vehicle or operating machinery
- alcohol, sedatives, and tranquilizers may increase drowsiness

Stop use and ask a doctor if
- pain or cough gets worse or lasts more than 7 days

Continued on next page

Vicks Nyquil LiquiCaps—Cont.

- fever gets worse or lasts more than 3 days
- redness or swelling is present
- new symptoms occur
- cough comes back or occurs with rash or headache that lasts.

These could be signs of a serious condition.

If pregnant or breast-feeding, ask a health professional before use.

Keep out of reach of children.

Overdose warning: Taking more than the recommended dose can cause serious health problems. In case of overdose, get medical help or contact a Poison Control Center right away. Quick medical attention is critical for adults as well as for children even if you do not notice any signs or symptoms.

Directions:
- take only as recommended - see Overdose warning
- use dose cup or tablespoon (TBSP)
- do not exceed 4 doses per 24 hours

adults and children 12 years and over	2 TBSP (30 ml) every 6 hours
children 2 to under 12 yrs	ask a doctor
children under 2 yrs	do not use

- **when using other DayQuil or NyQuil products, carefully read each label to insure correct dosing**

Other Information:
- **each tablespoon contains** sodium 18 mg [original] or 19 mg [cherry]
- store at room temperature

Inactive Ingredients [original] alcohol, citric acid, D&C Yellow No. 10, FD&C Green No. 3, FD&C Yellow No. 6, flavor, high fructose corn syrup, polyethylene glycol, propylene glycol, purified water, saccharin sodium, sodium citrate [cherry] alcohol, citric acid, FD&C Blue No. 1, FD&C Red No. 40, flavor, high fructose corn syrup, polyethylene glycol, propylene glycol, purified water, saccharin sodium, sodium citrate

Questions? 1-800-362-1683

How Supplied:
Available in 6, 10, 12 and 16 OZ, twin, triple and quad pack.
Shown in Product Identification Guide, page 504

UNKNOWN DRUG?
Consult the
Product Identification Guide
(Gray Pages)
for full-color photos of
leading over-the-counter
medications

Reese Pharmaceutical Company

**10617 FRANK AVENUE
CLEVELAND, OH 44106**

Direct Inquiries to:
Voice - (800) 321-7178
Fax - (216) 231-6444
http://www.reesepharmaceutical.com

REESE'S PINWORM TREATMENTS
[rēsĭs]

Directions for Use: For the treatment of pinworms. Read package insert carefully before taking this medication. Take according to directions. Do not exceed recommended dosage unless directed by a doctor. Medication should be taken only one time as a single dose: do not repeat treatment unless directed by a doctor. When one individual in a household has pinworms, the entire household should be treated unless otherwise advised. These products can be taken any time of day, with or without food. If you are pregnant, nursing a baby, or have liver disease, do not take this product unless directed by a doctor.

DOSAGE GUIDE		
under 25 lbs or 2 yrs of age, consult a doctor		
WEIGHT LBS.	**DOSAGE**	
	Teaspoons	**Caplets**
25–37	1/2	2
38–62	1	4
63–87	1-1/2	6
88–112	2	8
113–137	2-1/2	10
138–162	3	12
163–187	3-1/2	14
188 & over	4	16

Warnings: Keep this and all drugs out of the reach of children. In case of accidental overdose, seek professional assistance or contact a poison control center immediately.

How Supplied:
Oral Suspension Liquid
NDC: 10956-618-01
Each 1 mL contains: pyrantel pamoate 144mg
(equivalent of 50 mg pyrantel base)
Pre-Measured Caplet
NDC: 10956-658-24
Packaged in boxes of 24 caplets.
Each caplet contains: pyrantel pamoate 180mg
(equivalent of 62.5 mg pyrantel base)
Shown in Product Identification Guide, page 504

Hyland's, A Division of Standard Homeopathic Company

**210 WEST 131ST STREET
BOX 61067
LOS ANGELES, CA 90061**

Direct Inquiries to:
Jay Borneman
(800) 624-9659 Ext. 20

HYLAND'S BACKACHE WITH ARNICA

Active Ingredients: BENZOICUM ACIDUM 3X HPUS, COLCHICUM AUTUMNALE 3X HPUS, SULPHUR 3X HPUS, ARNICA MONTANA 6X HPUS, RHUS TOXICODENDRON 6X HPUS.

Inactive Ingredients: Lactose, N.F.

Indications: A homeopathic medicine for the temporary relief of symptoms of low back pain due to strain or overexertion.

Directions: Adults and children over 12 years of age: Take 1-2 caplets with water every 4 hours or as needed.

Warnings: Do not use if imprinted cap band is broken or missing. If symptoms persist for more than seven days or worsen, contact a licensed health care professional. As with any drug, if you are pregnant or nursing a baby, seek the advice of a licensed health care professional before using this product. Keep this and all medications out of the reach of children. In case of accidental overdose, contact a poison control center immediately. In case of emergency, the manufacturer may be reached 24 hours a day, 7 days a week at 800/624-9659.

How Supplied: Bottles of 40 5.5 grain caplets (NDC 54973-2965-2). Store at room temperature.

HYLAND'S CALMS FORTÉ™

Active Ingredients: *Passiflora* (Passion Flower) 1X triple strength HPUS, *Avena Sativa* (Oat) 1X double strength HPUS, *Humulus Lupulus* (Hops) 1X double strength HPUS, *Chamomilla* (Chamomile) 2X HPUS, *Calcarea Phosphorica* (Calcium Phosphate) 3X HPUS, *Ferrum Phosphorica* (Iron Phosphate) 3X HPUS, *Kali Phosphoricum* (Potassium Phosphate) 3X HPUS, *Natrum Phosphoricum* (Sodium Phosphate) 3X HPUS, *Magnesia Phosphoricum* (Magnesium Phosphate) 3X HPUS.

Inactive Ingredients: Lactose, N.F., Calcium Sulfate, Starch (Corn and Tapiocal), Magnesium Stearate.

Indications: Temporary symptomatic relief of simple nervous tension and sleeplessness.

Directions: Adults: As a relaxant: Swallow 1–2 tablets with water as needed, three times daily, preferably before meals. For insomnia: 1 to 3 tablets 1/2 to 1 hour before retiring. Repeat as needed without danger of side effects. Children: As a relaxant: Swallow 1 tablet with water as needed, three times daily, preferably before meals. For insomnia: 1 to 2 tablets ½ to 1 hour before retiring. Repeat as needed without danger of side effects.

Warning: Do not use if imprinted cap band is broken or missing. If symptoms persist for more than seven days or worsen, consult a licensed health care professional. As with any drug, if you are pregnant or nursing a baby, seek the advice of a licensed health care professional before using this product. Keep this and all medications out of the reach of children. In case of accidental overdose, contact a Poison Control Center immediately. In case of emergency, the manufacturer may be reached 24 hours a day, 7 days a week by calling 800/624-9659.

How Supplied: Bottles of 100 4-grain tablets (NDC 54973-1121-02), 50 4-grain tablets (NDC 54973-1121-01) and 32 5.5-grain caplets (NDC 54973-1121-68). Store at room temperature.

HYLAND'S CALMS FORTÉ 4 KIDS

Active Ingredients: ACONITUM NAP. 6X HPUS, CALC. PHOS. 12X HPUS, CHAMOMILLA 6X HPUS, CINA 6X HPUS, LYCOPODIUM 6X HPUS, NAT. MUR. 6X HPUS, PULSATILLA 6X HPUS, SULPHUR 6X HPUS

Inactive Ingredients: Lactose, N.F.

Indications: Temporarily relieves the symptoms restlessness, sleeplessness, night terrors, growing pains, causeless crying, occasional sleeplessness due to travel and lack of focus in children.

Directions: Children ages 2–5: dissolve 2 tablets under tongue every 15 minutes for up to 8 doses until relieved; Then every 4 hours as required.
Children ages 6–11: Dissolve 3 tablets under tongue every 15 minutes for up to 8 doses until relieved; Then every 4 hours as required.
Children 12 years and over: Dissolve 4 tablets under tongue every 15 minutes for up to 8 doses until relieved; then every 4 hours as are required or as recommended by a health care professional

Warnings: Ask a doctor before use if: pregnant or nursing, child is taking any prescription medications. If symptoms don't improve within 7 days, discontinue use and seek the advice of a licensed medical practitioner.

Keep this and all medications out of reach of children. Do not use if imprinted tamper band is broken or missing. In case of accidental overdose, contact a poison control center immediately. In case of emergency, the manufacturer may be contacted 24 hours a day, 7 days a week at 800/624-9659.

How Supplied: Bottles of 125 1 grain tablets (NDC 54973-7518-03). Store at room temperature.

HYLAND'S COLIC TABLETS

Active Ingredient: *Dioscorea* 3X HPUS, *Chamomilla* 3X HPUS, *Colocynthis* 3X HPUS

Inactive Ingredients: Lactose N.F.

Indications: Temporarily relieves the symptoms of colic and gas pains caused by irritating food, feeding too quickly, swallowing air and similar conditions during teething, colds and other minor upset periods in children.

Directions: For Children up to 2 years: Dissolve 2 tablets on tongue every 15 minutes for up to 8 doses until relieved; then every 2 hours as required. For Children over 2 years: Dissolve 3 tablets as above or as recommended by a licensed health care professional. If you prefer, tablets may be dissolved in a teaspoon of water and then given to the child. Colic Tablets are very soft and dissolve almost instantly under the tongue. Please note: if your baby has been crying or is very upset, your baby may fall asleep after using this product because the pain has been relieved and your child can rest.

Warnings: Ask a doctor before use if pregnant or nursing. Consult a physician if symptoms persist for more than 7 days or worsen. Keep out of the reach of children. Do not use if imprinted tamper band is broken or missing. In case of accidental overdose, contact a Poison Control Center immediately. In case of emergency, the manufacturer may be contacted 24 hours a day, 7 days a week at 800/624-9659.

How Supplied: Bottle of 125 one-grain, sublingual tablets (NDC 54973-7502-1)

HYLAND'S COUGH SYRUP WITH HONEY

Active Ingredients: *Ipecacuanha* 6X HPUS, *Aconitum Napellus* 6X HPUS, *Spongia Tosta* 6X HPUS, *Antimonium Tartaricum* 6X HPUS.

Inactive Ingredients: Orange Honey, Purified Water USP, Cane Sugar, Vegetable Glycerine USP, Sodium Benzoate USP.

Indications: Temporarily relieves symptoms of simple, dry, tight or tickling coughs due to colds in children.

Directions: Adults and children over 12 years: 3 to 4 teaspoonfuls as required. May be taken with or without water. Repeat as often as necessary to relieve symptoms. Children 1 to 12 years: 1 to 3 teaspoonfuls as required. Children under 1 year of age: Consult a licensed health care professional before using this product.

Warnings: Ask a doctor before use if pregnant or nursing. Consult a physician if: symptoms persist for more than 7 days, cough tends to recur or is accompanied by a high fever, rash or persistent headache. Keep this and all medications out of the reach of children. Do not use this product for persistent or chronic cough such as occurs with asthma, smoking or emphysema; or if cough is accompanied with excessive mucous, unless directed by a licensed health care professional. A persistent cough may be the sign of a serious condition. Do not use if imprinted tamper band is broken or missing. In case of accidental overdose, contact a poison control center immediately. In case of emergency, the manufacturer may be contacted 24 hours a day, 7 days a week at 800/624-9659.

How Supplied: Bottle of 4 Fluid oz (NDC 54973-7503-1)

HYLAND'S EARACHE DROPS

Active Ingredients:
Pulsatilla 30C HPUS, Chamomilla 30C HPUS, Sulphur 30C HPUS, Calc Carb 30C HPUS, Belladonna 30C HPUS, Lycopodium 30C HPUS.

Inactive Ingredients:
Citric Acid USP, Purified Water, Sodium Benzoate USP, Vegetable Glycerin USP.

Indications:
Temporarily relieves the symptoms of fever, pain, irritability and sleeplessness associated with earaches after diagnosis by a physician. Relieves common pain and itching of "swimmer's ear." If symptoms persist for more than 48 hours, or if there is a discharge from the ear, discontinue use and contact your physician.

Directions:
Adults and children of all ages: Tilt head sideways and apply 3–4 drops into involved ear 4 times daily or as needed. Tilt ear upward for at least 2 minutes after application or gently place cotton in ear to keep drops in.

Warnings:
Keep away from eyes. Do not take by mouth. Earache drops are only to be used in the ears. Tip of applicator should not enter ear canal. Ask a doctor before use if pregnant or nursing. Consult a physician if symptoms persist for more than 48 hours or if there is discharge from the ear. Keep this and all medications out of reach of children. Do not use

Continued on next page

Hyland's Earache Drops—Cont.

if imprinted tamper band is broken or missing. In case of accidental overdose, contact a poison control center immediately. In case of emergency, the manufacturer may be contacted 24 hours a day, 7 days a week at 800/624-9659.

How Supplied: Bottle of .33 ounce (NDC 54973-7516-1)

HYLAND'S EARACHE TABLETS

Active Ingredients: Pulsatilla (Wind Flower) 30C, HPUS; Chamomilla (Chamomile) 30C, HPUS; Sulphur 30C, HPUS; Calcarea Carbonica (Carbonate of Lime) 30C, HPUS; Belladonna 30C, HPUS; (3×10^{-60} % Alkaloids) and Lycopodium (Club Moss) 30C, HPUS.

Inactive Ingredients: Lactose NF

Indications: For the relief of symptoms of fever, pain, irritability and sleeplessness associated with earaches in children after diagnosis by a physician. If symptoms persist for more than 48 hours or if there is a discharge from the ear, discontinue use and contact your health care professional.

Directions: Dissolve 4 tablets under the tongue 3 times per day for 48 hours or until symptoms subside. If you prefer, tablets may be dissolved in a teaspoon of water and then given to the child. Earache Tablets are very soft and dissolve almost instantly under the tongue.

Warnings: Do not use if imprinted blisters are broken or damaged. If symptoms persist for more than 48 hours, or if there is a discharge from the ear, discontinue use and consult a licensed health care professional. As with any drug, if you are pregnant or nursing a baby, seek the advice of a licensed health care professional before using this product. Keep this and all medications out of the reach of children. In case of accidental overdose, contact a poison control center immediately. In cases of emergency, the manufacturer may be contacted 24 hours a day, 7 days a week at 800/624-9659.

How Supplied: Blister pack of 40 tablets (NDC 54973-7507-1). Store at room temperature.

HYLAND'S LEG CRAMPS WITH QUININE

Active Ingredients: Cinchona Officinalis 3X, HPUS (Quinine); Viscum Album 3X, HPUS; Gnaphalium Polycephalum 3X, HPUS; Rhus Toxicodendron 6X, HPUS; Aconitum Napellus 6X, HPUS; Ledum Palustre 6X, HPUS; Magnesia Phosphorica 6X, HPUS.

Inactive Ingredients: Lactose, N.F.

Indications: Hyland's Leg Cramps is a traditional homeopathic formula for the relief of symptoms of cramps and pains in lower back and legs often made worse by damp weather. Working without contraindications or side effects, Hyland's Leg Cramps stimulates your body's natural healing response to relieve symptoms. Hyland's Leg Cramps is safe for adults and can be used in conjuction with other medications.

Directions: Adults: Dissolve 2–3 tablets under tongue every 4 hours as needed.

Warnings: Do not use if imprinted cap band is missing or broken. If symptoms persist for more than seven days or worsen, contact a licensed health care professional. As with any drug, if you are pregnant or nursing a baby, seek the advice of a licensed health care professional before using this product. Do not use if pregnant, sensitive to quinine or under 12 years of age. Keep this and all medications out of the reach of children. In case of accidental overdose, contact a poison control center immediately. In case of emergency, the manufacturer may be reached 24 hours a day, 7 days a week at 800-624-9659.

How Supplied: Bottles of 100 three-grain sublingual tablets (NDC 54973-2956-02), Bottles of 50 three-grain sublingual tablets (NDC 54973-2956-01), Bottles of 40 5.5 grain caplets (NDC 54973-2956-68). Store at room temperature.

HYLAND'S NERVE TONIC

Active Ingredients: Calcarea Phosphorica (Calcium Phosphate) 3X HPUS; Ferrum Phosphorica (Iron Phosphate) 3X HPUS; Kali Phosphoricum (Potassium Phosphate) 3X HPUS; Natrum Phosphoricum (Sodium Phosphate) 3X HPUS; Magnesia Phosphoricum (Magnesium Phosphate) 3X HPUS.

Inactive Ingredients: Lactose, N.F.

Indications: Temporary symptomatic relief of simple nervous tension and stress.

Directions: Adults take 2–6 tablets before each meal and at bedtime. Children: 2 tablets. In severe cases take 3 tablets every 2 hours.

Warnings: Do not use if imprinted cap band is broken or missing. If symptoms persist for more than seven days or worsen, contact a licensed health care professional. As with any drug, if you are pregnant or nursing a baby, seek the advice of a licensed health care professional before using this product. Keep this and all medications out of the reach of children. In case of accidental overdose, contact a poison control center immediately. In cases of emergency, the manufacturer may be contacted 24 hours a day, 7 days a week at 800/624-9659.

How Supplied: Bottles of 32 caplets (NDC 54973-1129-68), Bottles of 500 tablets (NDC 54973-1129-1), Bottles of 100 tablets (NDC 54973-3014-02)

HYLAND'S RESTFUL LEGS

Active Ingredients: ARSENICUM ALBUM 12X HPUS, LYCOPODIUM 6X HPUS, PULSATILLA 6X HPUS, RHUS TOXICODENDRON 6X HPUS, SULPHUR 6X HPUS, ZINC METALLICUM 12X HPUS.

Inactive Ingredients: Lactose, N.F.

Indications: Temporarily relieves the symptoms of the compelling urge to move legs to relieve sensations of itching, tingling, crawling, and restlessness of legs. Symptoms may occur while sitting or lying down, and improve with activity.

Directions: Adults dissolve 2–3 quick dissolving tablets under tongue every 4 hours or as needed. Children ages 6–12 ½ adult dose.

Warnings: Ask a doctor before use if pregnant or nursing a baby. Consult a physician if symptoms persist for more than 7 days. Keep this and all medications out of reach of children. Do not use if imprinted tamper band is broken or missing. In case of accidental overdose, contact a poison control center immediately. In case of emergency, the manufacturer may be contacted 24 hours a day, 7 days a week at 800/624-9659.

How Supplied: Bottles of 50 3 grain tablets (NDC 54973-2966-1). Store at room temperature.

SMILE'S PRID®

Ingredients: Acidum Carbolicum 2X HPUS, Ichthammol 2X HPUS, Arnica Montana 3X HPUS, Calendula Off 3X HPUS, Echinacea Ang 3X HPUS, Sulphur 12X HPUS, Hepar Sulph 12X HPUS, Silicea 12X HPUS, Rosin, Beeswax, Petrolatum, Stearyl Alcohol, Methyl & Propyl Paraben.

Indications: Temporary topical relief of pain symptoms associated with boils, minor skin eruptions, redness and irritation. Also aids in relieving the discomfort of superficial cuts, scratches and wounds.

Directions: Wash affected parts with hot water, dry and apply PRID® twice daily on clean bandage or gauze. Do not squeeze or pressure irritated skin area. After irritation subsides, repeat application once a day for several days. Children under two years: consult a physician.
CAUTION: If symptoms persist for more than seven days or worsen, or if fever occurs, contact a licensed health care professional. Do not use on broken skin. Keep out of reach of children. In case of accidental ingestion, seek professional

assistance or contact a poison control center. For external use only. Avoid contact with eyes.

How Supplied: 18GM tin (NDC 0619-4202-54). Keep in a cool dry place.

HYLAND'S SNIFFLES'N SNEEZES 4 KIDS

Active Ingredients: ACONITUM NAPELLUS 6X HPUS, ALLIUM CEPA 6X HPUS, ZINCUM GLUCONICUM 2X HPUS, GELSENIUM SEMPERVIRENS 6X HPUS.

Inactive Ingredients: Lactose, N.F.

Indications: Temporarily relieves the symptoms of the common cold.

Directions: Children ages 2–5: dissolve 2 tablets under tongue every 15 minutes for up to 8 doses until relieved; then every 4 hours as required. Children ages 6–11: dissolve 3 tablets under tongue every 15 minutes for up to 8 doses until relieved; then every 4 hours as required. Children 12 years and older: dissolve 4 tablets under tongue every 15 minutes for up to 8 doses until relieved; then every 4 hours as required or as recommended by a health care professional.

Warnings: Ask a doctor before use if pregnant or nursing. Consult a physician if: symptoms persist for more than 7 days or worsen. Inflammation, fever or infection develops. Symptoms are accompanied by high fever. (over 101° F) Keep this and all medications out of the reach of children. Do not use if imprinted tamper band is broken or missing. In case of accidental overdose, contact a poison control center immediately. In case of emergency, the manufacturer may be contacted 24 hours a day, 7 days a week at 800/624-9659.

How Supplied: Bottles of 125 1 grain tablets (NDC 54973-7519-1). Store at room temperature.

HYLAND'S TEETHING GEL

Active Ingredients: Calcarea Phosphorica (Calcium Phosphate) 12X, HPUS; Chamomilla (Chamomile) 6X, HPUS; Coffea Cruda (Coffee) 6X, HPUS; and Belladonna 6X, HPUS (Alkaloids 0.0000003%)

Inactive Ingredients: Deionized water, Vegetable Glycerin, Hydroxyethyl Cellulose, Methyl Paraben and Propyl Paraben.

Indications: A homeopathic combination for the temporary relief of symptoms of simple restlessness and wakeful irritability due to cutting teeth.

Directions: Apply to gums as necessary. If symptoms persist for more than seven days or worsen, discontinue use and contact your health care profes-

sional. Please note, if your baby has been crying or has been very upset, your baby may fall asleep after using this product because the pain has been relieved and your child can rest.

Warnings: Do not use if tube tip is broken or missing. If symptoms persist for more than seven days or if irritation persists, inflammation develops or fever or infection develop, discontinue use and consult a licensed health care professional. As with any drug, if you are pregnant or nursing a baby, seek the advice of a licensed health care professional before using this product. Keep this and all medications out of the reach of children. In case of accidental overdose, contact a poison control center immediately. In case of emergency, the manufacturer may be contacted 24 hours a day, 7 days a week at 800/624-9659.

How Supplied: Tubes of 1/3 OZ. (NDC 54973-7504-3). Store at room temperature.

HYLAND'S TEETHING TABLETS

Active Ingredients: *Calcarea Phosphorica* (Calcium Phosphate) 3X HPUS, *Chamomilla* (Chamomile) 3X HPUS, *Coffea Cruda* (Coffee) 3X HPUS, *Belladonna* 3X HPUS (Alkaloids 0.0003%).

Inactive Ingredients: Lactose N.F.

Indications: A homeopathic combination for the temporary relief of symptoms of simple restlessness and wakeful irritability due to cutting teeth.

Directions: Dissolve 2 to 3 tablets under the tongue 4 times per day. If you prefer, tablets may first be dissolved in a teaspoon of water and then given to the child. If the child is restless or wakeful, 2 tablets every hour for 6 doses or as recommended by a licensed health care professional. Teething Tablets are very soft and dissolve almost instantly under the tongue. Please note, if your baby has been crying or has been very upset, your baby may fall asleep after using this product because the pain has been relieved and your child can rest.

Warnings: Do Not use if imprinted cap band is broken or missing. If symptoms persist for more than seven days, or if irritation persist, inflammation develops or fever or infection develop, discontinue use and consult a licensed health care professional. As with any drug, if you are pregnant or nursing a baby, seek the advice of a health care professional before using this product. Keep this and all medications out of the reach of children. In case of accidental overdose, contact a poison control center immediately. In case of emergency, the manufacturer may be contacted 24 hours a day, 7 days a week at 800/624-9659.

How Supplied: Bottles of 125—one grain sublingual tablets (NDC 54973-7504-1). Store at room temperature

IVYBLOCK®

Active Ingredient: *Bentoquatam* 5% (skin protectant)

Inactive Ingredients: *Bentonite, Benzyl Alcohol, Diisopropyl Adipate, Methylparaben, Purified Water, SDA 40 Denatured Alcohol* (25% By Weight)

Indications: Helps prevent poison ivy, oak and sumac rash when applied before exposure.

Directions: Shake well before use. Apply 15 minutes before risk of exposure. Avoid intentional contact with poison ivy, oak, and sumac. For adults and children 6 and older: apply every 4 hours for continued protection or sooner if needed. For children under 6 years: ask a doctor before use. Remove with soap and water after risk of exposure.

Warnings: For external use only. Keep away from fire or flame. Do not use if you are allergic to any ingredients, or have an open rash. When using this product, do not get into eyes. If contact occurs, rinse eyes thoroughly with water. Keep out of reach of children. If swallowed, get medical help or contact a Poison Control Center right away.

How Supplied: Bottle of 4 ounces (NDC 62333-111-40)

Topical BioMedics, Inc.
PO BOX 494
RHINEBECK, NY 12572-0494

Direct Inquiries to:
Professional Services
Phone: (845) 871-4900 ext. 1115
Fax: (845) 876-0818
E-mail:
info@topicalbiomedics.com

TOPRICIN®

Key Facts: Topricin® is an odorless non-irritating anti-inflammatory pain relief cream that provides excellent adjunctive support in medical treatments such as post surgical, physical and occupational therapy, chiropractic. Greaseless and contains no lanolin, menthol, capsaicin, or fragrances.

Active Ingredients: (HPUS) Arnica Montana 6X, Echinacea 6X, Aesculus 6X, Ruta Graveolens 6X, Lachesis 8X, Rhus Tox 6X Belladonna 6X, Crotalus 8X, Heloderma 8X, Naja 8X, Graphites 6X. Fomitopsis officinalis IX.

Major Uses: Topical relief of inflammation & pain, and a healing treatment for soft tissue & trauma/sports injuries.

Benefits: relieves swelling, stiffness, numbness, tingling and burning pain as-

Continued on next page

Topricin—Cont.

sociated with these soft tissue ailments: carpal tunnel syndrome, other neuropathic pain, arthritis, lower back pain, muscle spasm of the back, neck, legs, and feet, muscle soreness, crushing injury, and sprains. First aid: bruises, minor burns. Use before and after exercise

Directions: Apply generously 3–4 times a day or more often if needed making sure to cover the entire joint or area of pain. Massage in until absorbed. Reapply before bed and at the start of the day for best results.

For further information go to www.topicalbiomedics.com

Safety Information: For external use only, use only as directed, if pain persists for more that 7 days or worsens, Consult a doctor. This homeopathic medicine has no known side effects or contraindications. Complies with FDA standards as an OTC medicine. Safe to use for children, adults, pregnant women and the elderly. Paraben free.

Inactive Ingredients: purified water, highly refined vegetable oils, glycerin, medium-chain-triglyceride.

How Supplied:
Consumer size 4 oz jar or 2 oz tube or 8 oz pump
For professional use only: 16 oz or 32 oz pump bottle
Shown in Product Identification Guide, page 504

Upsher-Smith Laboratories, Inc
**6701 EVENSTAD DRIVE
MAPLE GROVE, MN 55369**

Direct Inquiries to:
Medical Information
(800) 654-2299

AMLACTIN® MOISTURIZING BODY LOTION AND CREAM
[ăm-lăk-tĭn]
Cosmetic Lotion and Cream

Description: AMLACTIN® Moisturizing Lotion and Cream are special formulations of 12% lactic acid neutralized with ammonium hydroxide to provide a lotion or cream pH of 4.5-5.5. Lactic acid, an alpha-hydroxy acid, is a naturally occurring humectant for the skin. AMLACTIN® moisturizes, exfoliates and softens rough, dry skin.

How Supplied: 225g (7.9oz) plastic bottle: List No. 0245-0023-22

400g (14.1oz) plastic bottle: List No. 0245-0023-40

140g (4.9oz) tube: List No. 0245-0024-14

AMLACTIN AP® Anti-Itch Moisturizing Cream
[ăm-lăk'-tĭn]
1% Pramoxine HCl

Description: AMLACTIN AP® Anti-Itch Moisturizing Cream is a special formulation containing 12% lactic acid neutralized with ammonium hydroxide to provide a cream pH of 4.5-5.5 with pramoxine HCl. Lactic acid, an alpha-hydroxy acid, is a naturally occurring humectant which moisturizes and softens rough, dry skin. Pramoxine HCl, USP, 1% is an effective antipruritic ingredient used to relieve itching associated with dry skin.

How Supplied: 140g (4.9oz) tube: NDC No. 0245-0025-14

AMLACTIN XL®
[ăm-lăk'-tĭn]
**Moisturizing Lotion
ULTRAPLEX® Formulation**

Description: AmLactin XL® Moisturizing Lotion is a clinically proven moisturizer which provides powerful mosturizing for rough, dry skin. AmLactin XL® Moisturizing Lotion contains ULTRAPLEX® formulation, a proprietary blend of alpha-hydroxy moisturizing compounds.

How Supplied: 160g (5.6oz) tube: List No. 0245-0022-16

SECTION 8

DIETARY AND HERBAL SUPPLEMENT INFORMATION

This section presents information on natural remedies and nutritional supplements marketed under the Dietary Supplement Health and Education Act of 1994. It is made possible through the courtesy of the manufacturers whose products appear on the following pages. The information concerning each product has been prepared, edited, and approved by the manufacturer's professional staff.

Products found in this section include vitamins, minerals, herbs and other botanicals, amino acids, other substances intended to supplement the diet, and concentrates, metabolites, constituents, extracts, and combinations of these ingredients. The descriptions of these products are designed to provide all information necessary for informed use, including, when applicable, active ingredients, inactive ingredients, actions, warnings, cautions, interactions, symptoms and treatment of oral overdosage, dosage and directions for use, and how supplied. Descriptions in

this section must be in full compliance with the Dietary Supplement Health and Education Act, which permits claims regarding a product's effect on the structure or functioning of the body, but forbids claims regarding a product's ability to treat, diagnose, cure, or prevent any specific disease. Descriptions of products marketed under the act do not receive formal evaluation or approval from the Food and Drug Administration.

In compiling this section, the publisher has emphasized the necessity of describing products comprehensively. The descriptions seen here include all information made available by the manufacturer. The publisher does not warrant or guarantee any product described here, and does not perform any independent analysis of the information provided. Inclusion of a product in this book does not represent an endorsement, and the publisher does not necessarily advocate the use of any product listed.

A&Z Pharmaceutical Inc.
**180 OSER AVENUE, SUITE 300
HAUPPAUGE, NY 11788**

Direct Inquiries to:
(631) 952-3800

D-CAL™
**Calcium Supplement with Vitamin D
Chewable Caplets**

Ingredients: Calcium Carbonate, Vitamin D, Sorbitol, Flavor, D&C Red #27 Lake, Magnesium Stearate. No sugar, No salt, No lactose, No preservative.
Supplement Facts
Serving Size One Caplet

Each Caplet Contains	% Daily Value	
Calcium (as calcium carbonate)	300 mg	30%
Vitamin D	100 IU	25%

Recommended Intake: Take two caplets daily for adult and one caplet for child, or as directed by your physician.

Warnings: KEEP OUT OF REACH OF CHILDREN. Do not accept if safety seal under cap is broken or missing.

Actions: D-Cal™ provides a concentrated form of calcium to help build healthy bones. It contains Vitamin D to help the body absorb calcium. D-Cal™ can also help prevent osteoporosis. It is helpful to pregnant and nursing women, children's growth, and calcium deficiency at all ages.

How Supplied: Bottles of 30 and 60 caplets

Awareness Corporation dba Awareness Life
**25 SOUTH ARIZONA PLACE
SUITE 500
CHANDLER, AZ 85225**

Direct Inquiries to:
1-800-69AWARE
Website: http://www.awarenesslife.net

AWARENESS CLEAR®

Description: May help with general digestion.*

Ingredients: Proprietary blend of Oregano Leaf, Clove Flowers, Black Walnut Seed Husk, Peppermint Leaf, Nigella, Grapefruit, Winter Melon Seed, Gentian, Hyssop Leaf, Crampbark, Thyme Leaf, Fennel.

Directions: Take 2 capsules a day each morning on an empty stomach, 1–2 hours before eating with 1 glass of water

Warnings: Do not use if Pregnant or Breastfeeding. Keep out of reach of children.

How Supplied: 90 Vegetarian Capsules per Bottle

---

*These statements have not been evaluated by the Food and Drug Administration. These products are not intended to diagnose, treat, cure, or prevent any disease.

AWARENESS FEMALE BALANCE®   OTC

Description: For the temporary relief of Menopausal and PMS symptoms like water gain, bloating, swelling, pain, cramps, etc.
Ingredients: Proprietary blend of Angelica Root, Yarrow Root, Chinese Peony Root, Damiana Leaf, Peppermint Leaf, Passionflower, Hemidesmus Indicus, Cramp Bark, Partridge Berry, Polygonatum, Valerian root, Dandelion Root, Chaste Tree Fruit, Rosemary Leaf, Caraway Seed, Black Cumin Seed, Queen of the Meadow Leaf, Herba Epimedii Leaf, Ligusticum Wallichii, Schisandra Berry, Raspberry Leaf.

Directions: To start take 1 capsule with water for the first 2 days. You may take either in the morning or the evening. Do not exceed 1 to 2 capsules twice a day. Take during your cycle when PMS symptoms are present.

Warnings: Do not use if pregnant or breast-feeding. Keep out of reach of children.

How Supplied: 60 vegetarian capsules per bottle.
Shown in Product Identification Guide, page 503

DAILY COMPLETE®

Description: Liquid Supplement. 100% vegetarian ingredients delivers 241 vitamins, minerals, Organic antioxidants, enzymes, Organic fruits and Organic vegetables, amino acids and herbs, in one ounce liquid a day (great orange taste) Helps to Provide Energy & Reduce Stress Levels*.

Ingredients: Rich in Vitamins & Minerals, Ionic Plant Minerals, Botanical Organic Antioxidants with Phenalgin™, Organic Fruit & Organic Vegetable Whole Juice Complex, Whole Superfood Green complex, 34 Mediterranean Herbs, Essential Fatty Acid Complex, Special Ocean Vegetable Blend

Directions: Take 1 ounce (30 ml) per day, during or immediately after a meal

Warnings: Do not use if pregnant or breast-feeding. Keep out of reach of children.

How Supplied: 30 ounces per Bottle, Clinically Tested Ingredients.
Shown in Product Identification Guide, page 503

EXPERIENCE®

Description: Promotes Regularity & Cleanses the Colon*

Ingredients: Proprietary Blend of Senna, Blonde Psyllium Seed Husk, Fennel Seed, Cornsilk, Solomon's seal, Rhubarb Root, Kelp

Directions: Take 1 to 2 Capsules before bedtime with a full glass of water.

Warnings: Do not use if pregnant or breast-feeding or if you have colitis. Keep out of reach of children

How Supplied: 90 Capsules per bottle, Clinically tested
Shown in Product Identification Guide, page 503

PURE GARDENS CREAM®

Description: Natural botanical cream may help to improve appearance of dry skin, fine lines and helps to tone the skin.

Ingredients: Apple oil, vitamin C, vitamin E, Aloe Vera Leaf, Almond Oil, Cold Press Virgin Olive Oil, Sesame Oil, Chamomile Flowers Oil, Calendula Officinalis Oil, Beeswax, Jojoba Oil, Linseed Oil.

Directions: Application for both face and body. External use only

How Supplied: 2 ounce jar, Clinically tested

PURETRIM® MEDITERRANEAN WELLNESS SHAKE

Description: Vegetarian Natural Wholefood High Protein Low Carb Energy Shake. No Dairy, No Soy

Ingredients: Vegetable Pea & Brown Rice Protein, Antioxidants, Prebiotics, Essential Fatty Acids & Enzyme Active Greens

Directions: Mix contents in 10 oz. of cold water.

Warnings: Not for use by pregnant or lactating women. Must be 18 years or older to use.

How Supplied: 10 Packets (Net Wt 500 g)
Shown in Product Identification Guide, page 503

SYNERGYDEFENSE® CAPSULES

Description: Improves Digestion, Boosts the Immune System, & strengthens the body's natural defenses*.

Ingredients: Proprietary Blend of Enzymes, Probiotics, Antioxidants, Prebiotics

Directions: Take 1 capsule with a glass of water during or before your largest meal of the day. Take once or twice a daily.

Warnings: Do not use if pregnant or lactating. If under 18, consult a physician before use.

How Supplied: 30 Vegetarian Capsules individually sealed

---

*These statements have not been evaluated by the Food and Drug Administration. These products are not intended to diagnose, treat, cure, or prevent any disease.

Shown in Product Identification Guide, page 503

Beach Pharmaceuticals
Division of Beach Products, Inc.
5220 SOUTH MANHATTAN AVENUE
TAMPA, FL 33611

Direct Inquiries to:
Richard Stephen Jenkins
(813) 839-6565
FAX (813) 837-2511

BEELITH TABLETS
magnesium supplement with pyridoxine HCl

Description: Each tablet contains magnesium oxide 600 mg and pyridoxine hydrochloride (Vitamin B_6) 25 mg equivalent to Vitamin B_6 20 mg.

Supplement Facts
Serving Size: 1 Tablet

	Amount Per Tablet	% Daily Value
Vitamin B_6 (pyridoxine HCl)	20 mg	1000%
Magnesium (from magnesium oxide)	362 mg	90%

Inactive Ingredients: FD&C Yellow No. 6, hydroxypropyl methylcellulose, magnesium stearate, microcrystalline cellulose, polyethylene glycol, sodium starch glycolate, titanium dioxide. May also contain D&C Yellow No. 10, FD&C Yellow No. 5 (Tartrazine), hydroxypropyl cellulose, polydextrose, stearic acid and/or triacetin.

J.R. Carlson Laboratories, Inc.
15 COLLEGE DRIVE
ARLINGTON HEIGHTS, IL
60004-1985

Direct Inquiries to:
Customer Service
(888) 234-5656
FAX: (847) 255-1605
www.carlsonlabs.com
For Medical Information Contact:
In Emergencies:
Customer Service
(888) 234-5656
FAX: (847) 255-1605

E-GEMS®   OTC

Description: 100% natural-source vitamin E (d-alpha tocopheryl acetate) soft gels. Available in 8 strengths: 30 IU, 100 IU, 200 IU, 400 IU, 600 IU, 800 IU, 1000 IU, 1200 IU.

How Supplied: Supplied in a variety of bottle sizes.

MED OMEGA™ FISH OIL 2800 OTC
[mĕd ōmĕga]
Balanced Concentrate
DHA 1200 mg & EPA 1200 mg
Professional Strength Dietary Supplement

Description: From Norway: The finest fish oil from deep, cold ocean-water fish. Concentrated to supply 2800 mg (2.8 grams) of total omega 3's per teaspoonful. Bottled in Norway to ensure maximum freshness. Refreshing natural orange taste.

Supplement Facts

Serving Size 1 Teaspoonful (5 ml)	Servings Per Container 20	
Each Teaspoonful Contains		% D.V.
Omega-3 Fatty Acids	2.8 g (2800 mg)	*
EPA (eicosapentaenoic acid)	1.2 g (1200 mg)	*
DHA (docosahexaenoic acid)	1.2 g (1200 mg)	*
Other Omega-3 Fatty acids	.4 g (400 mg)	*
Vitamin E (d-Alpha Tocopherol)	10 IU	33%

This product is regularly tested (using AOAC international protocols) for freshness, potency and purity by an independent, FDA-registered laboratory and has been determined to be fresh, fully-potent and free of detectable levels of mercury, cadmium, lead, PCB's and 28 other contaminants.
Other Ingredients: Natural orange flavor, rosemary extract, ascorbyl palmitate, natural tocopherols.

How Supplied: Supplied in 100 mL (3.35 Fl. oz.) bottles. Orange Flavor.

CARLSON NORWEGIAN COD LIVER OIL   OTC

Each Teaspoonful of Carlson Norwegian Cod Liver Oil provides:

		% DV
Total Omega 3 Fatty Acids	1100 mg to 1250 mg**	*
DHA (Docosahexaenoic Acid)	500 mg to 590 mg**	*
EPA (Eicosapentaenoic Acid)	360 mg to 500 mg**	*
ALA (Alpha-linolenic Acid)	40 mg to 60 mg**	*
Vitamin A	700 IU to 1,200 IU**	14% to 24%
Vitamin D	400 IU	100%
Vitamin E	10 IU	33%
Norwegian Cod Liver Oil	4.6 g	*

**Naturally Occurring Variations.

Description: Carlson Norwegian Cod Liver Oil comes from the livers of fresh cod fish found in the arctic coastal waters of Norway.
Suggested Use: Take one teaspoonful daily at mealtime.

Indications (continued from middle column):

Indications: As a dietary supplement for patients with magnesium and/or Vitamin B_6 deficiencies resulting from malnutrition, alcoholism, magnesium depleting drugs, chemotherapy, and inadequate nutritional intake or absorption. Also, increases urinary magnesium levels.

Dosage: One tablet daily or as directed by a physician.

Warnings: Do not take this product if you are presently taking a prescription drug without consulting your physician or other health professional. If you have kidney disease, take only under the supervision of a physician. Excessive dosage may cause laxation. If pregnant or breast-feeding, ask a health professional before use.
KEEP OUT OF THE REACH OF CHILDREN.

How Supplied: Golden yellow, film-coated tablet with the letters **BP** and the number **132** imprinted on each tablet. Packaged in bottles of 100 (Item No. 0486-1132-01) tablets.

Continued on next page

Cod Liver Oil—Cont.

This product is regularly tested (using AOAC international protocols) for freshness, potency, and purity by an independent, FDA-registered laboratory and has been determined to be fresh, fully-potent and free of detectable levels of mercury, cadmium, lead, PCB's and 28 other contaminants.

How Supplied: Supplied in bottles of 250ml and 500ml. Lemon or regular flavor.

SUPER OMEGA-3   OTC

Description: Carlson Super Omega-3 soft gels contain a special concentrate of fish body oils from deep cold-water fish, which are rich in EPA & DHA.
Each soft gelatin capsule provides 1000 mg of omega-3 fish oils consisting of:

		% U.S. RDA
EPA (eicosapentaenoic acid)	300 mg	*
DHA (docosahexaenoic acid)	200 mg	*
Other Omega-3's	100 mg	*
Vitamin E (d-alpha tocopherol)	10 IU	33%

This product is regularly tested (using AOAC international protocols) for freshness, potency and purity by an independent, FDA-registered laboratory and has been determined to be fresh, fully-potent and free of detectable levels of mercury, cadmium, lead, PCB's and 28 other contaminants.

How Supplied: In bottles of 50, 100, 250.

Eniva Nutraceutics

9702 ULYSSES STREET NE
MINNEAPOLIS, MN 55434

Direct Inquiries to:
Phone: 763-795-8870
Fax: 763-795-8890
www.eniva.com

EFACOR®
Omega-3 Essential Fatty Acids - Dietary Supplement
(Concentrated EPA and DHA)

Description: ENIVA EFACOR® provides pharmaceutical-grade ingredients independently tested for purity in a specialized, natural Omega-3 EFA dietary supplement containing high-dose EPA and DHA. Its formula provides these strongly researched substances with a synergistic blend of other Omega-3 derivatives in a pleasant tasting lemon-lime softgel. Manufactured under strict GMP standards, ENIVA EFACOR® is ultra-pure and free of environmental contaminants.

Uses: Omega-3s, especially EPA and DHA, have been shown to support:
• Cardiovascular Function*
• Neurologic Function and Mood*
• Immune and Joint Function*
• Vision and Ocular Function*
• Weight Management and Skin*†

ENIVA EFACOR® (2 gelcaps) meets the American Heart Association's (AHA) recommendation of providing 1,000 mg of EPA and DHA daily for cardiovascular health and the FDA's requirement for supporting the statement: Daily intake of Omega-3 in the form of EPA and DHA may reduce the risk of coronary heart disease. FDA evaluated the data and determined that, although there is scientific evidence supporting the claim, the evidence is not conclusive.
* This statement has not been evaluated by the Food and Drug Administration. This product is not intended to diagnose, treat, cure, or prevent any disease.
† Along with a proper diet and exercise, ENIVA EFACOR® is meant to assist the body's efforts in weight management and does not guarantee weight loss.
[See table above]

Ingredients: Ingredients: Highly refined and concentrated omega-3 fish oil, capsule (gelatin, glycerin and purified water), natural lemon and lime flavor, proprietary antioxidant blend (consisting of rosemary extract, ascorbyl palmitate and natural tocopherols).

Dosing: Adult Directions: Two softgels daily, preferably 10 minutes before a meal. Do not exceed 8 softgels daily.
Children (4+) Directions: One softgel daily.

Safety Information: As with all dietary supplements, contact your doctor before use, especially if you are pregnant or lactating, suspect a medical condition or are taking prescription drugs. Do not consume if you are allergic to fish, fish components or any substance in the ingredient listing. Although ENIVA EFACOR® is manufactured from natural and safe pharmaceutical-grade ingredients, rare sensitivity may develop; should this occur, discontinue use. ENIVA EFACOR® is not habit forming. Keep this and all dietary supplements out of the reach of children.

Supplement Facts
Serving Size: 2 Softgels
Servings Per Container: 30

	Amount Per Serving	% Daily Value*
Calories (energy)	20	
Calories From Fat	20	
Total Fat	2 g	3%
Saturated Fat	0 g	0%
Polyunsaturated Fat	1.5 g	†
Monounsaturated Fat	0 g	†
Cholesterol	0 mg	0%
Omega-3 Fatty Acids	1,120 mg	†
EPA (Eicosapentaenoic Acid)	680 mg	†
DHA (Docosahexaenoic Acid)	340 mg	†
Other Omega-3s (includes DPA/ETA)	100 mg	†

* Percent Daily Values are based on a 2,000 calorie diet.
† Daily Values not established.

ENIVA EFACOR® Quality Tested

ENIVA EFACOR® carries the Consumer Labs official seal of Approved Quality on the bottle to designate it has passed the required parameters for CL testing. Users of ENIVA EFACOR® can be assured the product incorporates the highest standards of QUALITY and SAFETY.

ConsumerLab.com
OMEGA-3 from EPA & DHA
Be Sure It's CL Approved

Data on file, Eniva Nutraceutics, 2008.

How Supplied: Vegetable gel capsule – translucent yellow. Capsule can be bitten to access liquid if person has difficulty swallowing capsule. Lemon-lime flavor. Bottle of 60 softgel capsules. Bottle opens with a tear-off, tamper-resistant plastic cap and contains an inner safety seal. Do not consume if seals are not secure.

Storage: Best if refrigerated upon receipt and after opening. Avoid freezing and excessive heat.
Eniva Nutraceutics, Minneapolis, MN 55434 USA

Shown in Product Identification Guide, page 503

VIBE®
Liquid Multi-Nutrient Supplement

Description: Leading medical researchers and clinicians recommend individuals ingest a multi-nutrient dietary supplement on a daily basis. The ENIVA VIBE® liquid nutraceutical not only meets medical recommendations in terms of nutrient content, but it has been specifically formulated for rapid absorption and bioavailability due to the predigested nature of its pharmaceutical-grade liquid contents.

Uses/Mechanism: Due to the predigested nature of the vitamins and minerals in the ENIVA VIBE® nutraceutical, nutrient absorption and cellular bioavailability of nutrients appear to be enhanced. This results in the support of body structure and function.* Through mechanisms not fully elucidated, the antioxidant capacity of ENIVA VIBE® appears to have an impact on free radicals and their associated metabolism.*

- Scientific evidence suggests consumption of antioxidant vitamins may reduce the risk of certain forms of cancer. However, FDA has determined this evidence is limited and not conclusive.
- As part of a well-balanced diet that is low in saturated fat and cholesterol, Folic Acid, Vitamin B6 and B12 may reduce the risk of vascular disease. However, the FDA has determined this evidence is limited and not conclusive.
- ENIVA VIBE® does NOT contain Vitamin K due to Vitamin K's ability to interfere with anti-coagulation medications.

Supplement Facts

Serving Size: 1 Fluid Ounce

Servings Per Container: 32

	Amount Per Serving	% Daily Value
Calories	30	
Total Carbohydrate	6 g	2%**
Sugars	4 g	†
Vitamin A	2,000 IU	40%
Vitamin C	120 mg	200%
Vitamin D	500 IU	125%
Vitamin E	30 IU	100%
Thiamin Vitamin B1	1.5 mg	100%
Riboflavin Vitamin B2	1.7 mg	100%
Niacin	18 mg	90%
Vitamin B6	2 mg	100%
Folic Acid	400 mcg	100%
Vitamin B12	12 mcg	200%
Biotin	300 mcg	100%
Pantothenic Acid	10 mg	100%
Calcium	100 mg	10%
Phosphorus	20 mg	2%
Iodine	150 mcg	100%
Magnesium	155 mg	39%
Zinc	5 mg	33%
Selenium	25 mcg	36%
Copper	.5 mg	25%
Manganese	1.8 mg	90%
Chromium	120 mcg	100%
Potassium	175 mg	5%

Proprietary Trace 37 mg †
Mineral Blend
Boron, Germanium, Sulfur, Vanadium

AntiOX2®* 6,500 mg †
Phytonutrient Proprietary Blend
Natural Extracts: Cranberry, Raspberry, Blueberry, Blackberry, Strawberry, Cherry, Carrot, Acai Berry, Elderberry, Hibiscus (flower), Lemon, Lime, Apple, Orange, Blackcurrant, Oregano, Chokeberry, Grape, Pumpkin, Tomato, Pomegranate, Wolfberry (gojiberry), Stevia (leaf), Grape Seed Extract; Citrus Bioflavonoids

HeartPRO™* 280 mg †
Proprietary Blend
D-Ribose, CoQ10, L-Carnitine, Malic Acid, Isolated Soy Lecithin, Mixed Tocopherols

CollaMAX®* 3,500 mg †
Proprietary Blend
Green Tea Leaf Extract (water decaffeinated), L-Lysine, L-Proline, Aloe Vera Gel (containing Alanine, Valine, Isoleucine, Glycine, Leucine), Glucosamine HCl (vegetable)

** Percent Daily Values are based on a 2,000 calorie diet.
† Daily Value not established.

Ingredients: Purified water, natural extracts and flavors (from blackberry, and/or apple, and/or chokeberry, and/or elderberry, and/or blueberry, and/or blackcurrant, and/or stevia [leaf], and/or oregano, and/or tomato, and/or hibiscus, and/or carrot, and/or pumpkin, and/or cherry, and/or grape, and/or cranberry, and/or green tea leaf extract [water decaffeinated], and/or lemon, and/or lime, and/or aloe vera gel, and/or grape seed extract, and/or pomegranate, and/or wolfberry [gojiberry], and/or acai berry, and/or strawberry, and/or raspberry, and/or orange), natural sugars (beet and/or molasses), magnesium (from magnesium citrate, and/or magnesium malate, and/or magnesium sulfate, and/or magnesium glycerophosphate, and/or magnesium chloride), citric acid, malic acid, potassium (from potassium citrate, and/or potassium chloride, and/or potassium iodide, and/or potassium lactate), calcium (from calcium citrate, and/or calcium malate, and/or calcium chloride, and/or calcium glycerophosphate), ascorbic acid, l-lysine, l-proline, d-alpha-tocopherol acetate (with mixed tocopherols), sorbic and/or benzoic acid(s) (protect freshness), d-ribose, niacin (from nicotinic acid), zinc (from zinc sulfate, and/or zinc chloride), l-carnitine fumarate, calcium panthothenate, boron (from sodium borate), glucosamine hcl (vegetable), vitamin A palmitate, natural gums (xanthan, guar, arabic), folic acid, manganese (from manganous chloride, and/or manganese sulfate), pyridoxine hcl, riboflavin phosphate, thiamin hcl, copper (from copper sulfate, and/or copper gluconate), cholecalciferol, isolated soy lecithin, chromium (from chromium chloride), biotin, sorbimacrogol, CoQ10 (ubiquinone), glycerin (vegetable), germanium (from germanium sesquioxide), selenium (from sodium selenate, and/or selenium chloride), vanadium (from vanadyl sulfate), cyanocobalamin, n-methylcobalamin. May contain rosemarinic acid.

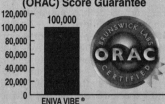

ENIVA VIBE® Antioxidant Capacity (ORAC) Score Guarantee

ORAC Score Per 32 Ounces, 2008

VIBE® provides patients a certified Antioxidant Assurance Rating of at least 100,000 ORAC units (ORAC = Oxygen Radical Absorbance Capacity) per 32 ounces during shelf-life based on peroxyl radical; total broad-spectrum antioxidant activity may be higher.

Predigested Liquid Formula

VIBE® promotes rapid absorption and bioavailability through its PREDIGESTED LIQUID formula to support proper body function.*

ENIVA VIBE® Certified Safety Assurance Testing
- Heavy Metals
- Pesticides / Herbicides
- Full Microbiologic, Including Mold & Yeast
- Fungal Toxin Screen (mycotoxin)
- Allergen & Food Additive Screening
- GMO Testing

Data on file, Eniva Nutraceutics, 2008.

ENIVA VIBE® Quality Testing
- Ingredient Potency Testing & Verification
- Antioxidant ORAC Analysis
- Shelf-Life Stability
- Biomass Assays
- Particle Size Analysis

Data on file, Eniva Nutraceutics, 2008.

- No Stimulants • No Artificial Colors
- No Artificial Flavors
- VIBE® is a Decaffeinated Product
- Vegetarian Friendly • No Fish Ingredients

Dosing: Adults: Ingest 1-2 ounces daily. Recommended to not exceed daily: 3 ounces—men, 2 ounces—women. For best results: Split dosing evenly between a.m. and p.m. hours, unless otherwise directed by a physician. May combine dose with 8 ounces of water/juice.
Children 14+: One ounce daily. It is recommended children under 14 years take ENIVA® KID'S VIBE®.
Pregnant/Lactating Women: Contact your doctor before use. Recommended to not exceed 2 ounces per day.

Safety Information: As with all dietary supplements, contact your doctor before use, especially if you are pregnant or lactating, suspect a medical condition or are taking prescription drugs. Do not consume if you are allergic to any substance in the ingredient listing. Although ENIVA VIBE® is manufactured from natural and safe pharmaceutical-grade ingredients, rare sensitivity may develop; should this occur, discontinue use. ENIVA VIBE® is not habit forming. Keep

Continued on next page

Vibe—Cont.

this and all dietary supplements out of the reach of children.

Storage: Keep refrigerated upon receipt and after opening. Avoid freezing and excessive heat. Due to natural contents, product should be consumed within 40 days after opening. It is normal and expected with natural extracts and ingredients some settling may occur. Shake well before using.

[See figure at top of previous page]
* This statement has not been evaluated by the Food and Drug Administration. This product is not intended to diagnose, treat, cure, or prevent any disease. Eniva Nutraceutics, Minneapolis, MN 55434 USA

Shown in Product Identification Guide, page 503

4Life Research USA, LLC

**9850 S. 300 W
SANDY, UT 84070**

Direct Inquiries to:
Ph: (801) 562-3600
Fax: (801) 562-3699
Email: productsupport@4life.com
Website: www.4life.com

4LIFE TRANSFER FACTOR PLUS® TRI-FACTOR™ FORMULA

4Life® specializes in the research, development, and manufacturing of immune system support supplements.

Product Description: 4Life Transfer Factor Plus Tri-Factor Formula combines scientifically studied ingredients to educate, boost, and balance immune cell response (such as T-cells and Natural Killer cells). Among its ingredients are Transfer Factor E-XF™, NanoFactor™, and a Cordyvant™ blend.

Supplement Facts

Serving Size: One (1) Capsule
Servings Per Container: 60

Amount Per Capsule		% DV*
Zinc (as Zinc Methionine)	5 mg	33%
4Life Tri-Factor™ Formula	150 mg	**
Transfer Factor E-XF™ A patented concentrate of transfer factors from cow colostrum and egg yolk.		
NanoFactor™ A proprietary concentrate of nano-filtered cow colostrum.		
Cordyvant Proprietary Polysaccharide Complex	440 mg	**
IP-6 (Inositol hexaphosphate)		
β-Sitosterol, other phytosterols		
Cordyceps sinensis (7% cordyceptic acids)		
Beta-Glucan (from baker's yeast) (Saacharomyces cerevisiae)		
Beta-Glucan (from Oat) (Avena sativa)		
Agaricus blazeii Extract		
Mannans (from Aloe vera) (leaf)		
Olive Leaf Extract (Olea europaea)		
Maitake Mushroom (Grifola frondosa)		
Shiitake Mushroom (Lentinus edodes)(5:1 extract)		
Lemon peel		

*Reference Daily Intake (RDI)
**Daily Value (DV) not established
Other Ingredient: Gelatin capsule.

Transfer factors: Transfer factors, discovered in 1949 by NYU immunolo-

gist Dr. H. Sherwood Lawrence, are messenger molecules that transfer immunity information from one entity to another, such as between a breastfeeding mother and her newborn infant. Defined as small peptides (proteins) and other compounds isolated from cow colostrum and chicken egg yolks, transfer factors have a molecular weight less than 10 kilodaltons. 4Life's patented Transfer Factor E-XF blend combines transfer factors from these two sources for a synergistic effect.

Nanofraction molecules: 4Life Research developed the isolation process and tested the immune activity of nanofraction molecules from cow colostrum and egg yolk. These nanofraction molecules are very small—a molecular weight of less than 3 kilodaltons. Nanofraction molecules regulate immune system function, educating immune cells on when to respond, how to respond, and when to rest. NanoFactor is 4Life's proprietary extract of nanofraction molecules from cow colostrum.

Cordyvant blend: This proprietary blend features known immune-supporting ingredients such as maitake and shiitake mushrooms, cordyceps, inositol hexaphosphate, beta glucans, beta sitosterol, and olive leaf extract.

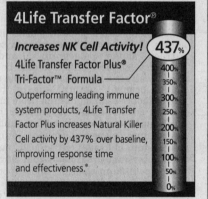

*Blind independent studies conducted by Dr. Anatoli Vorobiev, head of Immunology, at the Russian Academy of Medical Science.

4Life Transfer Factor Plus Tri-Factor Formula is protected by US patents 6,468,534 and 6,866,868, with other patents pending.

Major Uses: Provides immune system support through education, enhancement, and balanced immune cell activity; support for healthy energy levels; balance for over- or under-active immune systems; and support for healthy inflammation levels. In addition, 4Life's Targeted Transfer Factor® products provide specific support for healthy structures and functions throughout the body, including: support for healthy memory and cognitive function; cardiovascular, nervous, metabolic, endocrine, and urinary system support; male prostate support; and female breast and gynecologic health support.

Recommended Dose: 600mg daily. No toxicity level of 4Life Transfer Factor

Plus Tri-Factor Formula has been found. See www.4life.com for more information on 4Life Transfer Factor products. There is also a database of studies relating to transfer factors available on www.pubmed.org.

Greek Island Labs

**7620 E. MCKELLIPS ROAD
SUITE 4 PMB 86
SCOTTSDALE, AZ 85257**

Direct Inquiries to:
Website:
http://www.greekislandlabs.com
(888) 841-7363

NATURALJOINT®
dietary supplement

Description: Natural Dietary Supplement that Promotes Healthy Joints Supports Flexibility & Mobility*

Ingredients: Proprietary Greek Blend of 37 Natural Ingredients

Directions: 1 Capsule daily with meal

Warnings: Keep out of reach of children. Consult your doctor prior to using this product if you are taking any prescription medication

How Supplied: 30 Capsules (Vegetarian) Per Box

*The statements have not been reviewed or approved by the Food & Drug Administration. This product is not intended to diagnose, treat, cure or prevent any disease

PROSTATE COMPLETE™
Dietary supplement

Description: Supports healthy prostate function.

Ingredients: Proprietary Greek blend of Fruits, Vegetables and Herbs.

Directions: 1 Capsule twice a day with meal

Warnings: Keep out of reach of children. Consult your doctor prior to using this product if you are taking any prescription medication

How Supplied: 60 Capsules per box

**IF YOU SUSPECT
AN INTERACTION. . .**
The 1,800-page
PDR Companion Guide™ can help.
Use the order form
in the front of this book.

Legacy For Life, LLC

P.O. BOX 410376
MELBOURNE, FL 32941-0376

DIRECT INQUIRIES TO:
(800) 557-8477
(321) 951-8815
TECHNICAL INQUIRIES:
(800) 746-0300
info@legacyforlife.net
www.legacyforlife.com

i²⁶®

Description: i²⁶ ("hyperimmune" egg) is powdered whole egg from hens stimulated with >26 inactivated bacteria.

Clinical Background: i²⁶ passively transfers a variety of naturally-enriched immune factors that helps the body support immune, joint, digestive, and cardiovascular health [HyperimmuneEgg.org]. i²⁶ has been clinically proven to contribute to sports performance. i²⁶ does not *boost* immune function, rather it helps the body *balance* the immune system affecting autoimmune and excessive responsiveness. i²⁶ may be used concomitantly with prescription medications.

Precautions: Those with allergies to eggs should consult with a health practitioner.
Note: i²⁶ is not intended to diagnose, treat, cure or prevent disease. These statements have not been evaluated by the Food and Drug Administration.

How Supplied: Each serving (4.5g) of i²⁶ is available as: pure hyperimmune (HIE) egg powder, capsules (9/serving), and as chewable tablets (3/serving). A serving of COMPLETE Support®, contains 4.5g of HIE+ vitamins and minerals. The high protein and fiber, low carbohydrate BALANCE Shake with 4.5g HIE is utilized by athletes and for weight management.

Memory Secret

1221 BRICKELL AVENUE
SUITE 1540
MIAMI, FL 33131

Direct Inquiries to:
(866) 673-2738
Fax: (305) 675-2279
email: intelectol@memorysecret.net
www.memorysecret.net
www.intelectol.com

INTELECTOL® MEMORY ENHANCER VINPOCETINE TABLETS MEMORY SECRET

Description: INTELECTOL® is the purest form of Vinpocetine available.

Vinpocetine is a derivative of Vincamine, which is extracted from the Periwinkle plant (*Vinca Minor, Vinca Pervinca*). Research suggests that Vinpocetine helps to maintain healthy blood circulation in the brain and supports certain neurotransmitters in the memory process.* Vinpocetine supports and protects brain blood vessel health and aids mental function.*

Directions: As a dietary supplement, take 2 tablets twice daily with meals. Vinpocetine should be taken as part of an on-going regimen with exercise, a healthy diet and keeping active the mind.

Cautions: Take product with food to avoid stomach upset. Not recommended for use by pregnant women, nursing mothers or anyone under 18 years old. Consult a doctor or health care professional before use if you have any medical condition or if taking any medication. Not recommended for use by anyone with hemophilia, heart problems or low blood pressure. **Keep out of reach of children.** Store in a cool, dry place.

Supplement Facts
Serving Size 2 tablets
Servings Per Container: 25

	Amount Per Serving	% DV
Vinpocetine (from Periwinkle seed extract)	10 mg	*

*Daily Value not established.

Other Ingredients: Lactose, hydroxypropylcellulose, magnesium stearate and talc.

> *** These statements have not been evaluated by the Food & Drug Administration. This product is not intended to diagnose, treat, cure, or prevent any disease.**

Distributed by: The Memory Secret, Inc.
1221 Brickell Ave., Suite 1540, Miami, FL 33131/USA
memorysecret™
www.memorysecret.net
www.intelectol.com
Shown in Product Identification Guide, page 504

UNKNOWN DRUG?
Consult the
Product Identification Guide
(Gray Pages)
for full-color photos of
leading over-the-counter
medications

Mission Pharmacal Company

10999 IH 10 WEST, SUITE 1000
SAN ANTONIO, TX 78230-1355

Direct Inquiries to:
P.O. Box 786099
San Antonio, TX 78278-6099
(800) 292-7364; (210) 696-8400

CALCET® TRIPLE CALCIUM + VITAMIN D
Dietary Supplement

Description: For low-calcium Leg cramps* and to help reduce the risk of osteoporosis.
*The unique triple calcium formula found in Calcet is recommended by doctors and pharmacists for the relief of leg cramps in pregnancy, leg cramps in athletes and occasional leg cramps people get at night. Calcet is ideal if you need additional calcium to help fight osteoporosis or because of a milk allergy. Regular exercise and a healthy diet with enough calcium helps teens and young adult white and Asian women maintain good bone health and may reduce their high risk of osteoporosis later in life. Adequate calcium intake is important, but daily intakes above about 2,000 mg are not likely to provide any additional benefit.

*These statements have not been evaluated by the Food and Drug Administration. This product is not intended to diagnose, treat, cure or prevent any disease.

Supplement Facts

Serving Size: 2 tablets

	Amount Per Serving	% Daily Value
Vitamin D₃ (as cholecalciferol)	200 IU	50%
Calcium (as calcium carbonate, calcium gluconate, calcium lactate)	300 mg	30%

Ingredients: Calcium carbonate, calcium gluconate, calcium lactate, polyethylene glycol, hydroxypropyl methylcellulose, croscarmellose sodium, color added, magnesium stearate, FD & C Yellow 5 lake, magnesium silicate, vitamin D₃.

Directions for Use: Take two tablets at bedtime and two tablets upon waking. Do not exceed 4 tablets a day except on the advice or recommendation of your physician, pharmacist or health professional.

Warnings: KEEP THIS PRODUCT OUT OF THE REACH OF CHILDREN.

Continued on next page

Calcet—Cont.

How Supplied: 100 coated tablets, UPC 0178-0251-01.
STORE AT ROOM TEMPERATURE.

NOSMO Co., Ltd.

8414 DONG-EUI INSTITUTE OF TECHNOLOGY, SAN72 YANGJUNG-DONG, BUSANJIN-GU, BUSAN SOUTH KOREA

Direct Inquiries to:
Tel: 82-51-851-7688
www.nosmo.co.kr

NOSMO[KING]®
(Stop Smoking Aid)

DESCRIPTION
NOSMO[KING]® is a stop-smoking aid made from medicinal herbs showing high antioxidant activities. NOSMO[KING]® can scavenge reactive oxygen species generated from cigarette smoking, the major causes of aging and diseases, and decompose nicotine efficiently. The advantages of this tablet type NOSMO[KING]® are on the greatly reducing effects of smoking withdrawal symptoms which are major causes hampering stop-smoking. The principle of NOSMO[KING]® is accelerating nicotine metabolism and excreting it in urine rapidly to relieve nicotine-addiction. NOSMO[KING]® is a unique natural product supplement, which is intended to provide an alternative to the health risks of continued smoking of tobacco. NOSMO[KING]® contains many natural ingredients and is not pharmaceutical in nature, thereby giving it the added advantage of being safe to use as in any smoking cessation application, but provides a sense of well being and lessens the dependency on the need to smoke when taken as directed. The active ingredient of NOSMO[KING]® is NPL-X, which is made of eleven kinds of medicinal herbs such as *Ligusticum tenuissimum*, *Platycodon grandiflorum*, *Raphani sativus*, *Crataegus pinnatifida*, *Aloe arborescens*, *Acathopanax sessiliflorus*, *Polygonum multiflorum*, *Arctium lappa*, *Glycyrrhiza uralensis*, *Eugenia aromaticum*, and *Citrus reticulata*.
Drug Facts:
ACTIVE INGREDIENT
(in each tablet)   *Purpose*
NPL-X 750.0mg .... smoking deterrent
(Ligusticum tenuissimum 15.0mg, Platycodon grandiflorum 37.5mg, Raphani sativus 30.0mg, Crataegus pinnatifida 15.0mg, Aloe arborescens 202.5mg, Acathopanax sessiliflorus 15.0mg, Polygonum multiflorum 18.75mg, Arctium lappa 150.0mg, Glycyrrhiza uralensis 172.5mg, Eugenia aromaticum 18.75mg, Citrus reticulata 75.0mg)
EFFECT
Smoking Deterrent, Stop Smoking Aid, Remove Nicotine, Restrain withdrawal symptoms

WARNINGS
Allergy: There are very few associated risks with NOSMO[KING]®, as there may be with other similar systems. The only known risk to the end user of NOSMO[KING]® is the very unlikely occurrence of an allergic reaction. In the event that there is an allergic reaction, the reaction will be very mild due to the nature of the ingredients and is easily remedied by stopping use.
Recovering phenomenon: You may experience Recovering phenomenon such as dizziness and diarrhea within the first week of taking this product. These minor reactions usually resolve in a few days. This is one of the symptoms that show a turn for the better, which means a transient phenomenon in the process of constitution improvement, so it is different from side effects.
Rejection symptoms: If you continue to smoke while taking NOSMO[KING]®, you may feel Rejection symptoms with respect to smoking such as dizziness, headache, and vomiting. Therefore, you had better not continue to smoke while taking NOSMO[KING]®.
Do not use with other prescription medicine: Inform your healthcare professional if you have or have had kidney or heart disease or if you are taking any prescription medicine.
Do not take if you are pregnant or breast feeding.

DIRECTIONS
- take a tablet four times a day for 4-5 weeks
- after a meal, or upon feeling the urge to smoke, take NOSMO[KING] with water
- start the very first medication in the evening after dinner
OTHER INFORMATION
- avoid exposing the product directly to sunlight, high temperatures and humidity
- keep in a cool place
- keep out of reach of children
INACTIVE INGREDIENTS
Vitamin A, Vitamin C, Vitamin E, Magnesium Stearate, Magnesium aluminum metasilicate, Flavor.

HOW SUPPLIED
In packs of 2 BLISTER packs (NDC #34605-1001-1) each pack contains 10 oblong shaped NOSMO[KING]® tablets, each containing 750mg NPL-X
NOSMO Co., Ltd.
#8414 Dong-eui Institute of Technology, San72
Yangjung-dong, Busanjin-gu, Busan, SOUTH KOREA
82-51-851-7688 www.nosmo.co.kr
These statements have not been evaluated by the Food & Drug Administration. This product is not intended to diagnose, treat, cure or prevent any disease.

Procter & Gamble
P.O. BOX 559
CINCINNATI, OH 45201

Direct Inquiries to:
Consumer Relations
(800) 832-3064

ALIGN DAILY PROBIOTIC SUPPLEMENT

Description: Align contains Bifantis (*Bifidobacterium infantis* 35624), a purified strain of healthy (probiotic) bacteria. Align is a daily dietary supplement that works naturally to help build and maintain a healthy, balanced digestive system. Align comes as an easy-to-swallow capsule that, when taken just once a day, every day, provides a natural defense against episodic constipation, diarrhea, urgency, gas, and bloating. Each capsule of Align contains 1×10^9 (one billion) live bacteria when manufactured, and continues to provide an effective level until at least the "best by" date. Align capsules are calorie-free, and contain no artificial sweeteners, gluten or lactose. Align with Bifantis is clinically proven and is recommended by some of the world's leading gastroenterologists.

Uses: Align Daily Probiotic Supplement helps build and maintain a strong and healthy digestive system. Align may be especially helpful for people who desire a natural defense against episodes of digestive upsets such as constipation, diarrhea, urgency, gas and bloating. Taking Align daily can help restore the natural balance of healthy bacteria in the digestive system.

Warnings: Keep out of reach of children. In case of accidental ingestion, contact your doctor or contact a Poison Control Center.

Directions: Take one capsule daily. Keep capsules in original packaging for best results. Store at room temperature.

How Supplied: 28 capsules.

Other ingredients: microcystalline cellulose, hydroxypropylmethylcellulose capsule USP grade, magnesium stearate, sugar, sodium caseinate, sodium citrate dihydrate, propyl gallate, FD&C blue #2. Align contains milk and soy ingredients. Align is lactose free.
Questions? 1-800-208-0112 or AlignGI.com
Shown in Product Identification Guide, page 504

METAMUCIL® DIETARY FIBER SUPPLEMENT
[*met uh-mū sil*]
(psyllium husk)
Also see Metamucil Fiber Laxative in Nonprescription Drugs section

Description: Metamucil contains psyllium husk (from the plant *Plantago*

Metamucil Dietary Fiber Supplements

Versions/Flavors	Ingredients (alphabetical order)	Sodium mg/dose	Calcium mg/dose	Potas-sium mg/dose	Calories kcal/dose	Total Carbo-hydrate g/dose	Dietary Fiber/ (Soluble) g/dose	Serving (Weight in gms)	How Supplied
Capsules plus Calcium	Psyllium husk, Calcium carbonate, Geltain, Crosprovidone, Titanium dioxide, Polysorbate 80, Caramel color, Red 40 Lake, Blue 1 Lake, Yellow 6 Lake	0	300	30	10	12	3 (2.4)	5 capsules (2.6)	Bottles: 75 ct, 120 ct, 150 ct.
Smooth Texture Orange Flavor Metamucil Powder	Citric Acid, FD&C Yellow #6, Natural and Artificial Flavor, Psyllium Husk, Sucrose	5	7	30	45	12	3 (2.4)	1 rounded tablespoon ~12g	Canisters: Doses: 48, 72, 114, 188; Cartons: 30 single-dose packets.
Smooth Texture Sugar-Free Orange Flavor Metamucil Powder	Aspartame, Citric Acid, FD&C Yellow #6, Maltodextrin, Natural and Artificial Flavor, Psyllium Husk	5	7	30	20	5	3 (2.4)	1 rounded teaspoon ~5.8g	Canisters: Doses: 30, 48, 72, 114, 180, 220; Cartons: 30 single-dose packets.
Smooth Texture Sugar-Free Unflavored Metamucil Powder	Citric Acid, Maltodextrin, Psyllium Husk	4	7	30	20	5	3 (2.4)	1 rounded teaspoon ~5.4g	Canisters: Doses: 48, 72 114.
Smooth Texture Sugar-Free Berry Bust	Psyllium Husk, Maltodextrin, Natural And Artificial Flavor, Citric Acid, Malic Acid, Acesulfame Potassium, Aspartame, FD&C Red No. 40, FD&C Blue No. 1	5	7	30	20	5	3 (2)	1 rounded teaspoon (5.8g)	Canisters: 48, 72, 114.
Coarse Milled Unflavored Metamucil Powder	Psyllium Husk, Sucrose	3	6	30	25	7	3 (2.4)	1 rounded teaspoon ~7g	Canisters: Doses: 48, 72 114.
Coarse Milled Orange Flavor Metamucil Powder	Citric Acid, FD&C Yellow #6, Natural and Artificial Flavor, Psyllium Husk, Sucrose	5	6	30	40	11	3 (2.4)	1 rounded tablespoon ~11g	Canisters: Doses: 48,72 114.
Metamucil Capsules	Caramel color, FD&C Blue No. 1 Aluminum Lake, FD&C Red No. 40 Aluminum Lake, FD&C Yellow No. 6 Aluminum Lake, gelatin, polysorbate 80, psyllium husk	0	5	30	10	3	3 (2.4)	6 capsules 3.2g	Bottles: 100 ct, 160 ct, 300 ct
Wafers **Apple** Metamucil Wafers	(1)	20	14	60	120	17	6	2 wafers 24 g	Cartons: 12 doses
Cinnamon Metamucil Wafers	(2)	20	14	60	120	17	6	2 wafers 24 g	Cartons: 12 doses

(1) ascorbic acid, brown sugar, cinnamon, corn oil, corn starch, fructose, lecithin, molasses, natural and artificial flavors, oat hull fiber, psyllium husk, sodium bicarbonate, sucrose, water, wheat flour

(2) ascorbic acid, cinnamon, corn oil, corn starch, fructose, lecithin, molasses, natural and artificial flavors, nutmeg, oat hull fiber, oats, psyllium husk, sodium bicarbonate, sucrose, water, wheat flour

Continued on next page

Metamucil—Cont.

ovata), a concentrated source of soluble fiber which can be used to increase one's dietary fiber intake. When used as part of a diet low in saturated fat and cholesterol, 7g per day of soluble fiber from psyllium husk (the amount in 3 doses of Metamucil) may reduce the risk of heart disease by lowering cholesterol. Each dose of Metamucil powder and Metamucil Fiber Wafers contains approximately 3.4 grams of psyllium husk (or 2.4 grams of soluble fiber). A listing of ingredients and nutrition information is available in the listing of Metamucil Fiber Laxative in the Nonprescription Drug section. Metamucil Smooth Texture Sugar-Free Unflavored, Metamucil capsules and Metamucil plus Calcium capsules contains no sugar and no artificial sweeteners. Metamucil Plus Calcium Capsules also helps build strong bones. Metamucil Smooth Texture Sugar-Free Orange Flavor and Berry Burst Flavor contains aspartame (phenylalanine content of 25 mg and 16 mg per dose respectively). Metamucil powdered products are gluten-free.
[See table on previous page]

Uses: Metamucil Dietary Fiber Supplement can be used as a concentrated source of soluble fiber to increase the dietary intake of fiber. Diets low in saturated fat and cholesterol that include 7 grams of soluble fiber per day from psyllium husk, as in Metamucil, may reduce the risk of heart disease by lowering cholesterol. One adult dose of Metamucil has 2.4 grams of this soluble fiber. Consult a doctor if you are considering use of this product as part of a cholesterol-lowering program.

Warnings: Read entire Drug Facts section in listing for Metamucil Fiber Laxative in the Nonprescription Drug section.

Directions: Adults 12 yrs. & older: 1 dose in 8 oz of liquid 3 *times daily*.
Capsules: 2–6 capsules for increasing daily fiber intake; 6 capsules for cholesterol lowering use. Up to three times daily. Under 12 yrs.: Consult a doctor. See mixing directions in Drug Facts in listing for Metamucil Fiber Laxative in the Nonprescription Drug section.
NOTICE: Mix this product with at least 8 oz (a full glass) of liquid. Taking without enough liquid may cause choking. Do not take if you have difficulty swallowing.
Capsules plus Calcium: 2–5 capsules as an easy way to increase daily fiber and calcium intake. May be taken up to 4 times daily. Under 12 yrs: Consult a doctor.
Fibersure: Stir 1 heaping teaspoon briskly in 8 oz or more water or other beverages. Product dissolves best in room temperature or warmer liquid. Not recommended for carbonated beverages. Add desired amount directly to foods as you prepare them. For best results use in moist foods or recipes.
For listing of ingredients and nutritional information for Metamucil Di-etary Fiber Supplement, and for laxative indications and directions for use, see Metamucil Fiber Laxative in the Nonprescription Drug section.
Notice to Health Care Professionals: To minimize the potential for allergic reaction, health care professionals who frequently dispense powdered psyllium products should avoid inhaling airborne dust while dispensing these products.
Handling and Dispensing: To minimize generating airborne dust, spoon product from the canister into a glass according to label directions.

How Supplied: Powder: canisters and cartons of single-dose packets. Capsules: 100 and 160 count bottles. For complete ingredients and sizes for each version, see Metamucil Table 1, page 718, Nonprescription Drug section.
Questions? 1-800-983-4237
Shown in Product Identification Guide, page 504

Statacor Biosciences
**133 ROLLINS AVENUE
ROCKVILLE, MD 20852**

1-888-782-8226

OMEGA 3–10®
[ō-mā-gǎ]
High Potency Omega-3 Fish Oil *plus* Coenzyme Q10

Description: Omega 3-10® is a high potency Omega-3 Fish Oil plus Coenzyme Q10 cardiovascular nutritional supplement.
Research has shown that omega-3 fatty acids: decrease risk of arrhythmias, which can lead to sudden cardiac death; decrease growth rate of atherosclerotic plaque; decrease triglyceride levels; and slightly lower blood pressure. Randomized clinical trials have shown that omega-3 supplements can reduce cardiovascular events (death, non-fatal heart attacks, non-fatal strokes).
Coenzyme Q10 (CoQ10) is a potent lipophilic antioxidant that is essential for the production of ATP in the mitochondria. CoQ10 and ATP levels have been shown to decrease during statin therapy as a pleiotropic side effect; this may result in varying degrees of fatigue, muscle weakness, and elevated transaminase (liver enzyme) levels. CoQ10 supplementation has been shown to replenish ATP levels during statin therapy without interfering with the cholesterol lowering benefits of statins.
Origin: Omega 3–10® is manufactured in the USA.

Directions: As a dietary supplement, take two capsules once a day.
Ingredients: Marine lipid concentrate, Gelatin, Glycerin, Coenzyme-Q10, Purified Water, Yellow Beeswax, Silica, Annatto, Lecithin, Zinc Oxide, Hypromellose Phthalate-NF, Polyethylene Glycol-NF.

How Supplied: 30-day calendar pack contains 60 softgels, 31-day calendar pack contains 62 softgels.
These statements have not been evaluated by the Food & Drug Administration. This product is not intended to diagnose, treat, cure or prevent any disease.

Tahitian Noni International
**333 WEST RIVER PARK DRIVE
PROVO, UT 84604 USA**

Direct Inquiries to:
Phone: (801) 234-1000
Website: http://www.tahitiannoni.com

TAHITIAN NONI® Leaf Serum
TAHITIAN NONI® Leaf Serum Soothing Gel

Description: In an exclusive process known only to Tahitian Noni International, we've extracted the juice of the long-treasured noni leaf and made it into a soothing balm. Especially for skin that's been exposed to the elements, this serum will condition and revitalize irritated, wind-chaffed, or sunburned skin with lasting relief.

Ingredients: TAHITIAN NONI® Exclusive Noni Leaf Formula [Purified Water, *Morinda citrifolia* (Noni) Leaf Juice, *Morinda citrifolia* (Noni) Leaf Extract, *Vanilla tahitensis* (Tahitian Vanilla) Fruit Extract], Pentylene Glycol, Propylene Glycol, SD Alcohol 40-B, PEG-400 Laurate and Laureth-4, Sodium Dehydroacetate, Disodium EDTA, Phenoxyethanol, Fragrance, Acrylates/C10-30 Alkyl Acrylate Crosspolymer, Potassium Hydroxide.

Suggested Use: Smooth over irritated skin as needed.

Storage: Keep tightly closed in a dry place; do not expose to excessive heat.

How Supplied:
1, 3 and 6 packs of cream, 1 oz/30 ml Packaged for Tahitian Noni International, a subsidiary of Morinda, Inc. Provo, UT 84604. USA.

References
Su C, Palu 'AK et al., TNI Patent Pending.
A noni leaf ethanolic extract demonstrated significant wound healing effects in the mouse cutaneous assay by doubling the wound closure rate with 5.4 CT_{50}.
Nayak BS et al., Evaluation of the wound-healing activity of ethanolic extract of *Morinda citrifolia* L. leaf. *eCAM* 2007, 1–6.

The ethanolic extract from the noni leaf significantly enhanced wound contraction, decreased epithilialization time, and increased hydorxyproline suggesting that noni leaf extract has wound healing effects.

Su C, Palu 'AK et al., TNI Patent Pending

Noni leaf extracts and noni leaf juice inhibited the proliferation of a human epidermoid carcinoma cell line, A431, with an IC_{50} 76 ug/mL and 0.2% respectively.

Mannetje L. *Morinda citrifolia* L. in: Plant-Resources of South-East Asia (Edit.: E. Westphal, P. and C. M. Jansen). Pudoc Wageningen 1989, p. 185–187.

A noni leaf preparation is used as a tonic and antiseptic. Leaves are placed directly on wounds and the leaf juice produces pain-killing effects.

Saludes JP et al., Antitubercular consituents from the hexane fraction of *Morinda citrifolia* Linn. (Rubiaceae). Phytother. Res. 2002. (16): 683–685

Ethanol and hexane fractions from *Morinda citrifolia* leaf showed antitubercular activity by killing 89% of the bacteria *in vitro*, comparable to 97% kill by the anti-TB drug Rifampicin at the same concentration.

Zin ZM et al., Antioxidant activities of chromatographic fractions obtained from roots, fruit and leave of Mengkudu (*Morinda citrifolia* L.). Food Chemistry 2006. 94: 169–178.

Methanol fractions from defatted noni leaf juice showed strong antioxidant activities comparable to that of alpha-tocopherol.

---

* This statement has not been evaluated by the Food and Drug Administration. This product is not intended to diagnose, treat, cure or prevent any disease

---

Shown in Product Identification Guide, page 504

TAHITIAN NONI® LIQUID DIETARY SUPPLEMENT

Description: TAHITIAN NONI® Juice has a heritage, a pedigree that distinguishes it from every other product on the market. This pedigree extends back 2,000 years to the people who used the noni fruit for its benefits. The countless benefits of this unique fruit can only be enjoyed if the fruit is revealed in its most pure form. Our proprietary formulation captures this precisely. It's no wonder that TAHITIAN NONI Juice touches the lives of millions worldwide. You'll find 2,000 years of goodness in every bottle of TAHITIAN NONI Juice! Always look for the TAHITIAN NONI Juice Footprint: Your only assurance of quality, purity, and authenticity.

Supplement Facts

Serving Size: 1 fluid ounce (30 ml)

Servings Per Container 33

Amount Per Serving	%Daily Value*
Calories 13	
Total Carbohydrate 3g	1%
Surgars 2g	†

*Percent Daily Values are based on a 2,000 calorie diet.
† Daily Value not established.

Ingredients: Reconstituted *Morinda citrifolia* fruit juice from pure juice puree from French Polynesia, natural grape juice concentrate, natural blueberry juice concentrate, and natural flavors. Not made from dried or powdered *Morinda citrifolia*.

How Supplied: 1 FL. OZ./30 mL daily. Preferably before meals
Shake well before using and refrigerate after opening
Do not use if seal around cap is broken
Packaged by Tahitian Noni International, a subsidiary of Morinda, Inc. Provo, UT 84604. USA.

References
A single centre, double-blind, three dose level, parallel group, and placebo controlled safety study with TAHITIAN NONI® Juice in healthy subjects. Mugglestone et al., BIBRA International LtD, Clinical Studies Department. Woodmansterne Road, Carshalton UK. 2003
Drinking up to 750 ml TAHITIAN NONI® Juice per day found to be safe in a human clinical safety study involving 96 subjects.
***Morinda citrifolia* L., Noni has Cholesterol Lowering Potential. Palu et al., The 47th Annual Meeting of Society for Economic Botany. Chiang Mai, Thailand June 5–9, 2006.**
Bioassay showed TAHITIAN NONI® Juice (TNJ) inhibited HMG-CoA Reductase, an enzyme involved in human cholesterol biosynthesis by 50, 81 and 83%, respectively. This might explain how TNJ lowers cholesterol in smokers. Smokers drinking 4 ounces of TAHITIAN NONI® Juice daily for 4 weeks in a double blind placebo control clinical trial showed a decrease in averages of cholesterol from 235.2/dL to 190.2 mg/dL and triglycerides from 242.5 mg/dL to 193.5 mg/dL. **Wang et al., American Heart Association 46th Annual Conference on Cardiovascular Disease Epidemiology and Prevention Meeting Report. Phoenix, Ariz., March 2 2006.**
Noni modulates the immune system. Palu et al., J Ethnopharmacol. 2008, 115: 502–506.
TAHITIAN NONI® Juice was shown to modulate the immune system via a mechanism that suppresses IL-4, increases IFNγ, and activates CB_2 receptors.
***Morinda citrifolia* L. Noni: An angiotensin converting enzyme inhibitor. Palu et**

al., **The 232nd ACS National Meeting, San Francisco, CA, Sept. 10–14, 2006.**
TAHITIAN NONI® Juice inhibited ACE enzymes and blocked AT_1 and AT_2 receptors concentration-dependently. A pilot clinical study of 10 hypertensive subjects showed consuming 4 ounces of TNJ a day for 1 month lowered blood pressure from averages of 144/83 (pre-test) to 132/76 (post-test).
TAHITIAN NONI® Juice increases energy, combat fatigue, and improve endurance. Palu et al., CPAM, 2006. Ma et al., 2007, 21: 1100–1101.
TNJ was shown to inhibit PDE-3 enzymes which involves in processes leading to increases in energy. TNJ was shown in mice to increase their energy levels by 36–45%, and endurance by 59–128% compared to control.
TAHITIAN NONI® Juice Does Not Contain Athletic Banned Substances. http://www.consumerlab.com/bannedsub.asp
Analysis of TNJ revealed the absence of all performance-enhancing substances banned by the World Anti Doping Association.
Noni Juice Protect the Liver. West et al., Eur J Gastroenterol Hepatol. 2006 May; 18(5):575–7
Published safety data show that noni juice is not toxic to the liver. Studies demonstrate TNJ protects the liver in a CCl_4 model.
TAHITIAN NONI® Juice Is Safe for Human Consumption. The EFSA Journal 2006, 376: 1–12.
The European Food Safety Authority reports, "it is unlikely that consumption of noni juice, at the observed levels of intake, induces adverse human liver effects."
TAHITIAN NONI® Juice Not a Significant Source of Potassium.
A case report stated that the potassium content of noni juice was 56.3 mEq/L, or 65 mg/ounce, and may be a "surreptitious" source of potassium for patients with renal disease. **(Mueller et al. Am J. Kidney Dis. 2000 35: 330–2).** Mueller **USA Today, March 28, 2000)** clarified his research, stating he did not analyze TAHITIAN NONI® Juice, but rather a different brand of noni juice and that the amount of potassium was only "as much as you'd get in 2 inches of banana."
Quantitative ICP Mineral Analysis of TAHITIAN NONI® Juice. Tolson et al., Tahitian Noni International Research Center. American Fork, Utah. USA 84003. Internal Data.
Potassium content of TAHITIAN NONI® Juice is 40 mg per 1 ounce serving. Compared to Grape juice* 42 mg per 1 ounce serving, Banana* 102 mg per 1 ounce serving and Yogurt* 66 mg per 1 ounce.
Not all Liquid Dietary Supplements Are Created Equal. Palu 'AK et al., Am J Hematol 2005 79: 79–82.
TAHITIAN NONI® Juice does not contain any significant quantity of vitamin

Continued on next page

Tahitian Noni Liquid—Cont.

K. A case of coumadin resistance was reported in a patient drinking juice from the "Noni Juice 4 Everything" brand, which is fortified with vitamin K (**Carr ME et al., Coumadin Resistance and the Vitamin Supplement "Noni." Am J Hematol 2004 77:103–4**). This case of coumadin resistance is due to vitamin K and does not apply to the TAHITIAN NONI® Juice Brand.

* Source: USDA Nutrient Database for Standard Reference.

This statement has not been evaluated by the Food and Drug Administration.
This product is not intended to diagnose, treat, cure or prevent any disease

Shown in Product Identification Guide, page 504

TAHITIAN NONI® Seed Oil

Product Information
This exclusive oil delivers intense moisture and relief to dry or distressed skin. It is designed to help improve skin health issues that come from within.
The first and only essential oil derived from noni seeds. High in linoleic acid, a powerful ally in skin hydration and cellular health.
This world exclusive light oil delivers intense healing moisture and relief to rough, distressed skin. It takes over 50,000 seeds to make just one ounce of this rare and precious oil. Absorbs easily into skin.

Product Benefits
• Hydrates and softens skin to hasten the healing process of distressed skin
• Protects with valuable antioxidants
• An essential building block for healthy looking skin
• High in linoleic acid which helps relieve dry, flaky, or rough skin and helps maintain smooth, moist skin
• Won't clog pores

Featured Ingredients
Pure Noni Seed Oil
Hydrates and softens while protecting skin with valuable antioxidants
Recommended Use
Gently apply a small amount of Noni Seed Oil to distressed skin anywhere healing moisture can be beneficial.

How Supplied:
33 FL oz (10 ml) bottle
Packaged for Tahitian Noni International, a subsidiary of Morinda, Inc. Provo, UT 84604. USA.

References
West BJ, Palu 'AK, Jensen CJ. Noni Seed Oil Analysis. TNI Patent Pending. Noni seed oil analysis reveal that it has natural phytosterols, vitamin E and a significant source of omega-6 fatty acid, an essential fatty acid.
Palu 'AK, Zhou BN, West BJ et al. TNI Patent Pending. Noni seed oil can reduce pain and inflammation due to its selective, and significant inhibitions of COX-2 over 5-LOX enzymes.
Douglas M. Rope, M.D. Midwest Clinical Trials. A study to Asses the Comedogenicity of a Test Product When Applied-Topically to the Skin of Healthy Human Subjects 2004.
Noni seed oil significantly reduced the number of closed comedones (white heads) on the skin of 26 teenage volunteers during a clinical trial.

* Source: USDA Nutrient Database for Standard Reference.

This statement has not been evaluated by the Food and Drug Administration.
This product is not intended to diagnose, treat, cure or prevent any disease.

Shown in Product Identification Guide, page 504

UAS Laboratories
9953 VALLEY VIEW ROAD
EDEN PRAIRIE, MN 55344

Direct Inquiries to:
Dr. S.K. Dash
(952) 935-1707
FAX: (952) 935-1650

DDS®-ACIDOPHILUS
Capsule, Tablet & Powder
free of dairy products, corn, soy, and preservatives

Description: DDS®-Acidophilus is the source of a special strain of Lactobacillus acidophilus free of dairy products, corn, soy and preservatives. Each capsule or tablet contains 2.5 billion viable DDS®-1 L.acidophilus at the time of manufacturing. One gram of powder contains 5 billion viable DDS®-1 L.acidophilus.

Indications and Usages: An aid in implanting the gut with beneficial Lactobacillus acidophilus under conditions of digestive disorders, acne, yeast infections, and following antibiotic therapy.

Administration: One to two capsules or tablets twice daily before meals. One-fourth teaspoon powder can be substituted for two capsules or tablets.

How Supplied: Bottles of 100 capsules or tablets. 12 bottles per case. Powder is available in 2.5 oz. bottle; 12 bottles per case.

Storage: Keep refrigerated under 40°F.

EDUCATIONAL MATERIAL

DDS®-Acidophilus
Booklet describing superior-strain Acidophilus without dairy products, corn, soy, or preservatives. Five billion viable DDS®-1. L.acidopohilus per gram.

Wellness International Network, Ltd.®
5800 DEMOCRACY DRIVE
PLANO, TX 75024

Direct Inquiries to:
Product Inquiries
(972) 312-1100
E-mail: winproducts@winltd.com

ACCELERATOR™
Herbal & Amino Acid Formulation

Description: Accelerator™ is a unique blend of herbal extracts and amino acids that, when used in conjunction with BioLean II® or BioLean Free®, prolongs their adaptogenic and thermogenic properties while adding powerful restorative properties. The restorative properties of the amino acids and herbal extracts in Accelerator are a strong complement to the energetic and thermogenic properties of BioLean II and BioLean Free. When used together, these products provide a well-balanced approach to weight loss, increased energy and detoxification.

Directions: Accelerator was specifically designed to be used in conjunction with the other products in the BioLean System. Adults take one tablet in the morning with BioLean II or BioLean Free. Accelerator may also be taken in the afternoon with or without additional BioLean II or BioLean Free if desired. As with the other two supplements, maximum absorption will be attained if taken with low calorie food.
CAUTION PHENYLKETONURICS: Contains 200 mg phenylalanine per serving.
Not for use by children. Consult your physician before using this product if you are taking appetite suppressing drugs or antidepressants or if you are pregnant or lactating. If symptoms of allergy develop, discontinue use.

Ingredients: Proprietary herbal extract 250mg (Cuscuta Seed, Black Sesame Seed, Rehmannia Root, Achyranthes Root, Cornus Fruit, Chinese Yam, Eclipta Herb, Rosehips, Ligustrum Fruit, Mulberry Fruit, Polygonati Rhizome, Fo Ti, Poria Cocos, Euryale Seed, Alisma Rhizome, Moutan Bark, Phellodendron Bark, Anemarrhena Rhizome, Schisandra Berry, Royal Jelly), L-Phenylalanine 200mg, L-Tyrosine 200mg, Calcium

Carbonate, Calcium Phosphate Dibasic, Hydroxypropyl Cellulose, Croscarmelose Sodium, Magnesium Stearate, and Silicon Dioxide.

How Supplied: One bottle contains 56 tablets.

Additional Information: For additional information on ingredients or uses, please visit winltd.com.

These statements have not been evaluated by the Food & Drug Administration. This product is not intended to diagnose, treat, cure or prevent any disease.

BIOLEAN II®
Herbal & Amino Acid Dietary Supplement

Description: BioLean II® is a dietary supplement for weight loss, appetite suppression and increased energy without the side effects found in many supplements of this nature. BioLean II has a proprietary synergistic blend of natural herbal extracts and pharmaceutical-grade amino acids that promote a multifaceted approach to fat loss. Key ingredients such as Advantra Z®, guarana seed extract, green tea leaf extract and L-carnitine work together to increase the metabolic rate and encourage fat loss by elevating rates of thermogenesis and lipolysis. Our weight loss products work in conjunction with a sensible diet and moderate exercise.

Directions: Recommended Use: AM Serving - Take 1 white tablet and 2 green tablets with low calorie food. PM Serving - Take 1 green tablet with low calorie food. If using BioLean II for the first time, limit daily intake to 1 white tablet and 1 green tablet on days 1 and 2, and 1 white tablet and 2 green tablets on day 3. Needs may vary with each individual.

Warnings: CAUTION PHENYLKETONURICS: Contains 196mg phenylalanine per AM serving. Not for use by children under the age of 18, pregnant or lactating women. If you have heart disease, thyroid disease, diabetes, high blood pressure, depression or other psychiatric condition, glaucoma, difficulty urinating, prostate enlargement, seizure disorder, or if you are using a monoamine oxidase inhibitor (MAOI), consult a health professional before using this product. Exceeding recommended serving may cause serious adverse effects. Discontinue use and consult your health professional if dizziness, sleeplessness, severe headache, heart palpitations or other similar symptoms occur. The recommended dose of this product contains about as much caffeine as a cup of coffee. Limit the use of caffeine-containing medications, food, or beverages while taking this product because too much caffeine may cause nervousness, irritability, sleeplessness, and occasionally, rapid heart beat. BioLean II should not be taken on the same day as BioLean Free®.

Ingredients: Calcium (206.76mg per AM serving & 91.88mg per PM serving) (as calcium carbonate, calcium phosphate dibasic), Proprietary Blend (1661.68mg per AM serving & 830.34mg per PM serving): (Caffeine (167mg per AM serving & 83.5mg per PM serving) (as Guarana Seed 50% Extract, Yerba Mate Leaf 10% Extract, Green Tea Leaf 40% Extract), Citrus Aurantium Fruit 30% Extract (Advantra Z®), Schizandra Berry, Gymnema Sylvestre Leaf 25% Extract, Rehmannia Root, Hawthorne Berry Extract, Jujube Seed, Alisma Root, Angelicae dahuricae Radix, Epemidium grandiflorum Radix, Poria Cocos Mushroom, Rhubarb Root, Angelicae sinensis Radix, Codonopsis Root, Eucommia Bark, Panax notoginseng Radix), L-Tyrosine (196mg per AM serving), L-Phenylalanine (196mg per AM serving), L-Carnitine (8mg per AM serving) (as L-Carnitine Bitartrate). Herbal Blend: Calcium Carbonate, Starch, Stearic Acid, Cellulose, Hydroxypropylcellulose, Croscarmellose Sodium, Magnesium Stearate, Silicon Dioxide. Amino Acid: Calcium Phosphate Dibasic, Stearic acid, Silicon Dioxide, Croscarmellose Sodium, Hydroxypropylcellulose, Magnesium Stearate, Ethylcellulose. Advantra Z® - registered trademark of Nutratech, Inc./Zhishin, LLC licensor of U.S. Patents.

How Supplied: 28 Servings per Container. AM Serving Size 2 green tablets, 1 white tablet. PM Serving Size 1 green tablet

Additional Information: For additional information on ingredients or uses, please visit winltd.com.

These statements have not been evaluated by the Food & Drug Administration. This product is not intended to diagnose, treat, cure or prevent any disease.

BIOLEAN FREE®
Herbal & Amino Acid Dietary Supplement

Description: BioLean Free® is a dietary supplement designed to reduce body fat, suppress the appetite, provide a healthy feeling of fullness, and improve metabolism of dietary carbohydrates, fats, and proteins. BioLean Free utilizes a strategic blend of vitamins, minerals, amino acids and herbal extracts that enhance fat utilization and energy production through several metabolic pathways. Key ingredients such as quebracho, green tea leaf extract, yerba maté and spices such as ginger and tumeric work together to promote healthy lipolysis, curb cravings, stimulate thermogenesis and increase energy without disrupting the healthy sleep cycle.

Directions: As a dietary supplement, take 4 tablets in mid- to late-morning with low-calorie food. Some persons may require less than 4 tablets, or may prefer taking 3 tablets mid-morning and 1 additional tablet mid-afternoon to achieve optimum results. Do not exceed recommended daily amounts. Needs may vary with each individual.

Warnings: Not for use by children under the age of 18, pregnant or lactating women. Consult your physician before using this product if you are taking appetite suppressing drugs or cardiovascular medication. Consult your physician if you have hypertension, heart disease, arrhythmias, prostatic hypertrophy, glaucoma, liver disease, renal disease or diabetes. Do not use if you have hyperthyroidism, psychosis, Parkinson's Disease, or are taking monoamine oxidase inhibitors (MAOI). Limit the use of caffeine-containing medications, food, or beverages while taking this product because too much caffeine may cause nervousness, irritability, sleeplessness, and occasionally, rapid heart beat. If allergic symptoms develop, discontinue use immediately. BioLean Free® should not be taken on the same day as BioLean II®.

Ingredients: Niacin 40mg (as niacinamide), Vitamin B6 16mg (as pyridoxine HCL), Chromium 400mcg (as chromium Chelavite® chloride), Potassium 100mg (as potassium citrate), Standardized botanical extracts 2972mg (Caffeine 200mg (as Guarana seed 22%, Yerba mate leaf extract 10%, Green tea leaf extract 10%)), Korean ginseng root extract (4% ginsenosides), Uva ursi leaf (20% arbutin), Quebracho bark extract (10% quebrachine), non-irradiated pure herbs and thermogenic spices 1440mg (Gotu kola leaf (Centella asiatica), Ceylon cinnamon bark, Chinese horseradish root, Jamaican ginger root, Turmeric rhizome, Nigerian cayenne pepper (fruit), English mustard seed, Ho shou wu root, Ginkgo biloba leaf (24% ginkgoflavoneslycosides and 6% bilobalides)), L-Tyrosine 500mg, L-Methionine 100mg, Vanadium 400mcg (as BMOV), Dicalcium phosphate, Cellulose, Cellulose gum, Vegetable stearic acid, Silica, Vegetable magnesium stearate and Vegetable resin glaze.

How Supplied: One box contains 28 packets, 4 tablets per packet.

Additional Information: For additional information on ingredients or uses, please visit winltd.com.

These statements have not been evaluated by the Food & Drug Administration. This product is not intended to diagnose, treat, cure or prevent any disease.

Continued on next page

CLARITY®
Vitamin, Mineral and Amino Acid Supplement

Description: Clarity® contains specific vitamins, minerals, amino acids and nutrients important for memory and concentration. Key ingredients such as lecithin, glutamic acid and ginkgo biloba promote increased brain functioning. These nutrients provide fuel for the brain as well as increased blood flow to the entire central nervous system. These ingredients and their effects ensure that Clarity is a natural and effective way to better one's health.

Directions: Take 1 capsule 3 times daily with meals.

Warnings: CAUTION PHENYLKE-TONURICS: Contains 9.2mg phenylalanine per serving.

Ingredients: Proprietary blend (Lecithin (Soy), Bee Pollen, L-Glutamic Acid, Ribonucleic Acid Yeast, L-Aspartic Acid, L-Arginine HCL, L-Leucine, L-Lysine HCL, L-Phenylalanine, L-Serine, L-Proline, L-Valine, L-Isoleucine, L-Alanine, L-Glycine, L-Threonine, L-Tyrosine, L-Histidine, L-Cysteine HCL, L-Methionine, Adenosine Triphosphate, Ginkgo Biloba 50:1 Extract), Hydroxypropylmethylcellulose, DL-Alpha Tocopheryl Acetate, Ascorbic Acid, Niacinamide, Stearic Acid, Ethylcellulose, Vitamin A Acetate, D-Calcium Pantothenate, Thiamine HCL, Silicon Dioxide, Dicalcium Phosphate, Pyridoxine HCL, Riboflavin, Folic Acid, Cholecalciferol, Biotin, Cyanocobalamin.

How Supplied: One bottle contains 60 easy-to-swallow capsules.

Additional Information: For additional information on ingredients or uses, please visit winltd.com.

These statements have not been evaluated by the Food & Drug Administration. This product is not intended to diagnose, treat, cure or prevent any disease.

DHEA PLUS™
Herbal Supplement

Description: DHEA Plus™ uniquely combines dihydroxyepiandrosterone (DHEA), Bioperine® and ginkgo biloba leaf to safely and effectively provide antioxidants and support the body in a healthy aging process. DHEA, the primary ingredient, is used by the body to manufacture the sex hormones estrogen and testosterone. As DHEA levels decline with age, women produce less estrogen, which is essential for healthy heart function. Additionally, men lose the metabolic boost that testosterone provides and are at increased risk for fat accumulation. Supplemental DHEA can therefore slow this normal hormonal decline. In fact, scientific research has indicated that adequate levels of DHEA in the body can actually slow the normal aging process. A second key ingredient is Bioperine®, which enhances thermogenic activity and can lead to increases in fat mobilization and utilization. To further ward off the forgetfulness associated with the aging process, DHEA Plus includes gingko biloba to augment blood flow throughout the circulatory system and to the brain. Some improvement in cognitive abilities has been noted as well as inhibition of lipid peroxidation, thereby stabilizing the cell wall against free-radical attack.

Directions: Adults take 1 enteric-coated tablet daily with food.

Warnings: Not for use by children under the age of 18, pregnant or lactating women. Consult your physician before using this product if you are taking prescription medications. Persons with a history of prostate cancer should seek medical advice before using this product.

Ingredients: Dihydroxyepiandrosterone 50mg (DHEA), Ginkgo Biloba Leaf 25mg, Bioperine 5mg (Piper Nigrum L.), Calcium Phosphate Dibasic, Partially Hydrogenated Vegetable Oil, (cotton seed), Starch, Magnesium Stearate, Silicon Dioxide and Croscarmellose Sodium.

Bioperine is a registered trademark of Sabinsa Corporation.

How Supplied: One bottle contains 60 enteric-coated tablets.

Additional Information: For additional information on ingredients or uses, please visit winltd.com.

These statements have not been evaluated by the Food & Drug Administration. This product is not intended to diagnose, treat, cure or prevent any disease.

ELASTICITY®
Vitamin, Mineral and Amino Acid Supplement

Description: Elasticity® contains a scientifically balanced mixture of specific amino acids and nutrients important for skin tone and texture. Vitamin A and selenium, 2 key ingredients known for their antioxidant properties, help maintain the skin's youthful appearance and provide internal protection against the effects of sun exposure on the skin.

Directions: Take 1 capsule 3 times daily with meals.

Warnings: CAUTION: PHENYLKE-TONURICS: Contains 9.2mg phenylalanine per serving. Accidental overdose of iron-containing products is a leading cause of fatal poisoning in children under 6. Keep this product out of reach of children. In case of accidental overdose, call a doctor or poison control center immediately.

Ingredients: Proprietary Blend (Shavegrass Herb, L-Glutamic Acid, Bladderwrack Extract, Ribonucleic Acid Yeast, L-Aspartic Acid, L-Arginine HCL, L-Leucine, L-Lysine HCL, L-Phenylalanine, L-Serine, L-Proline, L-Valine, L-Isoleucine, L-Alanine, L-Glycine, L-Threonine, L-Tyrosine, L-Histidine, L-Cysteine HCL, L-Methionine, Adenosine Triphosphate), Hydroxypropylmethylcellulose, DL-Alpha Tocopheryl Acetate, Ascorbic Acid, Ethylcellulose, Stearic Acid, Silicon Dioxide, Calcium Amino Acid Chelate, Manganese Amino Acid Chelate, Iron Amino Acid Chelate, Magnesium Amino Acid Chelate, Zinc Amino Acid Chelate, Vitamin A Acetate, Selenium Amino Acid Chelate, Chromium Amino Acid Chelate.

How Supplied: One bottle contains 60 easy-to-swallow capsules.

Additional Information: For additional information on ingredients or uses, please visit winltd.com.

These statements have not been evaluated by the Food & Drug Administration. This product is not intended to diagnose, treat, cure or prevent any disease.

ELIXIR®
Vitamin, Mineral and Amino Acid Supplement

Description: Elixir® is formulated with an exclusive blend of vitamins, minerals and amino acids that provide an overall feeling of well-being and are an important component for healthy living. Key ingredients such as vitamin E and the amino acid cysteine have shown to protect the body from the effects of aging with their powerful antioxidant properties. These antioxidants help protect cells by preventing the damaging effects of free-radicals. Additionally, cysteine is an important component in assisting the body's normal detoxification process.

Directions: Take 1 capsule 3 times daily with meals.

Warnings: CAUTION PHENYLKE-TONURICS: Contains 6.9mg phenylalanine per serving. Accidental overdose of iron-containing products is a leading cause of fatal poisoning in children under 6. Keep this product out of reach of children. In case of accidental overdose, call a doctor or poison control center immediately.

Ingredients: Proprietary Blend (Isolated Soy Protein (Soy), Bee Pollen, Citric Acid, Malic Acid, Ribonucleic Acid Yeast, Ginkgo Biloba Leaf Extract, Adenosine Triphosphate), Hydroxypropylmethylcellulose, Zinc Amino Acid Chelate, Iron Amino Acid Chelate, DL-Alpha Tocopheryl Acetate, Starch, Ascorbic Acid, Calcium Carbonate, Niacinamide, D-Calcium Pantothenate, Vitamin A Acetate, Silicon Dioxide, Thiamine HCL, Dicalcium Phosphate, Pyridoxine HCL, Riboflavin, Folic Acid, Selenium Amino Acid Chelate, Cholecalciferol, Biotin, Cyanocobalamin.

How Supplied: One bottle contains 60 easy-to-swallow capsules.

Additional Information: For additional information on ingredients or uses, please visit winltd.com.

These statements have not been evaluated by the Food & Drug Administration. This product is not intended to diagnose, treat, cure or prevent any disease.

ESSENTIAL®
Herbal and Amino Acid Supplement

Description: **Essential®** contains specific vitamins, minerals, herbs and amino acids that are proactive to cardiovascular and circulatory management. Two primary ingredients, L-carnitine and vitamin E, provide increased energy utilization in the heart and skeletal muscles as well as protective antioxidant effects, thereby supporting the health of the entire circulatory system. Another key ingredient, linoleic acid, also supports heart health by improving blood flow and healthy cardiovascular levels.

Directions: Take 1 capsule 3 times daily with meals.

Warnings: CAUTION PHENYLKE-TONURICS: Contains 9.2mg phenylalanine per serving.

Ingredients: Proprietary Blend (Isolated Soy Protein (Soy), L-Carnitine Bitartrate, Bee Pollen, marine lipid concentrate (mussel), Ribonucleic Acid Yeast, Adenosine Triphosphate), Hydroxypropylmethylcellulose, Magnesium Amino Acid Chelate, Starch, D-Alpha Tocopheryl Succinate (Soy), Selenium Amino Acid Chelate, Silicon Dioxide.

How Supplied: One bottle contains 60 easy-to-swallow capsules.

Additional Information: For additional information on ingredients or uses, please visit winltd.com.

These statements have not been evaluated by the Food & Drug Administration. This product is not intended to diagnose, treat, cure or prevent any disease.

FEMININE®
Vitamin, Mineral and Amino Acid Supplement

Description: **Feminine®** contains selected vitamins, minerals and amino acids regarded as important to the ever-changing female body. This is achieved through such scientifically researched ingredients as magnesium and boron. Magnesium is important for regulating the flow of calcium between cells and is essential for adequate calcium uptake, which can lead to fewer PMS symptoms such as irritability, depression, headaches, backaches and menstrual cramps. Boron is vital at reducing excretion of both calcium and magnesium. This in turn assists in maintaining healthy bones.

Directions: Take 1 capsule 3 times daily with meals.

Warnings: CAUTION PHENYLKE-TONURICS: Contains 9.2mg phenylalanine per serving.

Ingredients: Proprietary blend (Isolated Soy Protein (soy), Magnesium Oxide, Ribonucleic Acid Yeast, Boron Aspartate, Adenosine Triphosphate), Hydroxypropylmethylcellulose, DL-Alpha Tocopheryl Acetate, Starch, Silicon Dioxide, Selenium Amino Acid Chelate.

How Supplied: One bottle contains 60 easy-to-swallow capsules.

Additional Information: For additional information on ingredients or uses, please visit winltd.com.

These statements have not been evaluated by the Food & Drug Administration. This product is not intended to diagnose, treat, cure or prevent any disease.

FLEXIBILITY®
Vitamin, Mineral and Amino Acid Supplement

Description: **Flexibility®** is rich in vitamins, minerals and amino acids recognized as beneficial to the health of joints and soft tissues. Two important amino acids utilized in Flexibility include glycine and histidine. These amino acids are known to promote neuromuscular control as well as maintain healthy, flexible joints. Boron, another key ingredient, is vital in protecting joints and vitamin E is added to soothe muscle cramps associated with heavy exercise or everyday exertions.

Directions: Take 1 capsule 3 times daily with meals.

Warnings: CAUTION PHENYLKE-TONURICS: Contains 9.2mg phenylalanine per serving.

Ingredients: Proprietary Blend (Boron Gluconate, L-Glutamic Acid, Ribonucleic Acid Yeast, L-Aspartic Acid, L-Arginine HCL, L-Leucine, L-Lysine HCL, Bee Pollen, L-Phenylalanine, L-Serine, L-Proline, L-Valine, L-Isoleucine, L-Alanine, L-Glycine, L-Threonine, L-Tyrosine, L-Histidine, L-Cysteine HCL, L-Methionine, Adenosine Triphosphate), Hydroxypropylmethylcellulose, Zinc Amino Acid Chelate, Calcium Amino Acid Chelate, Stearic Acid, Ascorbic Acid, Whey (Milk), D-Alpha Tocopheryl Succinate (Soy), Magnesium Stearate, Niacinamide, Silicon Dioxide, Cellulose, Vitamin A Palmi-

tate, D-Calcium Pantothenate, Thiamine HCL, Dicalcium Phosphate, Pyridoxine HCL, Riboflavin, Folic Acid, Selenomethionine, Cholecalciferol, Biotin, Cyanocobalamin.

How Supplied: One bottle contains 60 easy-to-swallow capsules.

Additional Information: For additional information on ingredients or uses, please visit winltd.com.

These statements have not been evaluated by the Food & Drug Administration. This product is not intended to diagnose, treat, cure or prevent any disease.

FOOD FOR THOUGHT®
Mental Performance Drink
Vitamin and Amino Acid Supplement

Description: **Food For Thought®**, ideal anytime peak mental performance is needed, contains a proprietary blend of amino acids and choline along with powerful antioxidants and B vitamins that are essential in the production of the acetylcholine, the most abundant neurotransmitter in the body. Adequate acetylcholine is vital because of its role in neuromuscular control and cognitive functioning. This neurotransmitter promotes concentration, good memory, and healthy sleep patterns. Food For Thought further enhances its effectiveness through the utilization of essential vitamins and minerals required for promoting the synthesis of the brain neurotransmitter serotonin, which is crucial for maintaining and regulating normal sleep patterns.

Directions: Add 1 packet of mix to 6 oz. of chilled water or fruit juice. Stir briskly. Consume 1–2 times per day.

Warnings: Not for use by pregnant or lactating women. Persons taking medications should seek medical advice before taking this product. Persons with ulcers or a history of ulcers should consult their physician before using a choline supplement. Do not consume more than four servings per day. Avoid the use of antacids containing aluminum with this product.

Ingredients: Carbohydrates 6g, Sugars 6g, Vitamin C 72mg (as Ascorbic Acid), Vitamin E 30IU (as DL-Alpha Tocopheryl Acetate), Thiamin 2.9mg (as Thiamin Mononitrate), Riboflavin 2.8mg, Niacin 73mg (as Niacinamide), Vitamin B6 4.7mg (as Pyridoxine HCL), Vitamin B12 100mcg (as Cyanocobalamin), Pantothenic Acid 380mg (as Calcium Pantothenate), Calcium 34mg (as Calcium Pantothenate), Zinc 2.9mg (as Zinc Gluconate), Copper 0.4mg (as Copper Gluconate), Chromium 250mcg (as Chromium Aspartate), Choline 770mg (as Choline Bitartrate), Glycine

Continued on next page

Food For Thought—Cont.

130mg, Lysine 35mg (as L-Lysine HCL), Fructose, Natural Flavors, and Silicon Dioxide.

How Supplied: One box contains 28 single serving packets.

Additional Information: For additional information on ingredients or uses, please visit winltd.com.

These statements have not been evaluated by the Food & Drug Administration. This product is not intended to diagnose, treat, cure or prevent any disease.

LIPOTRIM™
Chromium and Herbal Supplement

Description: LipoTrim™ contains 2 dynamic and powerful ingredients that synergistically reduce the storage of new fat and maintain healthy blood glucose levels to assist in weight loss. Garcinia cambogia extract and chromium polynicotinate help reduce the rate of lipogenesis and assist in maintaining healthy blood sugar levels, especially when used in conjunction with either BioLean II® or BioLean Free®. These potent ingredients combine to help discourage accumulation of body fat, as well as to produce an appetite suppressant effect that can contribute to weight loss.

Directions: Take 1 capsule 3 times daily, 30 minutes before each meal. Lipo-Trim should be used in conjunction with a healthy diet and exercise plan.

Warnings: Not for use by children under the age of 18, pregnant or lactating women. Consult your physician before using this product if your diet consists of less than 1,000 calories per day.

Ingredients: Chromium 100mcg (as Chromium Polynicotinate), Garcinia Cambogia Fruit Extract 500mg, Hydroxypropylmethylcellulose, Calcium Sulfate, Starch, and Silicon Dioxide.

How Supplied: One bottle contains 84 easy-to-swallow capsules.

Additional Information: For additional information on ingredients or uses, please visit winltd.com.

These statements have not been evaluated by the Food & Drug Administration. This product is not intended to diagnose, treat, cure or prevent any disease.

LOVPIL™
Vitamin, Herbal and Amino Acid Supplement

Description: Lovpil™ is a nutritional supplement formulated with vitamins, minerals, herbs and amino acids recognized as important for general health and sexual vitality. Damiana, typically thought of as an aphrodisiac by those familiar with its effects, is an important ingredient utilized in Lovpil and is known for its stimulating properties on male virility and libido. Two other key ingredients, arginine and vitamin C, are essential in maintaining healthy sperm counts and protecting sperm from oxidative DNA damage.

Directions: Take 1 capsule 3 times daily with meals.

Ingredients: Proprietary Blend (Damiana Leaf, Isolated Soy Protein (Soy), Ribonucleic Acid Yeast, Adenosine Triphosphate), Calcium Carbonate, Hydroxypropylmethylcellulose, Ascorbic Acid, Stearic Acid, Zinc Amino Acid Chelate, Magnesium Stearate, Manganese Amino Acid Chelate, Silicon Dioxide, Vitamin A Acetate, Dicalcium Phosphate, Cholecalciferol, Folic acid, Selenomethionine, Cyanocobalamin.

How Supplied: One bottle contains 60 easy-to-swallow capsules.

Additional Information: For additional information on ingredients or uses, please visit winltd.com.

These statements have not been evaluated by the Food & Drug Administration. This product is not intended to diagnose, treat, cure or prevent any disease.

MASCULINE®
Mineral, Herbal and Amino Acid Supplement

Description: Masculine® contains a special blend of nutrients with vitamins, minerals, herbs and amino acids shown to be essential for healthy male reproductive systems. Zinc, a key ingredient in Masculine, is important in maintaining healthy testosterone levels. Adequate zinc levels are essential to support the health of the male sex glands, increased sexual interest, mental alertness, emotional stability and a healthy, balanced appetite. In many normal males, zinc supplementation was accompanied by increases in sperm count and plasma testosterone.

Directions: Take 1 capsule 3 times daily with meals.

Ingredients: Proprietary Blend (L-Histidine, Bee Pollen, Parsley Leaf, Ribonucleic Acid, Adenosine Triphosphate), Calcium Carbonate, Zinc Amino Acid Chelate, Hydroxypropylmethylcellulose, Magnesium Amino Acid Chelate, Stearic Acid, Magnesium Stearate.

How Supplied: One bottle contains 60 easy-to-swallow capsules.

Additional Information: For additional information on ingredients or uses, please visit winltd.com.

These statements have not been evaluated by the Food & Drug Administration. This product is not intended to diagnose, treat, cure or prevent any disease.

MASS APPEAL™
Dietary Supplement

Description: Utilizing natural muscle-boosting, **Mass Appeal™** is specifically formulated to enhance athletic performance without side effects. Creatine, the primary ingredient in Mass Appeal, functions as a storage molecule for high-energy phosphate bonds. These high-energy bonds provide greater energy during exercise requiring short periods of intense activity, such as weight lifting, sprinting, and jumping. Creatine causes a "cell volumizing" effect within the muscle by forcing additional water into the muscle cells. This promotes an increase in protein synthesis within the muscle which facilitates growth while slowing down the destructive breakdown of muscle cells that occurs during normal exercise. Mass Appeal also contains the branched chain amino acids (BCAAs) L-leucine, L-valine and L-isoleucine, which also increase protein synthesis and are oxidized inside muscle cells leading to a protein-sparing effect which indirectly increases anabolism by reducing the muscle's need to burn its own proteins during strenuous exercise. Other key ingredients used to protect against muscle catabolism include alpha-ketoglutaric acid and L-glutamine. Inosine, an important compound within Mass Appeal, is known for its role in helping make ATP (adenosine triphosphate), the body's main form of usable energy. Additionally, it may augment oxygen utilization within red blood cells and increase flow of these cells into muscle tissue. Through supplementation, the normal catabolic breakdown of muscle can be minimized and the muscle tissue preserved.

Directions: Adults may take a loading dose of 3 packets in the morning and 2 packets in the late afternoon for one week. This loading dose may be repeated every 3 months. Following 1 week of the loading dose, begin the maintenance dose of 1 packet daily 2 hours after exercise. Needs may vary with each individual. For individuals desiring enhanced effects, increase the loading dose to 3–4 packets, 3 times per day (morning, afternoon and evening). Following 1 week of this enhanced loading dose, begin the enhanced maintenance dose of 2 packets in the morning and 2 packets in the late afternoon. It is recommended that one maintain a low-fat, high-protein diet; drink at least 8 glasses of water per day; and engage in 30-60 minutes of aerobic and anaerobic exercise 3–4 times per week. Phyto-Vite®, ProXtreme™ and Sure2Endure™ may be taken with this product for optimum results.

Warnings: Not for use by children under the age of 18, pregnant or lactating women. Consult your physician before using this product if you have any medical conditions. Do not take if you have kidney disease, muscle disease or are on a protein restricted diet. Discontinue immediately if allergic symptoms develop.

Ingredients: Proprietary Supplement Blend 3250 mg: (Creatine Monohydrate, Inosine (phosphate-bonded), L-Leucine, L-Valine, L-Isoleucine, Alpha-Ketoglutaric Acid, KIC (Calcium Keto-Isocaproate), L-Glutamine, Dicalcium Phosphate, Microcrystalline Cellulose, Stearic Acid, Croscarmellose Sodium, Silica, Magnesium Stearate and film coating (Hydroxypropyl Methylcellulose, Hydroxypropyl Cellulose, Polyethylene Glycol, Titanium Dioxide and Propylene Glycol).

How Supplied: One box contains 28 packets, 4 tablets per packet.

Additional Information: For additional information on ingredients or uses, please visit winltd.com.

These statements have not been evaluated by the Food & Drug Administration. This product is not intended to diagnose, treat, cure or prevent any disease.

PHYTO-VITE®
Advanced Antioxidant, Vitamin and Mineral Supplement

Description: Phyto-Vite® is a state-of-the-art nutritional supplement providing chelated minerals, vitamins and a diverse group of antioxidants. The antioxidant coverage provided by Phyto-Vite is both comprehensive and diverse. First, it includes optimal amounts of vitamins A, C, and E as well as the pro-vitamins alpha and beta carotene. The inclusion of these powerful antioxidants provides protection against the oxidative damage caused by free-radicals. Increased immune system support, increased protein and hormone synthesis, increased soft tissue integrity and improved circulation are just a few of the many effects of these antioxidants. Esterified vitamin C is used in Phyto-Vite to ensure quicker uptake and a decreased rate of excretion. Ginkgo biloba has been added to promote healthy brain function and circulation of blood to the brain, as well as to inhibit lipid peroxidation. A phytonutrient blend obtained from entire plant sources has been incorporated into Phyto-Vite to further enhance its antioxidant effects. Key phytonutrients included are lutein, lycopene, soy isoflavones, and allicin. To ensure optimum absorption and maximum antioxidant effects, Phyto-Vite includes the minerals copper, zinc, manganese and selenium in a chelated form. Phyto-Vite has several unique features such as the inclusion of canola oil to ensure proper absorption of fat-soluble vitamins even on an empty stomach, an extended-release formula-

tion to allow flexibility in serving size and a Betacoat™ casing. This is a beta carotene coating that is designed to provide antioxidant coverage to the tablet itself. This helps to protect the integrity and activity of the product.

Directions: Take 6 tablets per day.

Warnings: Accidental overdose of iron-containing products is a leading cause of fatal poisoning in children under 6. Keep this product out of reach of children. In case of accidental overdose, call a doctor or poison control center immediately. If pregnant or lactating, consult physician before using. Contains milk and soy.

Ingredients: Vitamin A (25,000IU), Vitamin C (500mg), Vitamin D (200IU), Vitamin E (400IU), Vitamin K (70mcg), Thiamin (15mg), Riboflavin (17mg), Niacin (100mg), Vitamin B6 (20mg), Folate (400mcg), Vitamin B12 (60mcg), Biotin (300mcg), Pantothenic Acid (75mg), Calcium (500mg), Iron (4mg), Phosphorus (250mg), Iodine (150mcg), Magnesium (400mg), Zinc (15mg), Selenium (200mcg), Copper (2mg), Manganese (5mg), Chromium (200mcg), Potassium (70mg), Phytonutrient Blend (800mg, alfalfa leaf, aged garlic bulb concentrate, Pur-Gar®A-10,000 (garlic bulb), soy protein isolate (soy), broccoli floret, cabbage leaf, cayenne pepper fruit, green onion bulb, parsley leaf, tomato, spirulina), canola oil concentrate (milk) (100mg), citrus bioflavonoid complex (50mg), rutin (26mg), quercetin dihydrate (24mg), choline (50mg), inositol (50mg), PABA (25mg), ginkgo biloba leaf standardized extract (20mg: 4.6mg ginkgo flavone glycosides; 1.2mg terpene lactones), bilberry fruit standardized extract (10mg: 2.5mg anthocyanosides), catalase enzymes (10mg), grape seed proanthocyanidins (5mg), red grape skin extract (5mg: 0.7-0.9mg total polyphenols), Boron (1mg), dicalcium phosphate, magnesium oxide, calcium carbonate, calcium ascorbate, microcrystalline cellulose, d-alpha-tocopheryl succinate (soy), croscarmellose sodium, stearic acid, potassium citrate, choline bitartrate, beta-carotene, niacinamide, silica, d-calcium pantothenate, magnesium stearate, copper Chelazome® glycinate, zinc Chelazome® glycinate, calcium citrate, calcium lactate, magnesium amino acid chelate, inositol, L-selenomethionine, kelp, manganese Chelazome® glycinate, biotin, pyridoxine HCL, Ferrochel® iron bisglycinate, boron chelate, riboflavin, magnesium citrate, thiamin mononitrate, retinyl palmitate, chromium Chelavite® glycinate, phylloquinone, cyanocobalamin, vanillin, cholecalciferol, folic acid.

How Supplied: One bottle contains 180 hypoallergenic Betacoat™ tablets. This hypoallergenic formula is free of yeast, wheat, sugar, starch, animal products, dyes, preservatives, artificial flavors and pesticide residues.

Additional Information: For additional information on ingredients or uses, please visit winltd.com.

These statements have not been evaluated by the Food and Drug Administration. This product is not intended to diagnose, treat, cure or prevent any disease.

PROTECTOR®
Immune Formula Herbal Supplement

Description: Protector® is a nutritional supplement that combines specific vitamins, minerals and amino acids recognized as important for the health of areas associated with the human immune system. Astragalus is a key ingredient known for improving immune system integrity by relieving stress-induced immune system suppression. Additionally, research indicates that kelp supplies dozens of important nutrients for optimal cardiovascular health and function.

Directions: As a dietary supplement, take 1 capsule 3 times daily with meals.

Warnings: CAUTION PHENYLKETONURICS: Contains 9.2mg phenylalanine per serving.

Ingredients: Proprietary Blend (Isolated Soy Protein (Soy), Astragalus Root, Bee Pollen, Kelp, Ribonucleic Acid Yeast, Adenosine Triphosphate), Hydroxypropylmethylcellulose, Cellulose, Stearic acid, Magnesium Stearate, Silicon Dioxide.

How Supplied: One bottle contains 60 easy-to-swallow capsules.

Additional Information: For additional information on ingredients or uses, please visit winltd.com.

These statements have not been evaluated by the Food & Drug Administration. This product is not intended to diagnose, treat, cure or prevent any disease.

PROXTREME™
Multi-Protein Dietary Supplement

Description: ProXtreme™ is a multi-protein formula containing a scientific blend of ion-exchange whey protein isolates, cross flow ultra filtration isolates, whey protein concentrates, hydrolyzed whey peptides, glutamine peptides and egg albumen. This combination of various protein sources provides 25g of protein per serving while only having 3g or less of carbohydrates. ProXtreme provides an ideal ratio of essential and nonessential amino acids in their most easily assimilated forms, while also providing high levels of the branched chain amino acids (BCAAs). To increase absorption and digestibility, the proteins in ProXtreme are enzymatically predigested. These proteins are further processed with whey protein to minimize protein crosslinking.

Continued on next page

Proxtreme—Cont.

Directions: Add 1 packet to 6–8 ounces of water, milk, or juice. Stir, shake, or blend for 20 seconds, or until completely dispersed, then drink immediately.

Ingredients: Total Fat 1g (Saturated Fat 0g, Sugar 1g), Potassium 240mg, Carbohydrate 3g or less, Cholesterol 13mg, Sodium 80mg, Protein 25g, Vitamin A 1,125IU, Vitamin C 27mg, Vitamin D 90IU, Vitamin E 14IU, Riboflavin 450mcg, Niacin 5mg, Vitamin B6 450mcg, Folic Acid 63mcg, Vitamin B12 1.4mcg, Biotin 68mcg, Pantothenic Acid 2mg, Calcium 185mg, Chromium 55mcg, Proprietary Amino Acid Blend 1g (Glutamine Peptides, L-Leucine, L-Isoleucine, L-Valine, Zytrix®* 100mg), **PROXTREME™ CHOCOLATE INGREDIENTS:** Protein Complex (Whey Protein Isolate, Whey Protein Concentrate, Egg Albumen, Whey Peptides, Glutamine Peptides), Cocoa, Natural and Artificial Flavor, Lecithin, Vitamin/Mineral Blend (Ascorbic Acid, Chromium GTF Polynicotinate, d-alpha Tocopheryl Succinate [Natural Vitamin E], diCalcium Phosphate, Biotin, Vitamin A Palmitate, Niacinamide, d-Calcium Pantothenate, Cholecalciferol, Folic Acid, Pyridoxine Hydrochloride, Riboflavin, Cyanocobalamin), Xanthan Gum, Acesulfame Potassium, Sodium Chloride, Sucralose. Contains Dairy and Soy. **PROXTREME™ VANILLA INGREDIENTS:** Protein Complex (Whey Protein Isolate, Whey Protein Concentrate, Egg Albumen, Whey Peptides, Glutamine Peptides), Natural and Artificial Flavor, Lecithin, Vitamin/Mineral Blend (Ascorbic Acid, Chromium GTF Polynicotinate, d-alpha Tocopheryl Succinate [Natural Vitamin E], diCalcium Phosphate, Biotin, Vitamin A Palmitate, Niacinamide, d-Calcium Pantothenate, Cholecalciferol, Folic Acid, Pyridoxine Hydrochloride, Riboflavin, Cyanocobalamin), Xanthan Gum, Acesulfame Potassium, Sodium Chloride, Sucralose. Contains Dairy and Soy.

*Zytrix® is a registered trademark of Custom Nutriceutical Laboratories.

How Supplied: One box contains 7 vanilla and 7 chocolate single serving packets.

Additional Information: For additional information on ingredients or uses, please visit winltd.com.

These statements have not been evaluated by the Food & Drug Administration. This product is not intended to diagnose, treat, cure or prevent any disease.

RELIEF®
Mineral, Herbal and Amino Acid Supplement

Description: Relief® is formulated with a special combination of nutrients, vitamins, minerals, amino acids and herbs recognized as important to the digestive and excretory systems. Parsley, a key ingredient in Relief, aids digestion with its carminative effects. Also included is psyllium, a gel-forming fiber that promotes both bowel regularity and helps maintain healthy, normal cholesterol levels.

Directions: Take 1 capsule 3 times daily with meals.

Ingredients: Proprietary Blend (Psyllium Seed Powder, L-Isoleucine, L-Leucine, L-Valine, Bee Pollen, Bladderwrack Herb 5:1 Extract, Parsley Leaf 4:1 Extract, Ribonucleic Acid Yeast, Adenosine Triphosphate), Hydroxypropylmethylcellulose, Starch, D-Calcium Pantothenate, Silicon Dioxide.

How Supplied: One bottle contains 60 easy-to-swallow capsules.

Additional Information: For additional information on ingredients or uses, please visit winltd.com.

These statements have not been evaluated by the Food & Drug Administration. This product is not intended to diagnose, treat, cure or prevent any disease.

SATIETÉ®
Herbal and Vitamin Supplement

Description: Satieté® has a synergistic blend of herbs and amino acids that promotes healthy regulation of the neurotransmitter serotonin, supports a healthy appetite and maintains healthy blood sugar levels. Satieté's key ingredient, 5-HTP, derived from griffonia seed extract, is a precursor to serotonin, which regulates normal mood, sleep, appetite and energy levels. Also included is gymnema sylvestre, an important ingredient which has an effect on the oral cavity that reduces appetite for sweets as well as an ability to reduce metabolism of simple carbohydrates in the gastrointestinal system, thus promoting healthy blood sugar levels. Additional ingredients included to improve energy levels and combat fatigue are St. John's Wort extract, malic acid, and magnesium. The combination of these ingredients provides a positive impact on serotonin function.

Directions: Begin dosage by taking 1 tablet 3 times per day 30–60 minutes before meals. If needed after 2 weeks of use, increase the serving size to 2 tablets 3 times per day. Do not exceed 9 tablets daily without medical supervision.

Warnings: If you are taking MAO inhibitors, tricyclic antidepressants, SSRI antidepressants (Prozac®, Paxil™, Zoloft®) or prescription diet drugs, do not take this product without medical supervision. If you suffer from liver or kidney diseases, serious gastrointestinal disorders or carcinoid syndrome, do not take this product without medical supervision. If gastrointestinal upset develops and persists, reduce dosage, take only with large meals or discontinue use.

Ingredients: Vitamin B-1 13mg, Vitamin B-2 13mg, Vitamin B-6 13mg, Niacinamide 13mg (as part of Niacin), Vitamin B-12 200mcg, Folic Acid 66mcg, Magnesium 110mg, (Oxide), Griffonia Seed Extract 100mg (5-Hydroxytryptophan (5-HTP) 27.5mg), Gymnema 66mg, Malic Acid 200mg, St. John's Wort Extract 100mg (Herb tops, flowers), Ginkgo Biloba Extract 40mg (Leaf), Microcrystalline Cellulose, Stearic Acid, Croscarmelose Sodium, Magnesium Stearate, Silicon Dioxide, Ethylcellulose and Hydroxypropylcellulose.

How Supplied: One bottle contains 84 hypoallergenic enteric-coated tablets.

Additional Information: For additional information on ingredients or uses, please visit winltd.com.

These statements have not been evaluated by the Food & Drug Administration. This product is not intended to diagnose, treat, cure or prevent any disease.

SLEEP-TITE™
Herbal Sleep Aid

Description: Sleep-Tite™ is a natural herbal sleep aid formulated to rejuvenate and restore by assisting the body in initiating and maintaining a deeper sleep. Sleep-Tite is a blend of 10 all-natural herbs, including California poppy, passion flower, valerian, and skullcap. These herbs help maintain healthy sleep cycles because of their calming effects and ability to relieve muscle tension. Additional ingredients, including hops, celery seed and chamomile all provide a generalized calming effect and are especially helpful for indigestion, gastrointestinal and smooth muscle relaxation. In addition to these calming herbs, Sleep-Tite also contains feverfew, an herb that reduces the body's production of prostaglandin and serotonin, hormones that can lead to the onset of everyday stress headaches. By utilizing this unique blend of herbs to aid in the effective initiation and maintenance of sleep patterns, Sleep-Tite can be consumed by adults, thereby promoting physical and emotional well-being in a safe, effective manner.

Directions: Take 2 tablets approximately 30–60 minutes prior to bedtime. Some persons may require less than 2 tablets to achieve optimum results. Do not exceed recommended nightly amounts. Needs may vary with each individual.

Warnings: This product contains chamomile and feverfew and should not be used by individuals with sensitivity to any plant from the Asteraceae family.

Not for use by children under the age of 18, pregnant or lactating women. Consult your physician before using this product if you have any medical condition or are taking antidepressants, sedatives or hypnotic medications. Do not take this product if using Monoamine Oxidase Inhibitors (MAOI). This product may cause drowsiness and should not be taken with alcohol or while operating a vehicle or other machinery. If allergic symptoms develop, discontinue use. Keep out of reach of children.

Ingredients: Proprietary Herbal concentrate 395 mg, (European Valerian Root 4:1 extract, Celery Seed 4:1 extract, Hops Strobile 4:1 extract, Passion Flower 4:1 extract (whole plant), California Poppy 5:1 extract (aerial parts), Chamomile Flower 5:1 extract, Chinese Fu Ling root 5:1 extract (Poria Cocos), Jujube Seed 5:1 extract, Feverfew 5:1 extract (aerial parts), Skullcap (aerial parts)), Dicalcium Phosphate, Microcrystalline Cellulose, Croscarmellose Sodium, Stearic Acid, Silica, Magnesium Stearate and Sugar Coat (calcium sulfate, sucrose, kaolin, talc, gelatin, shellac, titanium dioxide, anise oil, beeswax and carnauba wax).

How Supplied: One box contains 28 packets, 2 caplets per packet.

Additional Information: For additional information on ingredients or uses, please visit winltd.com.

These statements have not been evaluated by the Food & Drug Administration. This product is not intended to diagnose, treat, cure or prevent any disease.

SURE2ENDURE™
Endurance Formula Herbal Supplement

Description: Sure2Endure™ is formulated to enhance the body's endurance, stamina, and ability to recover after a workout through an innovative blend of herbs, vitamins and minerals. Among these specially selected ingredients is ciwujia, known to alleviate fatigue and support the immune system. This herb has been shown to improve overall performance in aerobic exercise, endurance activities and weight lifting without any stimulant side effects. Ciwujia increases fat metabolism during exercise by shifting toward the use of fat as an energy source instead of carbohydrates. Additionally, this herb improves endurance by reducing lactic acid production thereby delaying fatigue that can often lead to muscle pain and cramps after a normal workout. Sure2Endure also provides antioxidant coverage and enzyme cofactors to meet the high demands that exercise places on the body. These antioxidants and cofactors scavenge free radicals formed during exercise as well promote carbohydrate metabolism, fur-

ther leading to increased physical performance. To protect joints during exercise and ensure healthy connective tissue, glucosamine is a key ingredient in Sure2Endure. Since tissue stress and damage are often the result of strenuous exercise, it is important to maintain proper integrity and recovery of connective tissue. In addition to promoting healthy connective tissue, natural anti-inflammatory compounds bromelain and boswellia are included to further support the health of joints and soft tissues.

Directions: Adults and teens (13 years and older) may take 3 tablets 1 hour prior to exercise to achieve optimum performance. Needs may vary with each individual. To maximize this effect, you may wish to add BioLean II® or BioLean Free® 1 hour prior to exercise.

RECOMMENDATIONS: In addition to this supplement, it is recommended that you maintain a strict low-fat, high-protein diet, drink at least eight glasses of water daily, and engage in aerobic exercise three to four times per week at intervals of 30 to 60 minutes. Phyto-Vite® should be taken to maximize the antioxidant effect necessary with exercise. Pro-Xtreme™ and Mass Appeal™ may also be consumed for optimal results.

Warnings: Not for use by children under the age of 13, pregnant or lactating women. Consult your physician before using this product if you have any medical conditions. Discontinue immediately if allergic symptoms develop. Contains shellfish.

Ingredients: Vitamin C 500mg (as Ascorbic Acid), Vitamin E 100IU (as D-Alpha Tocopheryl Succinate), Thiamin 10mg (as Thiamin Mononitrate), Riboflavin 12mg, Vitamin B6 15mg (as Pyridoxine HCL), Vitamin B12 20mcg (as Cyanocobalamin), Chromium 200mcg (as patented Chelavite® Chromium Dinicotinate Glycinate), Proprietary Endurance, Stamina and Recovery Blend 1.01g (Eleuthero [Cijwujia], Magnesium L-aspartate, Potassium L-aspartate), Proprietary Joint and Connective Tissue Blend 300mg (Indian Frankincense [Boswelia], Bromelain [600GDU/g], Glucosamine HCL), Dicalcium Phosphate, Microcrystalline Cellulose, Croscarmellose Sodium, Stearic Acid, Silica, Magnesium Stearate and Sugar Coat (calcium sulfate, sucrose, kaolin, talc, gelatin, shellac, titanium dioxide, wintergreen oil, FD&C yellow #5, FD&C blue #1, beeswax and carnauba wax). Contains shrimp, crab, lobster and prawn (Glucosamine hydrochloride).

How Supplied: One box contains 28 packets, 3 tablets per packet.

Additional Information: For additional information on ingredients or uses, please visit winltd.com.

These statements have not been evaluated by the Food & Drug Administration. This product is not intended to diagnose, treat, cure or prevent any disease.

TRANQUILITY™
Vitamin, Mineral and Amino Acid Supplement

Description: Tranquility™ is a nutritional supplement which contains a blend of vitamins, minerals and amino acids recognized as important to areas involved in stress management. Two primary ingredients are myo-inositol and valerian root, both of which are beneficial in regulating the healthy sleep cycle and stress levels. Additionally, myo-inositol has been shown to support healthy triglyceride and cholesterol levels.

Directions: Take 1 capsule 3 times daily with meals.

Warnings: CAUTION PHENYLKETONURICS: Contains 9.2mg phenylalanine per serving.

Ingredients: Proprietary Blend (Isolated Soy Protein (Soy), Choline Bitartrate, Inositol, Lecithin (Soy), Ribonucleic Acid Yeast, Valerian Root Extract, Adenosine Triphosphate), Hydroxypropylmethylcellulose, DL-Alpha Tocopheryl Acetate, Calcium Aspartate, Silicon Dioxide, Ascorbic Acid, Stearic Acid, Niacinamide, Magnesium Amino Acid Chelate, Vitamin A Palmitate, Hydroxypropylcellulose, D-Calcium Pantothenate, Thiamine HCL, Dicalcium Phosphate, Pyridoxine HCL, Riboflavin, Folic Acid, Cholecalciferol, Biotin, Cyanocobalamin.

How Supplied: One bottle contains 60 easy-to-swallow capsules.

Additional Information: For additional information on ingredients or uses, please visit winltd.com.

These statements have not been evaluated by the Food & Drug Administration. This product is not intended to diagnose, treat, cure or prevent any disease.

WIN CoQ10™
High Absorption Coenzyme Q10 Dietary Supplement

Description: WIN CoQ10™ is a nutritional supplement containing ubiquinol, the reduced form of coenzyme Q10, which has been shown to help lower blood pressure and improve symptoms related to heart disease and may help improve brain functioning. Additionally, WIN CoQ10 may help restore coenzyme Q10 which can be lost when taking certain medications to lower cholesterol levels, such as statins, and dietary supplements containing red yeast rice. Maintaining coenzyme Q10 levels are

Continued on next page

WIN CoQ10—Cont.

essential as it is a critical component of energy metabolism at the cellular level. WIN CoQ10's protective effect on the heart may slow the aging of cells associated with the cardiovascular system.

Directions: Take 2 capsules per day with a meal. Some people may realize additional benefits with a higher dosage.

Warnings: This product contains soy. Do not consume if allergic to soy or soy-containing products. Not for use by children under the age of 18, pregnant or lactating women. In case of accidental overdose, call a doctor or poison control center immediately.

Ingredients: Ubiquinol 50mg (Kaneka QH™ reduced form of CoQ10), Canola Oil, Diglyceryl Monooleate, Gelatin, Glycerin, Lecithin (Soy), Beeswax, Purified Water, Caramel Color. Kaneka QH™ is a trademark of Kaneka Corporation.

How Supplied: One bottle contains 60 easy-to-swallow soft-gel capsules.

Additional Information: For additional information on ingredients or uses, please visit winltd.com.

These statements have not been evaluated by the Food & Drug Administration. This product is not intended to diagnose, treat, cure or prevent any disease.

WINOMEG3COMPLEX™
Highly Concentrated Molecularly Distilled Omega-3 Ethyl Esters Dietary Supplement

Description: WINOmeg3complex™ is a highly purified pharmaceutical-grade 88% omega-3 ethyl ester supplement, scientifically formulated to promote mood elevation, cardiac health, joint health, cognitive clarity, improved digestion and emotional well-being. WINOmeg3complex provides a high concentration of 60% EPA for maximum benefit to the body's normal inflammatory response. Free of dangerous toxins and clinically tested to surpass all international standards for freshness and purity, WINOmeg3complex has three times the EPA and DHA potency of health food grade fish oil. This high concentration and optimal EPA to DHA blend is enhanced with natural lemon oil in the soft gel capsule for great lemon taste. One WINOmeg3complex soft gel capsule supplies 540mg of EPA and 160mg of DHA. The ratio of EPA to DHA is 3.3 to 1; a balance many experts believe is optimal for good health.

Directions: Take 2 capsules per day with a meal. Some people may realize additional benefits with a higher dosage.

Warnings: If you are pregnant or on a blood thinner or other anticoagulant, consult your physician before taking this supplement.

Ingredients: Eicosapentaenoic acid 1080mg (EPA), docosahexaenoic acid 320mg (DHA), other omega-3 fatty acids 180mg, omega-6 fatty acids 60mg, other fatty acids 150mg, anchovies, gelatin, glycerine, natural flavor and mixed tocopherols.

How Supplied: One bottle contains 60 easy-to-swallow soft-gel capsules enhanced with natural lemon oil.

Additional Information: For additional information on ingredients or uses, please visit winltd.com.

These statements have not been evaluated by the Food & Drug Administration. This product is not intended to diagnose, treat, cure or prevent any disease.

WINRGY®
**Energy Drink
Vitamin and Mineral Supplement**

Description: Utilizing key ingredients such as riboflavin, vitamin B12, niacin and a proprietary blend of amino acids and caffeine, **Winrgy®** helps promote the alertness and energy required for an active lifestyle. Winrgy incorporates a unique blend of vitamins and minerals that are important in the creation of noradrenaline, a powerful neurotransmitter responsible for regulating alertness and the sleep-wakefulness cycle as well as being essential for memory and the learning process. Additionally, essential ingredients in Winrgy help the body convert energy from carbohydrates, protein, and fat, as well as combat daily physical and mental fatigue. Unlike caffeine alone, Winrgy offers the raw materials necessary to promote the body's normal production of noradrenaline and is ideal for anytime performance is required.

Directions: Add 1 packet of mix to 6 oz. of chilled water or fruit juice. Stir briskly. Consume 1–2 times per day.

Warnings: CAUTION PHENYLKE-TONURICS: Contains 570mg phenylalanine per serving. Not for use by children under the age of 13, pregnant or lactating women. Persons taking medications should seek medical advice before taking this product. Do not consume more than 4 servings per day. Avoid the use of antacids containing aluminum with this product.

Ingredients: Carbohydrates 11g, Sugars 10g, Vitamin C 150mg (as Ascorbic Acid), Vitamin E 30IU (as DL-Alpha Tocopheryl Acetate), Thiamin 1.5mg (as Thiamin Mononitrate), Riboflavin 3mg, Niacin 73mg (as Niacinamide), Vitamin B6 13mg (as Pyridoxine HCL), Folate 180mcg (as Folic Acid), Vitamin B12 19mcg (as Cyanocobalamin), Pantothenic Acid 48mg (as Calcium Pantothenate), Zinc 4.5mg (as Zinc Gluconate), Copper 0.62mg (as Copper Gluconate), Manganese 2.6mg (as Manganese Aspartate), Chromium 260mcg (as Chromium Aspartate), Potassium 25mg (as Potassium Aspartate), Phenylalanine 570mg (as L-phenylalanine), Taurine 180mg, Glycine 135mg, Caffeine 80mg, Fructose, Natural Flavor, Citric Acid and Silicon Dioxide.

How Supplied: One box contains 28 single serving packets.

Additional Information: For additional information on ingredients or uses, please visit winltd.com.

These statements have not been evaluated by the Food & Drug Administration. This product is not intended to diagnose, treat, cure or prevent any disease.

PRODUCT COMPARISON TABLES

This section provides a quick comparison of the ingredients and dosages of common brand-name drugs in 24 therapeutic classes. In addition, you will find a chart on page T-53 that will help you determine whether your symptoms are due to a cold, the flu, or an allergy.

- Acne Products
- Allergic Rhinitis Products
- Analgesic Products
- Antacid and Heartburn Products
- Antidiarrheal Products
- Antiflatulant Products
- Antifungal Products
- Anitpyretic Products
- Antiseborrheal Products
- Artificial Tear Products
- Canker and Cold Sore Products
- Contact Dermatitis Products
- Cough, Cold, and Flu Products
- Dandruff Products
- Headache/Migraine Products
- Hemorrhoidal Products
- Insomnia Products
- Laxative Products
- Nasal Decongestant/Moisturizing Products
- Ophthalmic Decongestant/Antihistamine Products
- Psoriasis Products
- Smoking Cessation Products
- Weight Management Products
- Wound Care Products

Table 1. ACNE PRODUCTS

BRAND	INGREDIENT/STRENGTH	DOSE
BENZOYL PEROXIDE		
Clean & Clear Continuous Control Acne Cleanser	Benzoyl Peroxide 10%	**Adults & Peds:** Use bid.
Clean & Clear Persa-Gel 10, Maximum Strength	Benzoyl Peroxide 10%	**Adults & Peds:** Use qd-tid.
Clearasil Daily Acne Stay Clear Cream	Benzoyl Peroxide 10%	**Adults & Peds:** Use qd-tid.
Clearasil Total Acne Control	Benzoyl Peroxide 10%	**Adults & Peds:** Use qd-tid.
Clearasil Acne Treatment Tinted Cream	Benzoyl Peroxide 10%	**Adults & Peds:** Use up to tid.
Clearasil Ultra Acne Treatment Vanishing Cream	Benzoyl Peroxide 10%	**Adults & Peds:** Use up to tid.
Neutrogena Clear Pore Cleanser Mask	Benzoyl Peroxide 3.5%	**Adults & Peds:** Use biw-tiw.
Neutrogena On-the-Spot Acne Treatment Vanishing Cream	Benzoyl Peroxide 2.5%	**Adults & Peds:** Apply qd initially, then bid-tid.
Oxy Chill Factor Daily Wash	Benzoyl Peroxide 10%	**Adults & Peds:** Use qd.
Oxy Maximum Daily Wash	Benzoyl Peroxide 10%	**Adults & Peds:** Use qd.
Oxy Spot Treatment	Benzoyl Peroxide 10%	**Adults & Peds:** Use qd-tid.
PanOxyl Aqua Gel Maximum Strength Gel	Benzoyl Peroxide 10%	**Adults & Peds:** Apply qd initially, then bid-tid.
PanOxyl Bar 10% Maximum Strength	Benzoyl Peroxide 10%	**Adults & Peds:** Apply qd initially, then bid-tid.
PanOxyl Bar 5%	Benzoyl Peroxide 5%	**Adults & Peds:** Use qd initially, then bid-tid.
ZAPZYT Maximum Strength Acne Treatment gel	Benzoyl Peroxide 10%	**Adults & Peds:** Use up to tid. If dryness occurs, use qd or qod.
ZAPZYT Treatment Bar	Benzoyl Peroxide 10%	**Adults & Peds:** Use qd initially, then bid-tid. If dryness occurs, use qd or qod.
SALICYLIC ACID		
Aveeno Clear Complexion Cleansing Bar	Salicylic Acid 0.5%	**Adults & Peds:** Use daily.
Aveeno Clear Complexion Foaming Cleanser	Salicylic Acid 0.5%	**Adults & Peds:** Use daily.
Aveeno Correcting Treatment, Clear Complexion	Salicylic Acid 1%	**Adults & Peds:** Use qd-tid.
Biore Blemish Fighting Cleansing Cloths	Salicylic Acid 2%	**Adults & Peds:** Use qd-tid.
Biore Blemish Fighting Ice Cleanser	Salicylic Acid 2%	**Adults & Peds:** Use qd.
Bye Bye Blemish Anti-Acne Serum	Salicylic Acid 1%	**Adults & Peds:** Use qd-tid.
Bye Bye Blemish Drying Lotion	Salicylic Acid 2%	**Adults & Peds:** Use pm.
Bye Bye Blemish Purifying Acne Mask	Salicylic Acid 0.5%	**Adults & Peds:** Use qd.
Clean & Clear Advantage Acne Cleanser	Salicylic Acid 2%	**Adults & Peds:** Use qd.
Clean & Clear Advantage Acne Spot Treatment	Salicylic Acid 2%	**Adults & Peds:** Use qd.
Clean & Clear Advantage Cleansing Pads	Salicylic Acid 2%	**Adults & Peds:** Use qd.
Clean & Clear Blackhead Clearing Astringent	Salicylic Acid 1%	**Adults & Peds:** Use qd.
Clean & Clear Blackhead Clearing Daily Cleansing Pads	Salicylic Acid 1%	**Adults & Peds:** Use qd.
Clean & Clear Blackhead Clearing Scrub	Salicylic Acid 2%	**Adults & Peds:** Use qd.

Table 1. ACNE PRODUCTS (cont.)

BRAND NAME	INGREDIENT/STRENGTH	DOSE
Clean & Clear Clear Advantage Daily Acne Control Moisturizer	Salicylic Acid 0.5%	**Adults & Peds:** Use qd.
Clean & Clear Continuous Control Acne Wash, Oil Free	Salicylic Acid 2%	**Adults & Peds:** Use qd-tid.
Clean & Clear Oil-Free Acne Moisturizer	Salicylic Acid 0.5%	**Adults & Peds:** Use qd-tid.
Clearasil Stay Clear Deep Cleanse Acne Fighting Cleansing Wipes	Salicylic Acid 2%	**Adults & Peds:** Use qd-tid.
Clearasil Stay Clear Skin Perfecting Wash	Salicylic Acid 2%	**Adults & Peds:** Use bid.
Clearasil Stay Clear Oil Free Gel Wash	Salicylic Acid 2%	**Adults & Peds:** Use bid.
Clearasil Stay Clear Daily Pore Cleansing Pads	Salicylic Acid 2%	**Adults & Peds:** Use qd-tid.
Clearasil Stay Clear Daily Facial Scrub	Salicylic Acid 2%	**Adults & Peds:** Use qd.
Clearasil Ultra Acne Clearing Gel Wash	Salicylic Acid 2%	**Adults & Peds:** Use qd.
Clearasil Ultra Daily Face Wash	Salicylic Acid 2%	**Adults & Peds:** Use qd.
Clearasil Ultra Acne Clearing Scrub	Salicylic Acid 2%	**Adults & Peds:** Use qd.
Clearasil Ultra Deep Pore Cleansing Pads	Salicylic Acid 2%	**Adults & Peds:** Use qd-tid.
L'Oreal Pure Pore-Clearing Cleanser	Salicylic Acid 1%	**Adults & Peds:** Use tid.
Neutrogena Advanced Solutions Acne Mark Fading Peel with CelluZyme	Salicylic Acid 2%	**Adults & Peds:** Use qw-tiw.
Neutrogena Blackhead Eliminating Astringent	Salicylic Acid 1%	**Adults & Peds:** Use qd-tid.
Neutrogena Blackhead Eliminating Daily Scrub	Salicylic Acid 2%	**Adults & Peds:** Use bid.
Neutrogena Blackhead Eliminating Foaming Pads	Salicylic Acid 0.5%	**Adults & Peds:** Use qd.
Neutrogena Body Clear Body Scrub	Salicylic Acid 2%	**Adults & Peds:** Use qd.
Neutrogena Oil Free Acne Wash Foam Cleanser	Salicylic Acid 2%	**Adults & Peds:** Use qd.
Neutrogena Clear Pore Oil-Eliminating Astringent	Salicylic Acid 2%	**Adults & Peds:** Use qd-tid.
Neutrogena Oil Free Acne Stress Control Power Clear Scrub	Salicylic Acid 2%	**Adults & Peds:** Use qd.
Neutrogena Oil Free Acne Stress Control Power Foam Wash	Salicylic Acid 0.5%	**Adults & Peds:** Use qd-tid.
Neutrogena Acne Stress Control 3-in-1 Hydrating Acne Treatment	Salicylic Acid 2%	**Adults & Peds:** Use qd-tid.
Neutrogena Oil Free Acne Wash Cleansing Cloths	Salicylic Acid 2%	**Adults & Peds:** Use qd.
Neutrogena Oil Free Acne Wash Cream Cleanser	Salicylic Acid 2%	**Adults & Peds:** Use qd-bid.
Neutrogena Rapid Clear Acne Defense Face Lotion	Salicylic Acid 2%	**Adults & Peds:** Use qd-tid.
Neutrogena Rapid Clear Acne Eliminating Spot Gel	Salicylic Acid 2%	**Adults & Peds:** Use qd-tid.
Neutrogena Skin Polishing Acne Cleanser	Salicylic Acid 0.5%	**Adults & Peds:** Use bid.
Neutrogena Oil-Free Anti-Acne Moisturizer	Salicylic Acid 0.5%	**Adults & Peds:** Use qd initially, then bid-tid. If dryness occurs, use qd or qod.
Noxzema Continuous Clean Deep Foaming Cleanser	Salicylic Acid 2%	**Adults & Peds:** Use qd.

Table 1. ACNE PRODUCTS (cont.)

BRAND NAME	INGREDIENT/STRENGTH	DOSE
Noxzema Triple Clean Anti-Blemish Astringent	Salicylic Acid 2%	**Adults & Peds:** Use qd-tid. If dryness occurs, use qd or qod.
Noxzema Triple Clean Anti-Blemish Pads	Salicylic Acid 2%	**Adults & Peds:** Use qd-tid.
Olay Daily Facials Lathering Cleansing Cloths-Clarifying for Combination/Oily Skin	Salicylic Acid (strength NA)	**Adults & Peds:** Apply qd.
Olay Regenerist Daily Regenerating Cleanser	Salicylic Acid	**Adults & Peds:** Use qd.
Olay Total Effects Plus Blemish Control Moisturizer	Salicylic Acid	**Adults & Peds:** Apply qd-tid.
Oxy Chill Cleansing Pads	Salicylic Acid 2%	**Adults & Peds:** Use qd-tid.
Oxy Chill Face Scrub	Salicylic Acid 2%	**Adults & Peds:** Use qd-tid.
Oxy Maximum Bar Soap	Salicylic Acid 0.5%	**Adults & Peds:** Use qd-tid.
Oxy Maximum Face Scrub	Salicylic Acid 2%	**Adults & Peds:** Use qd-tid.
Oxy Maximum Daily Cleansing Pads	Salicylic Acid 2%	**Adults & Peds:** Use qd-tid.
Oxy Body Wash	Salicylic Acid 2%	**Adults & Peds:** Use qd.
Phisoderm Anti-Blemish Body Wash	Salicylic Acid 2%	**Adults & Peds:** Use qd.
St. Ives Medicated Apricot Scrub	Salicylic Acid 2%	**Adults & Peds:** Use qd.
Stridex Facewipes to Go with Acne Medication	Salicylic Acid 0.5%	**Adults & Peds:** Use qd-tid.
Stridex Triple Action Acne Pads Maximum Strength, Alcohol Free	Salicylic Acid 2%	**Adults & Peds:** Use qd-tid.
Stridex Essential Care Pads with Salicylic Acid	Salicylic Acid 1%	**Adults & Peds:** Use qd-tid.
Stridex Triple Action Medicated Acne Pads, Sensitive Skin	Salicylic Acid 0.5%	**Adults & Peds:** Use qd-tid.
ZAPZYT Acne Wash Treatment For Face & Body	Salicylic Acid 2%	**Adults & Peds:** Use bid.
ZAPZYT Pore Treatment Gel	Salicylic Acid 2%	**Adults & Peds:** Use qd-tid.
TRICLOSAN		
Noxema Triple Clean Anti-Bacterial Cleanser	Triclosan 0.3%	**Adults & Peds ≥6 months:** Use qd each time skin is cleansed.

Table 2. ALLERGIC RHINITIS PRODUCTS

Brand	Ingredient/Strength	Dose
ANTIHISTAMINE		
Alavert Oral Disintegrating Tablets	Loratadine 10mg	**Adults & Peds: ≥6 yrs:** 1 tab qd. **Max:** 1 tab q24h.
Alavert 24-Hour Allergy Tablets	Loratadine 10mg	**Adults & Peds: ≥6 yrs:** 1 tab qd. **Max:** 1 tab q24h.
Benadryl Allergy Quick Dissolve Strips	Diphenhydramine HCl 25mg	**Adults & Peds: ≥12 yrs:** Dissolve 1-2 strips on tongue q4-6h. **Max:** 6 doses q24h.
Benadryl Allergy Capsules	Diphenhydramine HCl 25mg	**Adults & Peds: ≥12 yrs:** 1-2 caps q4-6h. **Peds: 6-12 yrs:** 1 cap q4-6h. **Max:** 6 doses q24h.
Benadryl Allergy Chewable Tablets	Diphenhydramine HCl 12.5mg	**Adults & Peds: ≥12 yrs:** 2-4 tabs q4-6h. **Peds: 6-12 yrs:** 1-2 tabs q4-6h. **Max:** 6 doses q24h.
Benadryl Allergy Liquid	Diphenhydramine HCl 12.5mg/5mL	**Adults & Peds: ≥12 yrs:** 2-4 tsp (10-20mL) q4-6h. **Peds: 6-12 yrs:** 1-2 tsp (5-10mL) q4-6h. **Max:** 6 doses q24h.
Benadryl Allergy Ultratab	Diphenhydramine HCl 25mg	**Adults & Peds: ≥12 yrs:** 1-2 tabs q4-6h. **Peds: 6-12 yrs:** 1 tab q4-6h. **Max:** 6 doses q24h.
Benadryl Children's Quick Dissolve Strips	Diphenhydramine HCl 12.5mg	**Adults & Peds: ≥12 yrs:** Dissolve 1 or 2 strips on tongue q4-6h. Allow first strip to dissolve before placing second strip on tongue. **Max:** 6 doses q24h.
Chlor-Trimeton 4-Hour Allergy Tablets	Chlorpheniramine Maleate 4mg	**Adults & Peds: ≥12 yrs:** 1 tab q4-6h. **Max:** 6 tabs q24h. **Peds: 6-12 yrs:** ½ tab q4-6h. **Max:** 3 tabs q24h.
Claritin 24 Hour Allergy Tablets	Loratadine 10mg	**Adults & Peds: ≥6 yrs:** 1 tab qd. **Max:** 1 tab q24h.
Claritin Children's Syrup	Loratadine 5mg/5mL	**Adults & Peds: ≥6 yrs:** 2 tsp qd. **Max:** 2 tsp q24h. **Peds: 2-6 yrs:** 1 tsp qd. **Max:** 1 tsp q24h.
Claritin RediTabs	Loratadine 10mg	**Adults & Peds: ≥6 yrs:** 1 tab qd. **Max:** 1 tab q24h.
Dimetapp ND Children's Allergy Tablets	Loratadine 10mg	**Adults & Peds: ≥6 yrs:** 1 tab qd. **Max:** 1 tab q24h.
Zyrtec Tablets	Cetirizine 10mg	**Adults: 18 yrs-64 yrs & Peds: ≥6 yrs:** 1 tab q24h. **Max:** 1 tab q24h.
Zyrtec Children's Syrup	Cetirizine 5mg/5mL	**Adults ≥65:** 1 tsp q24h. **Peds: 2-6 yrs:** ½ tsp (2.5mL) qd or bid. **≥6 to 12:** 1 or 2 tsp (5-10mL) qd. **Max: Adults: ≥65 & Peds: 2-6 yrs:** 1 tsp (5mL) q24h **≥6 to 12yrs:** 2 tsp (10mL) qd
Zyrtec Children's Chewables 5mg	Cetirizine 5mg	**Adults & Peds ≥6 yrs-64 yrs:** 1 tab q24h. **Adults ≥65 yrs:** 1 tab q24h. **Max:** 1 tab q24h.
Zyrtec Children's Chewables 10mg	Cetirizine 10mg	**Adults & Peds ≥6 yrs:** 1 tab q24h. **Adults ≥65 yrs:** Ask doctor. **Max:** 1 tab qd
Zyrtec Children's Hive Relief Syrup	Cetirizine 5mg/5mL	**Adults & Peds ≥6 yrs-64yrs:** 1-2 tsp (5-10ml) q24h. **Max:** 2 tsp (10ml) q24h. **Adults >65:** 1 tsp q24h. **Max:** 1 tsp (5ml) q24h.
ANTIHISTAMINE COMBINATIONS		
Advil Allergy Sinus Caplets	Chlorpheniramine Maleate/ Ibuprofen/Pseudoephedrine 2mg-200mg-30mg	**Adults & Peds: ≥12 yrs:** 1 tab q4-6h. **Max:** 6 tabs q24h.
Alavert D-12 Hour Allergy and Sinus Tablets	Loratadine/Pseudoephedrine Sulfate 5mg-120mg	**Adults & Peds: ≥12 yrs:** 1 tab q12h. **Max:** 2 tabs q24h.

Table 2. ALLERGIC RHINITIS PRODUCTS (cont.)

BRAND	INGREDIENT/STRENGTH	DOSE
Benadryl Allergy & Sinus Headache Caplets	Diphenhydramine HCl/Acetaminophen/ Phenylephrine HCl/ 12.5mg-325mg-5mg	**Adults & Peds: ≥12 yrs:** 2 caps q4h. **Max:** 12 caps q24h.
Benadryl Severe Allergy & Sinus Headache Caplets	Diphenhydramine HCl/Acetaminophen/ Phenylephrine HCl 25mg-325mg-5mg	**Adults & Peds: ≥12 yrs:** 2 tabs q4h. **Max:** 12 tabs q24h.
Benadryl-D Allergy & Sinus Liquid	Diphenhydramine HCl/ Phenylephrine 12.5mg-5mg/5mL	**Adults & Peds: ≥12 yrs:** 2 tsp q4h. **Peds: 6-12 yrs:** 1 tsp q4h. **Max:** 6 doses q24h.
Claritin-D 12 Hour Allergy & Congestion Tablets	Loratadine/Pseudoephedrine Sulfate 5mg-120mg	**Adults & Peds: ≥12 yrs:** 1 tab q12h. **Max:** 2 tabs q24h.
Claritin-D 24 Hour Allergy & Congestion Tablets	Loratadine/Pseudoephedrine Sulfate 10mg-240mg	**Adults & Peds: ≥12 yrs:** 1 tab q12h. **Max:** 1 tab q24h.
Drixoral Cold & Allergy Sustained Action Tablets	Dexbrompheniramine Maleate/Pseudoephedrine HCl 6mg-120mg	**Adults & Peds: ≥12 yrs:** 1 tabs q12h. **Max:** 2 tabs q24h.
Dimetapp Elixir Cold & Allergy	Brompheniramine/Phenylephrine 1mg-2.5mg/5ml	**Adults & Peds: ≥12 yrs:** 4 tsp (20mL) q4h. **Peds: 6-12 yrs:** 2 tsp (10mL) q4h. **Max:** 6 doses q24h.
Dimetapp Children's Chewable Tablets	Brompheniramine/Phenylephrine 1mg-2.5mg	**Peds: ≥6-12 yrs:** 2 tabs q4h. **Max:** 6 doses q24h
Sudafed Sinus & Allergy Tablets	Chlorpheniramine/ Pseudoephedrine 4mg-60mg	**Adults: ≥12 yrs:** 1 tab q4-6h. **Peds: 6-12 yrs:** 1/2 tab q4h-6h. **Max:** 4 doses q24h.
Tylenol Allergy Complete Multi-Symptom Cool Burst Caplets	Chlorpheniramine Maleate/ Acetaminophen/Phenylephrine HCl 2mg-325mg-5mg	**Adults & Peds: ≥12 yrs:** 2 tabs q4h. **Max:** 12 tabs q24h.
Tylenol Allergy Complete Nighttime Cool Burst Caplets	Diphenhydramine HCl/ Acetaminophen/Phenylephrine HCl 25mg-325mg-5mg	**Adults & Peds: ≥12 yrs:** 2 tabs q4h. **Max:** 12 tabs q24h.
Tylenol Severe Allergy Caplets	Diphenhydramine HCl/Acetaminophen 12.5mg-500mg	**Adults & Peds: ≥12 yrs:** 2 tabs q4-6h. **Max:** 8 tabs q24h.

TOPICAL NASAL DECONGESTANTS

BRAND	INGREDIENT/STRENGTH	DOSE
4-Way Fast Acting Nasal Decongestant Spray	Phenylephrine HCl 1%	**Adults & Peds: ≥12 yrs:** Instill 2-3 sprays per nostril q4h.
4-Way Mentholated Nasal Decongestant Spray	Phenylephrine HCl 1%	**Adults & Peds: ≥12 yrs:** Instill 2-3 sprays per nostril q4h.
Afrin No Drip Extra Moisturizing Nasal Spray	Oxymetazoline HCl 0.05%	**Adults & Peds: ≥6 yrs:** Instill 2-3 sprays per nostril q10-12h. **Max:** 2 doses q24h.
Afrin No Drip Sinus Nasal Spray	Oxymetazoline HCl 0.05%	**Adults & Peds: ≥6 yrs:** Instill 2-3 sprays per nostril q10-12h. **Max:** 2 doses q24h.
Afrin Original Nasal Spray	Oxymetazoline HCl 0.05%	**Adults & Peds: ≥6 yrs:** Instill 2-3 sprays per nostril q10-12h.
Afrin No Drip Original Pump Mist Nasal Spray	Oxymetazoline HCl 0.05%	**Adults & Peds: ≥6 yrs:** Instill 2-3 sprays per nostril q10-12h. **Max:** 2 doses q24h.
Afrin No Drip All Night 12 Hour Pump Mist	Oxymetazoline HCl 0.05%	**Adults & Peds: ≥6 yrs:** Instill 2-3 sprays per nostril q10-12h.
Benzedrex Inhaler	Propylhexedrine 250mg	**Adults & Peds: ≥6 yrs:** Inhale 2 sprays per nostril q2h
Dristan 12 Hour Nasal Spray	Oxymetazoline HCl 0.05%	**Adults & Peds: ≥12 yrs:** Instill 2-3 sprays per nostril q10-12h. **Max:** 2 doses q24h.
Neo-Synephrine 12 Hour Extra Moisturizing Nasal Spray	Oxymetazoline HCl 0.05%	**Adults & Peds: ≥6 yrs:** Instill 2-3 sprays per nostril q10-12h. **Max:** 2 doses per 24 hours.
Neo-Synephrine 12 Hour Nasal Decongestant Spray	Oxymetazoline HCl 0.05%	**Adults & Peds: ≥6 yrs:** Instill 2-3 sprays per nostril q10-12h.
Neo-Synephrine Extra Strength Nasal Decongestant Drops	Phenylephrine HCl 1%	**Adults & Peds: ≥12 yrs:** Instill 2-3 drops per nostril q4h.

Table 2. ALLERGIC RHINITIS PRODUCTS (cont.)

Brand	Ingredient/Strength	Dose
Neo-Synephrine Extra Strength Nasal Spray	Phenylephrine HCl 1%	**Adults & Peds: ≥6 yrs:** Instill 2-3 sprays per nostril q4h.
Neo-Synephrine Mild Formula Nasal Spray	Phenylephrine HCl 0.25%	**Adults & Peds: ≥6 yrs:** Instill 2-3 sprays per nostril q4h.
Neo-Synephrine Regular Strength Nasal Decongestant Spray	Phenylephrine HCl 0.5%	**Adults & Peds: ≥12 yrs:** Instill 2-3 sprays per nostril q4h.
Nostrilla 12 Hour Nasal Decongestant	Oxymetazoline HCl 0.05%	**Adults & Peds: ≥6 yrs:** Instill 2-3 sprays per nostril q10-12h. **Max:** 2 doses q24h.
Vicks Sinex 12 Hour Ultra Fine Mist For Sinus Relief	Oxymetazoline HCl 0.05%	**Adults & Peds: ≥6 yrs:** Instill 2-3 sprays per nostril q10-12h. **Max:** 2 doses q24h.
Vicks Sinex Long Acting Nasal Spray For Sinus Relief	Oxymetazoline HCl 0.05%	**Adults & Peds: ≥6 yrs:** Instill 2-3 sprays per nostril q10-12h. **Max:** 2 doses per day.
Vicks Sinex Nasal Spray For Sinus Relief	Phenylephrine HCl 0.5%	**Adults & Peds: ≥12 yrs:** Instill 2-3 sprays per nostril q4h.
Zicam Extreme Congestion Relief	Oxymetazoline HCl 0.05%	**Adults & Peds: ≥6 yrs:** Instill 2-3 sprays per nostril q10-12h. **Max:** 2 doses q24h.
Zicam Intense Sinus Relief	Oxymetazoline HCl 0.05%	**Adults & Peds: ≥12 yrs:** Instill 2-3 sprays per nostril q10-12h. **Max:** 2 doses q24h.

TOPICAL NASAL MOISTURIZERS

Brand	Ingredient/Strength	Dose
4-Way Saline Moisturizing Mist	Water, Boric Acid, Glycerin, Sodium Chloride, Sodium Borate, Eucalyptol, Menthol, Polysorbate 80, Benzalkonium Chloride	**Adults & Peds: ≥2 yrs:** Instill 2-3 sprays per nostril prn.
Ayr Baby's Saline Nose Spray, Drops	Sodium Chloride 0.65%	**Peds:** Instill 2 to 6 drops in each nostril.
Ayr Saline Nasal Gel With Soothing Aloe	Water, Methyl Gluceth 10, Propylene Glycol, Glycerin, Glyceryl Polymethacrylate, Triethanolamine, Aloe Barbadensis Leaf Juice (Aloe Vera Gel), PEG/PPG 18/18 Dimethicone, Carbomer, Poloxamer 184, Sodium Chloride, Xanthan Gum, Diazolidinyl Urea, Methylparaben, Propylparaben, Glycine Soja Oil (Soybean), Geraniuim Maculatum Oil, Tocopheryl Acetate, Blue 1	**Adults & Peds: ≥12 yrs:** Apply to nostril prn.
Ayr Saline Nasal Gel, No-Drip Sinus Spray	Water, Sodium Carbomethyl Starch, Propylene Glycol, Glycerin, Aloe Barbadensis Leaf Juice (Aloe Vera Gel), Sodium Chloride, Cetyl Pyridinium Chloride, Citric Acid, Disodium EDTA, Glycine Soja (Soybean Oil), Tocopheryl Acetate, Benzyl Alcohol, Benzalkonium Chloride, Geranium Maculatum Oil	**Adults & Peds: ≥12 yrs:** Instill 1 spray in each nostril prn.
Ayr Saline Nasal Mist	Sodium Chloride 0.65%	**Adults & Peds: ≥12 yrs:** Instill 2 sprays per nostril prn.
ENTSOL Mist, Buffered Hypertonic Nasal Irrigation Mist	Purified Water, Sodium Chloride, Sodium Phosphate Dibasic Edetate Disodium, Potassium Phosphate Monobasic, Benzalkonium Chloride	**Adults & Peds: ≥12 yrs:** Instill 1-2 sprays per nostril prn.
ENTSOL Single Use, Pre-Filled Nasal Wash Squeeze Bottle	Purified Water, Sodium Chloride, Sodium Phosphate Dibasic, Potassium Phosphate Monobasic	**Adults & Peds: ≥12 yrs:** Use as directed.
ENTSOL Spray, Buffered Hypertonic Saline Nasal Spray	Purified Water, Sodium Chloride Phosphate Dibasic, Potassium Phosphate Monobasic	**Adults & Peds: ≥12 yrs:** Instill 1 spray per nostril bid, 2-6 times daily

Table 2. ALLERGIC RHINITIS PRODUCTS (cont.)

BRAND	INGREDIENT/STRENGTH	DOSE
ENTSOL Nasal Gel with Aloe and Vitamin E	Water (Purified), Propylene Glycol, Aloe, Glycerin, Dimethicone Copolyol, Poloxamer 184, Methyl Gluceth 10, Triethanolamine, Carbomer, Sodium Chloride, Vitamin E, Disodium EDTA, Xanthan Gum, Benzalkonium Chloride	**Adults & Peds:** Use prn.
Little Noses Saline Spray/Drops, Non-Medicated	Sodium Chloride 0.65%	**Peds:** 2-6 drops or sprays per nostril as directed.
Ocean Premium Saline Nasal Spray	Sodium Chloride 0.65%	**Adults & Peds: ≥6 yrs:** Instill 2 sprays per nostril prn.
Simply Saline Sterile Saline Nasal Mist	Sodium Chloride 0.9%	**Adults & Peds: ≥12 yrs:** Use prn as directed.
SinoFresh Moisturizing Nasal & Sinus Spray	Purified water, Propylene Glycol, Monobasic Sodium Phosphate, Dibasic Sodium Phosphate, Sodium Chloride, Polysorbate 80, Sorbitol Solution, Essential Oil Blend (Wintergreen Oil, Spearmint Oil, Peppermint Oil, Eucalyptus Oil) Cetylpyridinium Chloride, Benzalkonium Chloride	Adults & Peds: ≥12 yrs: Instill 1-3 sprays per nostril bid.
MISCELLANEOUS		
NasalCrom Nasal Allergy Symptom Prevention and Controller, Nasal Spray	Cromolyn Sodium 5.2mg	**Adults & Peds: ≥2 yrs:** Instill 1 spray per nostril q4-6h. **Max:** 6 doses q24h.
Similasan Hay Fever Relief, Non-Drowsy Formula, Nasal Spray	Cardiospermum HPUS 6X, Galphimia Glauca HPUS 6X, Luffa Operculata HPUS 6X, Sabadilla HPUS 6x	**Adults & Peds:** Instill 1 to 3 sprays in each nostril prn.
Zicam Allergy Relief, Homeopathic Nasal Solution, Pump	Luffa Operculata 4x, 12x, 30x, Galphimia Glauca 12x, 30x, Histaminum Hydrochloricum 12x, 30x, 200x, Sulphur 12x, 30x, 200x	**Adults & Peds: ≥6 yrs:** Instill 1 spray per nostril q4h.

Table 3. ANALGESIC PRODUCTS

BRAND NAME	INGREDIENT/STRENGTH	DOSE
ACETAMINOPHEN		
Anacin Extra Strength Aspirin Free Tablets	Acetaminophen 500mg	**Adults & Peds: ≥12 yrs:** 2 tabs q6h. **Max:** 8 tabs q24h.
Feverall Childrens' Suppositories	Acetaminophen 120mg	**Peds: 3-6 yrs:** 1-2 Supp. q4-6h. **Max:** 6 supp. q24h.
Feverall Infants' Suppositories	Acetaminophen 80mg	**Peds: 3-11 months:** 1 supp. q6h. **12-36 months:** 1 supp. q4h. **Max:** 6 supp. q24h.
Feverall Jr. Strength Suppositories	Acetaminophen 325mg	**Peds: 6-12 yrs:** 1 supp. q4-6h. **Max:** 6 supp. q24h.
Tylenol 8 Hour Caplets	Acetaminophen 650mg	**Adults & Peds: ≥12 yrs:** 2 tabs q8h prn. **Max:** 6 tabs q24h.
Tylenol 8 Hour Geltabs	Acetaminophen 650mg	**Adults & Peds: ≥12 yrs:** 2 tabs q8h prn. **Max:** 6 tabs q24h.
Tylenol Arthritis Caplets	Acetaminophen 650mg	**Adults:** 2 tabs q8h prn. **Max:** 6 tabs q24h.
Tylenol Arthritis Geltabs	Acetaminophen 650mg	**Adults:** 2 tabs q8h prn. **Max:** 6 tabs q24h.
Tylenol Children's Meltaways Tablets	Acetaminophen 80mg	**Peds: 2-3 yrs (24-35 lbs):** 2 tabs **4-5 yrs (36-47 lbs):** 3 tabs. **6-8 yrs (48-59 lbs):** 4 tabs. **9-10 yrs (60-71 lbs):** 5 tabs. **11 yrs (72-95 lbs):** 6 tabs. May repeat q4h. **Max:** 5 doses q24h.
Tylenol Children's Suspension	Acetaminophen 160mg/5mL	**Peds: 2-3 yrs (24-35 lbs):** 1 tsp (5mL). **4-5 yrs (36-47 lbs):** 1.5 tsp (7.5mL). **6-8 yrs (48-59 lbs):** 2 tsp (10mL). **9-10 yrs (60-71 lbs):** 2.5 tsp (12.5mL). **11 yrs (72-95 lbs):** 3 tsp (15mL). May repeat q4h. **Max:** 5 doses q24h.
Tylenol Extra Strength Caplets	Acetaminophen 500mg	**Adults & Peds: ≥12 yrs:** 2 tabs q4-6h prn. **Max:** 8 tabs q24h.
Tylenol Extra Strength Cool Caplets	Acetaminophen 500mg	**Adults & Peds: ≥12 yrs:** 2 tabs q4-6h prn. **Max:** 8 tabs q24h.
Tylenol Extra Strength Gelcaps	Acetaminophen 500mg	**Adults & Peds: ≥ 12 yrs:** 2 caps q4-6h prn. **Max:** 8 caps q24h.
Tylenol Rapid Blast Liquid	Acetaminophen 500mg/15mL	**Adults & Peds: ≥12 yrs:** 2 tbl (30mL) q4-6h prn. **Max:** 8 tbl (120mL) q24h.
Tylenol Extra Strength EZ Tablets	Acetaminophen 500mg	**Adults & Peds: ≥12 yrs:** 2 tabs q4-6h prn. **Max:** 8 tabs q24h.
Tylenol Extra Strength Go Tablets	Acetaminophen 500mg	**Adults & Peds: ≥12 yrs:** 2 tabs q4-6h prn. **Max:** 8 tabs q24h.
Tylenol Infants' Suspension	Acetaminophen 80mg/0.8mL	**Peds: 2-3 yrs (24-35 lbs):** 1.6 mL q4h prn. **Max:** 5 doses (8mL) q24h.
Tylenol Junior Meltaways Tablets	Acetaminophen 160mg	**Peds: 6-8 yrs (48-59 lbs):** 2 tabs. **9-10 yrs (60-71 lbs):** 2.5 tabs. **11 yrs (72-95 lbs):** 3 tabs. **12 yrs (≥96 lbs):** 4 tabs. May repeat q4h. **Max:** 5 doses q24h.
Tylenol Regular Strength Tablets	Acetaminophen 325mg	**Adults & Peds: ≥12 yrs:** 2 tabs q4-6h prn. **Max:** 12 tabs q24h. **Peds: 6-11 yrs:** 1 tab q4-6h. **Max:** 5 tabs q24h.

Table 3. ANALGESIC PRODUCTS (cont.)

Brand Name	Ingredient/Strength	Dose
ACETAMINOPHEN COMBINATIONS		
Anacin Advanced Headache Tablets	Acetaminophen/Aspirin/Caffeine 250mg-250mg-65mg	**Adults & Peds: ≥12 yrs:** 2 tabs q6h. **Max:** 8 tabs q24h.
Excedrin Back & Body Caplets	Acetaminophen/Aspirin Buffered 250mg-250mg	**Adults & Peds: ≥12 yrs:** 2 tabs q6h **Max:** 8 tabs q24h.
Excedrin Extra Strength Caplets	Acetaminophen/Aspirin/Caffeine 250mg-250mg-65mg	**Adults & Peds: ≥12 yrs:** 2 tabs q6h. **Max:** 8 tabs q24h.
Excedrin Extra Strength Geltabs	Acetaminophen/Aspirin/Caffeine 250mg-250mg-65mg	**Adults & Peds: ≥12 yrs:** 2 tabs q6h. **Max:** 8 tabs q24h.
Excedrin Extra Strength Tablets	Acetaminophen/Aspirin/Caffeine 250mg-250mg-65mg	**Adults & Peds: ≥12 yrs:** 2 tabs q6h. **Max:** 8 tabs q24h.
Excedrin Migraine Caplets	Acetaminophen/Aspirin/Caffeine 250mg-250mg-65mg	**Adults:** 2 tabs prn. **Max:** 2 tabs q24h.
Excedrin Migraine Geltabs	Acetaminophen/Aspirin/Caffeine 250mg-250mg-65mg	**Adults:** 2 tabs prn. **Max:** 2 tabs q24h.
Excedrin Migraine Tablets	Acetaminophen/Aspirin/Caffeine 250mg-250mg-65mg	**Adults:** 2 tabs prn. **Max:** 2 tabs q24h.
Excedrin Sinus Headache Caplets	Acetaminophen/Phenylephrine HCl 325mg-5mg	**Adults & Peds: ≥12 yrs:** 2 tabs q4h. **Max:** 12 tabs q24h.
Excedrin Sinus Headache Tablets	Acetaminophen/Phenylephrine HCl 325mg-5mg	**Adults & Peds: ≥12 yrs:** 2 tabs q4h. **Max:** 12 tabs q24h.
Excedrin Tension Headache Caplets	Acetaminophen/Caffeine 500mg-65mg	**Adults & Peds: ≥12 yrs:** 2 tabs q6h. **Max:** 8 tabs q24h.
Excedrin Tension Headache Geltabs	Acetaminophen/Caffeine 500mg-65mg	**Adults & Peds: ≥12 yrs:** 2 tabs q6h. **Max:** 8 tabs q24h.
Excedrin Tension Headache Tablets	Acetaminophen/Caffeine 500mg-65mg	**Adults & Peds: ≥12 yrs:** 2 tabs q6h. **Max:** 8 tabs q24h.
Goody's Extra Strength Headache Powders	Acetaminophen/Aspirin/Caffeine 260mg-520mg-32.5mg	**Adults & Peds: ≥12 yrs:** 1 powder q4-6h. **Max:** 4 powders q24h.
Midol Menstrual Headache Caplets	Acetaminophen/Caffeine 500mg-65g	**Adults & Peds: ≥12 yrs:** 2 tabs q6h. **Max:** 8 tabs q24h.
Midol Menstrual Complete Caplets	Acetaminophen/Caffeine/Pyrilamine Maleate 500mg-60mg-15mg	**Adults & Peds: ≥12 yrs:** 2 tabs q6h. **Max:** 8 tabs q24h.
Midol Menstrual Complete Gelcaps	Acetaminophen/Caffeine/Pyrilamine Maleate 500mg-60mg-15mg	**Adults & Peds: ≥12 yrs:** 2 tabs q6h. **Max:** 8 tabs q24h.
Midol Teen Formula Caplets	Acetaminophen/Pamabrom 500mg-25mg	**Adults & Peds: ≥12 yrs:** 2 tabs q6h. **Max:** 8 tabs q24h.
Pamprin Multi-Symptom Caplets	Acetaminophen/Pamabrom/Pyrilamine 500mg-25mg-15mg	**Adults & Peds: ≥12 yrs:** 2 tabs q4-6h. **Max:** 8 tabs q24h.
Premsyn PMS Caplets	Acetaminophen/Pamabrom/Pyrilamine 500mg-25mg-15mg	**Adults & Peds: ≥12 yrs:** 2 tabs q4-6h. **Max:** 8 tabs q24h.
Tylenol Women's Menstrual Relief	Acetaminophen/Pamabrom 500mg-25mg	**Adults & Peds: ≥12 yrs:** 2 tabs q4-6h. **Max:** 8 tabs q24h.
Vanquish Caplets	Acetaminophen/Aspirin/Caffeine 194mg-227mg-33mg	**Adults & Peds: ≥12 yrs:** 2 tabs q6h. **Max:** 8 tabs q24h.
ACETAMINOPHEN/SLEEP AIDS		
Excedrin PM Caplets	Acetaminophen/Diphenhydramine 500mg-38mg	**Adults & Peds: ≥12 yrs:** 2 tabs qhs.
Excedrin PM Geltabs	Acetaminophen/Diphenhydramine citrate 500mg-38 mg	**Adults & Peds: ≥12 yrs:** 2 tabs qhs.
Excedrin PM Tablets	Acetaminophen/Diphenhydramine citrate 500mg-38 mg	**Adults & Peds: ≥12 yrs:** 2 tabs qhs.
Goody's PM Powder	Acetaminophen/Diphenhydramine 1000mg-76mg/dose	**Adults & Peds: ≥12 yrs:** 1 packet (2 powders) qhs.

Table 3. ANALGESIC PRODUCTS (cont.)

Brand Name	Ingredient/Strength	Dose
Tylenol PM Caplets	Acetaminophen/Diphenhydramine 500mg-25mg	**Adults & Peds: ≥12 yrs:** 2 tabs qhs.
Tylenol PM Rapid Release Gels	Acetaminophen/Diphenhydramine 500mg-25mg	**Adults & Peds: ≥12 yrs:** 2 caps qhs.
Tylenol PM Geltabs	Acetaminophen/Diphenhydramine 500mg-25mg	**Adults & Peds: ≥12 yrs:** 2 tabs qhs.
Tylenol PM Vanilla Liquid	Acetaminophen/Diphenhydramine 1000mg-50mg/30 mL	**Adults & Peds: ≥12 yrs:** 2 tbl (30mL) qhs. **Max:** 8 tbl (120mL) q24h.
NSAIDs		
Advil Caplets	Ibuprofen 200mg	**Adults & Peds: ≥12 yrs:** 1-2 tabs q4-6h. **Max:** 6 tabs q24h.
Advil Children's Chewable Tablets	Ibuprofen 50mg	**Peds: 2-3 yr (24-35 lb):** 2 tabs q6-8h. **4-5 yr (36-47 lb):** 3 tabs q6-8h. **6-8 yr (48-59 lb):** 4 tabs q6-8h. **9-10 yr (60-71 lb):** 5 tabs q6-8h. **11 yr (72-95 lb):** 6 tabs q6-8h. **Max:** 4 doses q24h
Advil Children's Suspension	Ibuprofen 100mg/5mL	**Peds: 2-3 yrs (24-35 lbs):** 1 tsp (5mL). **4-5 yrs (36-47 lbs):** 1.5 tsp (7.5mL). **6-8 yrs (48-59 lbs):** 2 tsp (10mL). **9-10 yrs (60-71 lbs):** 2.5 tsp (12.5mL). **11 yrs (72-95 lbs):** 3 tsp (15mL). May repeat q6-8h. **Max:** 4 doses q24h.
Advil Gel Caplets	Ibuprofen 200mg	**Adults & Peds: ≥12 yrs:** 1-2 caps q4-6h. **Max:** 6 caps q24h.
Advil Infants' Concentrated Drops	Ibuprofen 50mg/1.25mL	**Peds: 6-11 months (12-17 lbs):** 1.25mL. **12-23 months (18-23 lbs):** 1.875mL. May repeat q6-8h. **Max:** 4 doses q24h.
Advil Junior Strength Swallow Tablets	Ibuprofen 100mg	**Peds: 6-10 yrs (48-71 lbs):** 2 tabs. **11 yrs (72-95 lbs):** 3 tabs. May repeat q6-8h. **Max:** 4 doses q24h.
Advil Junior Strength Chewable Tablets	Ibuprofen 100mg	**Peds: 6-8 yrs (48-59 lbs):** 2 tabs. **9-10 yrs (60-71 lbs):** 2.5 tabs. **11 yrs (72-95 lbs):** 3 tabs. May repeat q6-8h. **Max:** 4 doses q24h.
Advil Liqui-Gels	Ibuprofen 200mg	**Adults & Peds: ≥12 yrs:** 1-2 caps q4-6h. **Max:** 6 caps q24h.
Advil Migraine Capsules	Ibuprofen 200mg	**Adults:** 2 caps prn. **Max:** 2 caps q24h.
Advil Tablets	Ibuprofen 200mg	**Adults & Peds: ≥12 yrs:** 1-2 tabs q4-6h. **Max:** 6 tabs q24h.
Aleve Caplets	Naproxen Sodium 220mg	**Adults: ≥65 yrs:** 1 tab q12h. **Max:** 2 tabs q24h. **Adults & Peds: ≥12 yrs:** 1 tab q8-12h. **Max:** 3 tabs q24h.
Aleve Liquid Gels	Naproxen Sodium 220mg	**Adults & Peds: ≥12 yrs:** 1 cap q8-12h. May take 1 additional tab within 1 hour of first dose. **Max:** 3 caps q24h.
Aleve Smooth Gels	Naproxen Sodium 220mg	**Adults & Peds: ≥12 yrs:** 1 cap q8-12h. May take 1 additional tab within 1 hour of first dose. **Max:** 3 caps q24h.
Aleve Tablets	Naproxen Sodium 220mg	**Adults & Peds: ≥12 yrs:** 1 tab q8-12h. May take 1 additional tab within 1 hour of first dose. **Max::** 3 tabs q24h.
Midol Cramps and Body	Ibuprofen 200mg	**Adults & Peds: ≥12 yrs:** 1-2 tabs q4-6h. **Max:** 6 tabs q24h.

Table 3. ANALGESIC PRODUCTS (cont.)

BRAND NAME	INGREDIENT/STRENGTH	DOSE
Midol Extended Relief Caplets	Naproxen Sodium 220mg	**Adults & Peds: ≥12 yrs:** 1-2 tabs q8-12h. **Max:** 3 tabs q24h.
Motrin Children's Suspension	Ibuprofen 100mg/5mL	**Peds: 2-3 yrs (24-35 lbs):** 1 tsp (5mL). **4-5 yrs (36-47 lbs):** 1.5 tsp (7.5mL). **6-8 yrs (48-59 lbs):** 2 tsp (10mL). **9-10 yrs (60-71 lbs):** 2.5 tsp (12.5mL). **11 yrs (72-95 lbs):** 3 tsp (15mL). May repeat q6-8h. **Max:** 4 doses q24h.
Motrin IB Caplets	Ibuprofen 200mg	**Adults & Peds: ≥12 yrs:** 1-2 tabs q4-6h. **Max:** 6 tabs q24h.
Motrin IB Gelcaps	Ibuprofen 200mg	**Adults & Peds: ≥12 yrs:** 1-2 tabs q4-6h. **Max:** 6 tabs q24h.
Motrin IB Tablets	Ibuprofen 200mg	**Adults & Peds: ≥12 yrs:** 1-2 tabs q4-6h. **Max:** 6 tabs q24h.
Motrin Infants' Drops	Ibuprofen 50mg/1.25mL	**Peds: 6-11 months (12-17 lbs):** 1.25mL. **12-23 months (18-23 lbs):** 1.875mL. May repeat q6-8h. **Max:** 4 doses q24h.
Motrin Junior Strength Caplets	Ibuprofen 100mg	**Peds: 6-8 yrs (48-59 lbs):** 2 tabs. **9-10 yrs (60-71 lbs):** 2.5 tabs. **11 yrs (72-95 lbs):** 3 tabs. May repeat q6-8h. **Max:** 4 doses q24h.
Motrin Junior Strength Chewable Tablets	Ibuprofen 100mg	**Peds: 6-8 yrs (48-59 lbs):** 2 tabs. **9-10 yrs (60-71 lbs):** 2.5 tabs. **11 yrs (72-95 lbs):** 3 tabs. May repeat q6-8h. **Max:** 4 doses q24h.
Pamprin All Day Caplets	Naproxen Sodium 220mg	**Adults & Peds: ≥12 yrs:** 1-2 tabs q8-12h. **Max:** 3 tabs q24h.
SALICYLATES		
Anacin 81 Tablets	Aspirin 81mg	**Adults & Peds: ≥12 yrs:** 2 tabs q6h. **Max:** 8 tabs q24h.
Aspergum Chewable Tablets	Aspirin 227mg	**Adults & Peds: ≥12 yrs:** 2 tabs q4h. **Max:** 16 tabs q24h.
Bayer Aspirin Extra Strength Caplets	Aspirin 500mg	**Adults & Peds: ≥12 yrs:** 1-2 tabs q4-6h. **Max:** 8 tabs q24h.
Bayer Aspirin Safety Coated Caplets	Aspirin 325mg	**Adults & Peds: ≥12 yrs:** 1-2 tabs q4h. **Max:** 12 tabs q24h.
Bayer Children's Aspirin Chewable Tablets	Aspirin 81mg	**Adults & Peds: ≥12 yrs:** 4-8 tabs q4h. **Max:** 48 tabs q24h.
Bayer Low Dose Aspirin Tablets	Aspirin 81mg	**Adults & Peds: ≥12 yrs:** 4-8 tabs q4h. **Max:** 48 tabs q24h.
Bayer Sugar Free Low Dose Aspirin Tablets	Aspirin 81mg	**Adults & Peds: ≥12 yrs:** 4-8 tabs q4h. **Max:** 48 tabs q24h.
Bayer Genuine Aspirin Tablets	Aspirin 325mg	**Adults & Peds: ≥12 yrs:** 1-2 tabs q4h or 3 tabs q6h. **Max:** 12 tabs q24h.
Bayer Extra-Strength Plus Caplets	Aspirin 500mg Buffered with Calcium Carbonate 500mg	**Adults & Peds: ≥12 yrs:** 1-2 tabs q4-6h. **Max:** 8 tabs q24h.
Doan's Caplets	Magnesium Salicylate Tetrahydrate 580mg	**Adults & Peds: ≥12 yrs:** 2 tabs q4h. **Max:** 12 tabs q24h.
Ecotrin Low Strength Tablets	Aspirin 81mg	**Adults:** 4-8 tabs q4h. **Max:** 48 tabs q24h.
Ecotrin Regular Strength Tablets	Aspirin 325mg	**Adults & Peds: ≥12 yrs:** 1-2 tabs q4h. **Max:** 12 tabs q24h.
Ecotrin Maximum Strength Tablets	Aspirin 500mg	**Adults & Peds: ≥12 yrs:** 2 tabs q6h. **Max:** 8 tabs q24h.

Table 3. ANALGESIC PRODUCTS (cont.)

BRAND NAME	INGREDIENT/STRENGTH	DOSE
Halfprin 162mg Tablets	Aspirin 162mg	**Adults & Peds: ≥12 yrs:** 2-4 tabs q4h. **Max:** 24 tabs q24h.
Halfprin 81mg Tablets	Aspirin 81mg	**Adults & Peds: ≥12 yrs:** 4-8 tabs q4h. **Max:** 48 tabs q24h.
St. Joseph Chewable Aspirin Tablets	Aspirin 81mg	**Adults & Peds: ≥12 yrs:** 4-8 tabs q4h. **Max:** 48 tabs q24h.
St. Joseph Enteric Safety-Coated Tablets	Aspirin 81mg	**Adults & Peds: ≥12 yrs:** 4-8 tabs q4h. **Max:** 48 tabs q24h.
SALICYLATES, BUFFERED		
Alka-Seltzer Original Effervescent Tablets	Aspirin/Citric Acid/Sodium Bicarbonate 325mg-1000mg-1916mg	**Adults & Peds: ≥12 yrs:** 2 tabs q4h. **Max:** 8 tabs q24h.
Alka-Seltzer Extra Strength Effervescent Tablets	Aspirin/Citric Acid/Sodium Bicarbonate 500mg-1000mg-1985mg	**Adults & Peds: ≥12 yrs:** 2 tabs q6h. **Max:** 7 tabs q24h.
Ascriptin Regular Strength Tablets	Aspirin Buffered with Maalox/Calcium Carbonate 325mg	**Adults & Peds: ≥12 yrs:** 2 tabs q4h. **Max:** 12 tabs q24h.
Bayer Extra Strength Plus Caplets	Aspirin Buffered with Calcium Carbonate 500mg	**Adults & Peds: ≥12 yrs:** 1-2 tabs q4-6h. **Max:** 8 tabs q24h.
Bufferin Extra Strength Tablets	Aspirin Buffered with Calcium Carbonate/Magnesium Oxide/Magnesium Carbonate 500mg	**Adults & Peds: ≥12 yrs:** 2 tabs q6h. **Max:** 8 tabs q24h.
Bufferin Tablets	Aspirin Buffered with Calcium Carbonate/Magnesium Oxide/Magnesium Carbonate 325mg	**Adults & Peds: ≥12 yrs:** 2 tabs q4h. **Max:** 12 tabs q24h.
SALICYLATE COMBINATIONS		
Alka-Seltzer Morning Relief Effervescent Tablets	Aspirin/Caffeine 500mg-65mg	**Adults & Peds: ≥12 yrs:** 2 tabs q6h. **Max:** 8 tabs q24h. **≥60 yrs: Max:** 4 tabs q24h.
Anacin Max Strength Tablets	Aspirin/Caffeine 500mg-32mg	**Adults & Peds: ≥12 yrs:** 2 tabs q6h. **Max:** 8 tabs q24h.
Anacin Tablets	Aspirin/Caffeine 400mg-32mg	**Adults & Peds: ≥12 yrs:** 2 tabs q6h. **Max:** 8 tabs q24h.
Bayer Back & Body Pain Caplets	Aspirin/Caffeine 500mg-32.5mg	**Adults & Peds: ≥12 yrs:** 2 tabs q6h. **Max:** 8 tabs q24h.
BC Arthritis Strength Powders	Aspirin/Caffeine/Salicylamide 742mg-38mg-222mg	**Adults & Peds: ≥12 yrs:** 1 powder q3-4h. **Max:** 4 powders q24h.
BC Original Formula Powders	Aspirin/Caffeine/Salicylamide 650mg-33.3mg-195mg	**Adults & Peds: ≥12 yrs:** 1 powder q3-4h. **Max:** 4 powders q24h.
SALICYLATE/SLEEP AID		
Alka-Seltzer PM Effervescent Tablets	Aspirin/Diphenhydramine Citrate 325mg-38 mg	**Adults & Peds: ≥12 yrs:** 2 tabs qhs.
Bayer PM Caplets	Aspirin/Diphenhydramine 500mg-38.3mg	**Adults & Peds: ≥12 yrs:** 2 tabs qhs.
Doan's Extra Strength PM Caplets	Magnesium Salicylate Tetrahydrate/Diphenhydramine 580mg-25mg	**Adults & Peds: ≥12 yrs:** 2 tabs qhs.

Table 4. ANTACID AND HEARTBURN PRODUCTS

BRAND	INGREDIENT/STRENGTH	DOSE
ANTACID		
Alka-Seltzer Gold Tablets	Citric Acid/Potassium Bicarbonate/ Sodium Bicarbonate 1000mg-344mg-1050mg	**Adults: ≥60 yrs:** 2 tabs q4h prn. **Max:** 6 tabs q24h. **Adults & Peds: ≥12 yrs:** 2 tabs q4h prn. **Max:** 8 tabs q24h. **Peds: ≤12 yrs:** 1 tab q4h prn. **Max:** 4 tabs q24h.
Alka-Seltzer Heartburn Relief Tablets	Citric Acid/Sodium Bicarbonate 1000mg-1940mg	**Adults: ≥60 yrs:** 2 tabs q4h prn. **Max:** 4 tabs q24h. **Adults & Peds: ≥12 yrs:** 2 tabs q4h prn. **Max:** 8 tabs q24h.
Alka-Seltzer Tablets, Original	Aspirin/Sodium Bicarbonate/Citric Acid 325mg-1916mg-1000mg	**Adults: ≥60 yrs:** 2 tabs q4h prn. **Max:** 4 tabs q24h. **Adults & Peds: ≥12 yrs:** 2 tabs q4h prn. **Max:** 8 tabs q24h.
Alka-Seltzer Tablets, Extra-Strength	Aspirin/Sodium Bicarbonate/Citric Acid 500mg-1985mg-1000mg	**Adults: ≥60 yrs:** 2 tabs q6h prn. **Max:** 3 tabs q24h. **Adults & Peds: ≥12 yrs:** 2 tabs q6h prn. **Max:** 7 tabs q24h.
Brioschi Powder	Sodium Bicarbonate/Tartaric Acid 2.69g-2.43g/dose	**Adults & Peds: ≥12 yrs:** 1 capful (6g) dissolved in 4-6 oz water q1h. **Max:** 6 doses q24h.
Gaviscon Extra Strength Liquid	Aluminum Hydroxide/Magnesium Carbonate 254mg-237.5mg/5mL	**Adults:** 2-4 tsp (10-20mL) qid.
Gaviscon Extra Strength Tablets	Aluminum Hydroxide/Magnesium Carbonate 160mg-105mg	**Adults:** 2-4 tabs qid. **Max:** 16 doses q24h.
Gaviscon Regular Strength Chewable Tablets	Aluminum Hydroxide/Magnesium Carbonate 80mg-20mg	**Adults:** 2-4 tabs qid. **Max:** 16 tabs q24h.
Gaviscon Regular Strength Liquid	Aluminum Hydroxide/Magnesium Carbonate 95mg-358mg/15mL	**Adults:** 1-2 tbl (15-30mL) qid.
Gaviscon Acid Breakthrough, Chewable Tablets	Calcium Carbonate 500mg	**Adults:** 2 tabs prn. **Max:** 15 tabs q24h.
Maalox Antacid Barrier Chewable Tablets	Calcium Carbonate 500mg	**Adults:** 2-4 tabs qid. **Max:** 16 tabs q24h.
Maalox Quick Dissolve Regular Strength Chewable Tablets	Calcium Carbonate 600mg	**Adults:** 1-2 tabs prn. **Max:** 12 tabs q24h.
Mylanta, Children's	Calcium Carbonate 400 mg	**Peds: 6-11 yrs (48-95 lbs):** Take 2 tab prn. **Max:** 6 tabs q24h. **Peds: 2-5 yrs (24-47 lbs):** Take 1 tab prn. **Max:** 3 tabs q24h.
Mylanta Ultimate Strength Liquid	Aluminum Hydroxide/Magnesium Hydroxide 500mg-500mg/5mL	**Adults & Peds ≥12 yrs:** 2-4 tsp (10-20mL) qid (between meals & hs). **Max:** 9 tsp (45mL) q24h for ≤2 weeks.
Mylanta Supreme Antacid Liquid	Calcium Carbonate/Magnesium Hydroxide 400mg-135mg/5mL	**Adults:** 2-4 tsp (10-20mL) qid. **Max:** 18 tsp (90mL) q24h.
Mylanta Ultimate Strength Chewable Tablets	Calcium Carbonate/Magnesium Hydroxide 700mg-300mg	**Adults:** 2-4 tabs qid. (between meals & hs). **Max:** 10 tabs q24h for ≤2 weeks.
Phillips Milk of Magnesia Liquid	Magnesium Hydroxide 400mg/5mL	**Adults & Peds: ≥12 yrs:** 30-60mL qd. **Peds: 6-11 yrs:** 15-30mL qd. **2-5 yrs:** 5-15mL qd.
Rolaids Extra Strength Softchews	Calcium Carbonate 1177mg	**Adults:** 2-3 chews q1h prn. **Max:** 6 chews q24h.
Rolaids Extra Strength Tablets	Calcium Carbonate/Magnesium Hydroxide 675mg-135mg	**Adults:** 2-4 tabs q1h prn. **Max:** 10 tabs q24h.
Rolaids Tablets	Calcium Carbonate/Magnesium Hydroxide 550mg-110mg	**Adults:** 2-4 tabs q1h prn. **Max:** 12 tabs q24h.
Titralac Chewable Tablets	Calcium Carbonate 420mg	**Adults:** 2 tabs q2-3h prn. **Max:** 19 tabs q24h.

Table 4. ANTACID AND HEARTBURN PRODUCTS (cont.)

BRAND	INGREDIENT/STRENGTH	DOSE
Tums Chewable Tablets	Calcium Carbonate 500mg	**Adults:** 2-4 tabs q1h prn. **Max:** 15 tabs q24h.
Tums E-X Chewable Tablets	Calcium Carbonate 750mg	**Adults:** 2-4 tabs prn. **Max:** 10 tabs q24h.
Tums E-X Sugar Free Chewable Tablets	Calcium Carbonate 750mg	**Adults:** 2-4 tabs prn. **Max:** 10 tabs q24h.
Tums Kids Chewable Tablets	Calcium Carbonate 750mg	**Peds: .4 yrs (.49 lbs):** Take 1 tab tid. **Max:** 4 tabs q24h. **Peds: 2-4 yrs (24-47 lbs):** Take ½ tab bid. **Max:** 2 tabs q24h.
Tums Smoothies Tablets	Calcium Carbonate 750mg	**Adults:** 2-4 tabs prn. **Max:** 10 tabs q24h.
Tums Ultra 1000 Chewable Tablets	Calcium Carbonate 1000mg	**Adults:** 2-4 tabs prn. **Max:** 7 tabs q24h for ≤2 weeks.

ANTACID/ANTIFLATULENT

BRAND	INGREDIENT/STRENGTH	DOSE
Gas-X with Maalox Capsules	Calcium Carbonate/Simethicone 250mg-62.5mg	**Adults:** 2-4 caps prn. **Max:** 8 caps q24h.
Gas-X Extra Strength with Maalox Capsules	Calcium Carbonate/Simethicone 500mg-125mg	**Adults:** 1-2 caps prn. **Max:** 4 caps q24h.
Gelusil Chewable Tablets	Aluminum Hydroxide/Magnesium Hydroxide/Simethicone 200mg-200mg-20mg	**Adults:** 2-4 tabs qid.
Maalox Max Liquid	Aluminum Hydroxide/Magnesium Hydroxide/Simethicone 400mg-400mg-40mg/5mL	**Adults & Peds: ≥12 yrs:** 2-4 tsp (10-20mL) qid. **Max:** 12 tsp (60mL) q24h.
Maalox Max Chewable Tablets	Calcium Carbonate/Simethicone 100mg-60mg	**Adults:** 1-2 tabs prn. **Max:** 8 tabs q24h.
Maalox Regular Strength Liquid	Aluminum Hydroxide/Magnesium Hydroxide/Simethicone 200mg-200mg-20mg/5mL	**Adults & Peds: ≥12 yrs:** 2-4 tsp (10-20mL) qid. **Max:** 12 tsp (60mL) q24h.
Mylanta Maximum Strength Liquid	Aluminum Hydroxide/Magnesium Hydroxide/Simethicone 400mg-400mg-40mg/5mL	**Adults & Peds: ≥12 yrs:** 2-4 tsp (10-20mL) qid. **Max:** 12 tsp (60mL) q24h.
Mylanta Regular Strength Liquid	Aluminum Hydroxide/Magnesium Hydroxide/Simethicone 200mg-200mg-20mg/5mL	**Adults & Peds: ≥12 yrs:** 2-4 tsp (10-20mL) qid. **Max:** 12 tsp (60mL) q24h.
Rolaids Multi-Symptom Chewable Tablets	Calcium Carbonate/Magnesium Hydroxide/Simethicone 675mg-135mg-60mg	**Adults:** 2 tabs qid prn. **Max:** 8 tabs q24h.
Titralac Plus Chewable Tablets	Calcium Carbonate/Simethicone 420mg-21mg	**Adults:** 2 tabs q2-3h prn. **Max:** 19 tabs q24h.

BISMUTH SUBSALICYLATE

BRAND	INGREDIENT/STRENGTH	DOSE
Maalox Total Stomach Relief Maximum Strength Liquid	Bismuth Subsalicylate 525mg/15mL	**Adults & Peds: ≥12 yrs:** 2 tbl (30mL) q1/2-1h. **Max:** 8 tbl (120mL) q24h.
Pepto Bismol Chewable Tablets	Bismuth Subsalicylate 262mg	**Adults & Peds: ≥12 yrs:** 2 tabs q1/2-1h. **Max:** 8 doses q24h.
Pepto Bismol Caplets	Bismuth Subsalicylate 262mg	**Adults & Peds: ≥12 yrs:** 2 tabs q1/2-1h. **Max:** 8 doses q24h.
Pepto Bismol Liquid	Bismuth Subsalicylate 262mg/15mL	**Adults & Peds: ≥12 yrs:** 2 tbl (30mL) q1/2-1h. **Max:** 8 doses (240mL) q24h.
Pepto Bismol Maximum Strengtth Liquid	Bismuth Subsalicylate 525mg/15mL	**Adults & Peds: ≥12 yrs:** 2 tbl (30mL) q1h. **Peds: 9-12 yrs:** 1 tbl (15mL) q1h. **6-9 yrs:** 2 tsp (10mL) q1h. **3-6 yrs:** 1 tsp (5mL). **Max:** 8 doses (240mL) q24h.

Table 4. ANTACID AND HEARTBURN PRODUCTS (cont.)

BRAND	INGREDIENT/STRENGTH	DOSE
H₂-RECEPTOR ANTAGONIST		
Pepcid AC Chewable Tablets	Famotidine 10mg	**Adults & Peds: ≥12 yrs:** 1 tab qd. **Max:** 2 tabs q24h.
Pepcid AC Gelcaps	Famotidine 10mg	**Adults & Peds: ≥12 yrs:** 1 tab qd. **Max:** 2 tabs q24h.
Pepcid AC Maximum Strength EZ Chews	Famotidine 20mg	**Adults & Peds: ≥12 yrs:** 1 tab qd. **Max:** 2 tabs q24h.
Pepcid AC Maximum Strength Tablets	Famotidine 20mg	**Adults & Peds: ≥12 yrs:** 1 tab qd. **Max:** 2 tabs q24h.
Pepcid AC Tablets	Famotidine 10mg	**Adults & Peds: ≥12 yrs:** 1 tab qd. **Max:** 2 tabs q24h.
Tagamet HB Tablets	Cimetidine 200mg	**Adults & Peds: ≥12 yrs:** 1 tab qd. **Max:** 2 tabs q24h.
Zantac 150 Tablets	Ranitidine 150mg	**Adults & Peds: ≥12 yrs:** 1 tab qd. **Max:** 2 tabs q24h.
Zantac 75 Tablets	Ranitidine 75mg	**Adults & Peds: ≥12 yrs:** 1 tab qd. **Max:** 2 tabs q24h.
H₂-RECEPTOR ANTAGONIST/ANTACID		
Pepcid Complete Chewable Tablets	Famotidine/Calcium Carbonate/ Magnesium Hydroxide 10mg-800mg-165mg	**Adults & Peds: ≥12 yrs:** 1 tab qd. **Max:** 2 tabs q24h.
PROTON PUMP INHIBITOR		
Prilosec OTC Tablets	Omeprazole 20mg	**Adults:** 1 tab qd x 14 days. May repeat 14 day course q 4 months.

Table 5. ANTIDIARRHEAL PRODUCTS

Brand Name	Ingredient/Strength	Dose
ABSORBENT AGENTS		
Equalactin Chewable Tablets	Calcium Polycarbophil 625mg	**Adults:** ≥12 yrs: 2 tabs q30min prn. **Max:** 8 tabs q24h. **Peds:** 6-12 yrs: 1 tab q30min. **Max:** 4 tabs q24h. **2 to ≥6 yrs:** 1 tab q30min. **Max:** 2 tabs q24h.
Fibercon Caplets	Calcium Polycarbophil 625mg	**Adults:** ≥12 yrs: 2 tabs qd. **Max:** 8 tabs q24h.
Konsyl Fiber Caplets	Calcium Polycarbophil 625mg	**Adults:** ≥12 yrs: 2 tabs qd. **Max:** 8 tabs q24h. **Peds:** 6-12 yrs: 1 tab qd. **Max:** 3 tabs q24h.
ANTIPERISTALTIC AGENTS		
Imodium A-D Caplet	Loperamide HCl 2mg	**Adults:** ≥12 yrs: 2 caplets after first loose stool; 1 caplet after each subsequent loose stool. **Max:** 4 caplets q24h. **Peds:** 9-11 yrs (60-95 lbs): 1 caplet after first loose stool; ½ caplet after each subsequent loose stool. **Max:** 3 caplets q24h. **6-8 yrs (48-59 lbs):** 1 caplet after first loose stool; ½ caplet after each subsequent loose stool. **Max:** 2 caplets q24h.
Imodium A-D E-Z Chews	Loperamide HCl 2mg	**Adults:** ≥12 yrs: 2 caplets after first loose stool; 1 caplet after each subsequent loose stool. **Max:** 4 caplets q24h. **Peds:** 9-11 yrs (60-95 lbs): 1 caplet after first loose stool; ½ caplet after each subsequent loose stool. **Max:** 3 caplets q24h. **6-8 yrs (48-59 lbs):** 1 caplet after first loose stool; ½ caplet after each subsequent loose stool. **Max:** 2 caplets q24h.
Imodium A-D Liquid	Loperamide HCl 1mg/7.5mL	**Adults:** ≥12 yrs: 30mL (6 tsp) after first loose stool; 15mL (3 tsp) after each subsequent loose stool. **Max:** 60mL (12 tsp) q24h. **Peds:** 9-11 yrs (60-95 lbs): 15mL (3 tsp) after first loose stool; 7.5mL (1½ tsp) after each subsequent loose stool. **Max:** 45mL (9 tsp) q24h. **6-8 yrs (48-59 lbs):**15 mL (3 tsp) after first loose stool; 7.5mL (1½ tsp) after each subsequent loose stool. **Max:** 30mL (6 tsp) q24h.
ANTIPERISTALTIC/ANTIFLATULENT AGENTS		
Imodium Advanced Caplet	Loperamide HCl/Simethicone 2mg-125mg	**Adults:** ≥12 yrs: 2 caplets after first loose stool; 1 caplet after each subsequent loose stool. **Max:** 4 caplets q24h. **Peds:** 9-11 yrs (60-95 lbs): 1 caplet after first loose stool; ½ caplet after each subsequent loose stool. **Max:** 3 caplets q24h. **6-8 yrs (48-59 lbs):** 1 caplet after first loose stool; ½ caplet after each subsequent loose stool. **Max:** 2 caplets q24h.
ANTIPERISTALTIC/ANTIFLATULENT AGENTS		
Imodium Advanced Chewable Tablet	Loperamide HCl/Simethicone 2mg-125mg	**Adults:** ≥12 yrs: 2 caplets after first loose stool; 1 caplet after each subsequent loose stool. **Max:** 4 caplets q24h. **Peds:** 9-11 yrs (60-95 lbs): 1 caplet after first loose stool; ½ caplet after each subsequent loose stool. **Max:** 3 caplets q24h. **6-8 yrs (48-59 lbs):** 1 caplet after first loose stool; ½ caplet after each subsequent loose stool. **Max:** 2 caplets q24h.
BISMUTH SUBSALICYLATE		
Kaopectate Caplets	Bismuth Subsalicylate 262mg	**Adults & Peds:** ≥12 yrs: 2 caplets q½-1h prn. **Max:** 8 doses q24h.
Kaopectate Extra Strength Liquid	Bismuth Subsalicylate 525mg/15mL	**Adults:** ≥12 yrs: 2 tbl (30mL). **Peds:** 9-12 yrs: 1 tbl (15mL) q1h prn. **6-9 yrs:** 2 tsp (10mL) q1h prn. **3-6 yrs:** 1 tsp (5mL) q1h prn. **Max:** 8 doses q24h.

Table 5. ANTIDIARRHEAL PRODUCTS (cont.)

BRAND NAME	INGREDIENT/STRENGTH	DOSE
Kaopectate Liquid	Bismuth Subsalicylate 262mg/15mL	**Adults: ≥12 yrs:** 2 tbl (30mL). **Peds: 9-12 yrs:** 1 tbl (15mL) q1h prn. **6-9 yrs:** 2 tsp (10mL) q1h prn. **3-6 yrs:** 1 tsp (5mL) q1h prn. **Max:** 8 doses q24h.
Pepto Bismol Chewable Tablets	Bismuth Subsalicylate 262mg	**Adults & Peds: ≥12 yrs:** 2 tabs q½-1h. **Max:** 8 doses (16 tabs) q24h.
Pepto Bismol Caplets	Bismuth Subsalicylate 262mg	**Adults & Peds: ≥12 yrs:** 2 tabs q½-1h. **Max:** 8 doses (16 caps) q24h.
Pepto Bismol Liquid	Bismuth Subsalicylate 262mg/15mL	**Adults & Peds: ≥12 yrs:** 2 tbl (30mL) q½-1h prn. **Max:** 8 doses (16 tbl) q24h.
Pepto Bismol Maximum Strength	Bismuth Subsalicylate 525mg/15mL	**Adults: ≥12 yrs:** 2 tbl (30mL) q1h prn. **Max:** 4 doses (8 tbl) q24h.

Table 6. ANTIFLATULANT PRODUCTS

BRAND NAME	INGREDIENT/STRENGTH	DOSE
ALPHA-GALACTOSIDASE		
Beano Food Enzyme Dietary Supplement Drops	Alpha-Galactosidase Enzyme 150 GalU	**Adults:** Add 5 drops before meals.
Beano Food Enzyme Dietary Supplement Tablets	Alpha-Galactosidase Enzyme 150 GalU	**Adults:** Take 3 tabs before meals.
ANTACID/ANTIFLATULENCE		
Gas-X with Maalox Capsules	Calcium Carbonate/Simethicone 250mg-62.5mg	**Adults:** 2-4 caps prn. **Max:** 8 caps q24h.
Gas-X Extra Strength with Maalox Capsules	Calcium Carbonate/Simethicone 500mg-125mg	**Adults:** 1-2 caps prn. **Max:** 4 caps q24h.
Gelusil Chewable Tablets	Aluminum Hydroxide/Magnesium Hydroxide/Simethicone 200mg-200mg-20mg	**Adults:** 2-4 tabs qid.
Maalox Max Liquid	Aluminum Hydroxide/Magnesium Hydroxide/Simethicone 400mg-400mg-40mg/5mL	**Adults & Peds: ≥12 yrs:** 2 -4 tsp (10-20mL) qid. **Max:** 12 tsp (60mL) q24h.
Maalox Max Chewable Tablets	Calcium Carbonate/Simethicone 100mg-60mg	**Adults:** 1-2 tabs prn. **Max:** 8 tabs q24h.
Maalox Regular Strength Liquid	Aluminum Hydroxide/Magnesium Hydroxide/Simethicone 200mg-200mg-20mg/5mL	**Adults & Peds: ≥12 yrs:** - 4 tsp (10-20mL) qid. **Max:** 12 tsp (60mL) q24h.
Mylanta Maximum Strength Liquid	Aluminum Hydroxide/Magnesium Hydroxide/Simethicone 400mg-400mg-40mg/5mL	**Adults & Peds: ≥12 yrs:** 2-4 tsp (10-20mL) qid. **Max:** 12 tsp (60mL) q24h.
Mylanta Regular Strength Liquid	Aluminum Hydroxide/Magnesium Hydroxide/Simethicone 200mg-200mg-20mg/5mL	**Adults & Peds: ≥12 yrs:** 2-4 tsp (10-20mL) qid. **Max:** 24 tsp (120mL) q24h.
Rolaids Antacid & Antigas Soft Chews	Calcium Carbonate/Simethicone 1177mg-80mg	**Adults:** 2-3 chews hourly prn.
Titralac Plus Chewable Tablets	Calcium Carbonate/Simethicone 420mg-21mg	**Adults:** 2 tabs q2-3h prn. **Max:** 19 tabs q24h.
SIMETHICONE		
GasAid Maximum Strength Anti-Gas Softgels	Simethicone 125mg	**Adults:** Take 1-2 caps prn and qhs. **Max:** 4 caps q24h.
Gas-X Infant Drops	Simethicone 20mg/0.3mL	**Peds: ≥2 yrs (≥24 lbs):** 0.6mL prn. **Peds: <2 yrs (<24 lbs):** 0.3mL prn. **Max:** 6 doses q24h.
Gas-X Children's Thin Strips	Simethicone 40mg hs.	**Peds: 2-12 yrs:** 1 strip prn and **Max:** 6 strips q24h.
Gas-X Thin Strips	Simethicone 62.5mg	**Adults:** Allow 2-4 strips to dissolve prn. **Max:** 8 strips q24h.
Gas-X Antigas Chewable Tablets	Simethicone 80mg	**Adults:** Take 1-2 caps prn and qhs. **Max:** 6 caps q24h.
Gas-X Extra Strength Antigas Softgels	Simethicone 125mg	**Adults:** Take 1-2 caps prn and qhs. **Max:** 4 caps q24h.
Gas-X Maximum Strength Antigas Softgels	Simethicone 166mg	**Adults:** Take 1-2 caps prn and qhs. **Max:** 3 caps q24h.
Little Tummys Gas Relief Drops	Simethicone 20mg/0.3mL	**Peds: ≥2 yrs (≥24 lbs):** 0.6mL prn (after meals & hs). **Peds: <2 yrs (<24 lbs):** 0.3mL prn (after meals & hs). **Max:** 12 doses q24h.
Mylanta Gas Maximum Strength Softgels	Simethicone 125mg	**Adults:** Chew 1-2 tabs (after meals & hs). **Max:** 4 tabs q24h.
Mylanta Gas Maximum Strength Chewable Tablets	Simethicone 125mg	**Adults:** Chew 1-2 tabs (after meals & hs). **Max:** 4 tabs q24h.
Mylicon Infant's Gas Relief Drops	Simethicone 20mg/0.3mL	**Peds: ≥2 yrs (≥24 lbs):** 0.6mL (after meals & hs). **Peds: <2 yrs (<24 lbs):** 0.3mL (after meals & hs). **Max:** 12 doses q24h.

Table 7. ANTIFUNGAL PRODUCTS

BRAND	INGREDIENT/STRENGTH	DOSE
BUTENAFINE		
Lotrimin Ultra Antifungal Cream	Butenafine HCl 1%	**Adults & Peds ≥12 yrs:** Use bid.
CLOTRIMAZOLE		
FungiCure Anti-Fungal Liquid Spray	Clotrimazole 1%	**Adults & Peds:** Use bid.
Lotrimin AF Antifungal Athlete's Foot Cream	Clotrimazole 1%	**Adults & Peds ≥2 yrs:** Use bid.
Lotrimin AF Antifungal Athlete's Foot Topical Solution	Clotrimazole 1%	**Adults & Peds ≥2 yrs:** Use bid.
Lotrimin AF For Her Antifungal Cream	Clotrimazole 1%	**Adults & Peds ≥2 yrs:** Use bid.
MICONAZOLE		
Clearly Confident Triple Action Fungus Treatment	Miconazole Nitrate 2%	**Adults:** Apply to affected area bid.
Desenex Antifungal Liquid Spray	Miconazole Nitrate 2%	**Adults:** Use bid.
Desenex Antifungal Powder	Miconazole Nitrate 2%	**Adults:** Use bid.
Desenex Antifungal Spray	Miconazole Nitrate 2%	**Adults:** Use bid.
DiabetAid Antifungal Foot Bath Tablets	Miconazole Nitrate 2%	**Adults & Peds ≥2 yrs:** Use prn.
Diabet-X Antifungal Skin Treatment Cream	Miconazole Nitrate 2%	**Adults & Peds ≥2 yrs:** Use prn.
Lotrimin AF Antifungal Aerosol Liquid Spray	Miconazole Nitrate 2%	**Adults & Peds ≥2 yrs:** Use bid.
Lotrimin AF Antifungal Jock Itch Aerosol Powder Spray	Miconazole Nitrate 2%	**Adults & Peds ≥2 yrs:** Use bid.
Lotrimin AF Antifungal Powder	Miconazole Nitrate 2%	**Adults & Peds ≥2 yrs:** Use bid.
Micatin Athlete's Foot Cream	Miconazole Nitrate 2%	**Adults:** Use bid.
Micatin Athlete's Foot Spray Liquid	Miconazole Nitrate 2%	**Adults:** Use bid.
Micatin Athlete's Foot Spray Liquid	Miconazole Nitrate 2%	**Adults:** Use bid.
Micatin Jock Itch Spray Powder	Miconazole Nitrate 2%	**Adults:** Use bid.
Micatin Jock Itch Antifungal Cream	Miconazole Nitrate 2%	**Adults:** Use bid.
Neosporin AF Antifungal Cream	Miconazole Nitrate 2%	**Adults & Peds ≥12 yrs:** Use bid.
Neosporin AF Athlete's Foot Antifungal Spray Liquid	Miconazole Nitrate 2%	**Adults & Peds ≥12 yrs:** Use bid.
Neosporin AF Athlete's Foot Antifungal Spray Powder	Miconazole Nitrate 2%	**Adults & Peds ≥12 yrs:** Use bid.
Neosporin AF Jock Itch Antifungal Cream	Miconazole Nitrate 2%	**Adults & Peds ≥12 yrs:** Use bid.
Zeasorb Super Absorbent Antifungal Powder	Miconazole Nitrate 2%	**Adults & Peds:** Use bid.
TERBINAFINE		
Lamisil AT Antifungal Cream	Terbinafine HCl 1%	**Adults & Peds ≥12 yrs:** Use bid.
Lamisil AT Antifungal Spray Pump	Terbinafine HCl 1%	**Adults & Peds ≥12 yrs:** Use qd or bid.
Lamisil AT Athlete's Foot Cream	Terbinafine HCl 1%	**Adults & Peds ≥12 yrs:** Use bid.
Lamisil AT Athlete's Foot Gel	Terbinafine HCl 1%	**Adults & Peds ≥12 yrs:** Use qd.
Lamisil AT Athlete's Foot Spray Pump	Terbinafine HCl 1%	**Adults & Peds ≥12 yrs:** Use bid.
Lamisil AT for Women Cream	Terbinafine HCl 1%	**Adults & Peds ≥12 yrs:** Use bid.
Lamisil AT Jock Itch Cream	Terbinafine HCl 1%	**Adults & Peds ≥12 yrs:** Use qd.
Lamisil AT Jock Itch Spray Pump	Terbinafine HCl 1%	**Adults & Peds ≥12 yrs:** Use qd.

Table 7. ANTIFUNGAL PRODUCTS (cont.)

BRAND	INGREDIENT/STRENGTH	DOSE
TOLNAFTATE		
Aftate Antifungal Liquid Spray for Athlete's Foot	Tolnaftate 1%	**Adults:** Use qd-bid
FungiCure Anti-Fungal Gel	Tolnaftate 1%	**Adults & Peds:** Use bid.
Gold Bond Antifungal Foot Swabs	Tolnaftate 1%	**Adults & Peds:** Use bid.
Miracle of Aloe Miracure Anti-Fungal	Tolnaftate 1%	**Adults & Peds ≥12 yrs:** Use bid.
Swabplus Foot Care Fungus Relief Swabs	Tolnaftate 1%	**Adults & Peds:** Use bid.
Tinactin Antifungal Deodorant Powder Spray	Tolnaftate 1%	**Adults & Peds:** Use bid.
Tinactin Antifungal Liquid Spray	Tolnaftate 1%	**Adults & Peds:** Use bid.
Tinactin Antifungal Powder Spray	Tolnaftate 1%	**Adults & Peds:** Use bid.
Tinactin Antifungal Cream	Tolnaftate 1%	**Adults & Peds:** Use bid.
Tinactin Antifungal Absorbent Powder	Tolnaftate 1%	**Adults & Peds:** Use qd-tid.
Tinactin Antifungal Jock Itch Powder Spray	Tolnaftate 1%	**Adults & Peds:** Use qd-tid.
UNDECYLENIC ACID		
Fungi Nail Anti-fungal Solution	Undecylenic Acid 25%	**Adults & Peds:** Use bid.
FungiCure Anti-fungal Liquid	Undecylenic Acid 10%	**Adults & Peds:** Use bid.
Tineacide Antifungal Cream	Undecylenic Acid 10%	**Adults & Peds ≥12 yrs:** Use bid.

Table 8. ANTIPYRETIC PRODUCTS

BRAND	INGREDIENT/STRENGTH	DOSE
ACETAMINOPHEN		
Anacin Aspirin Free Extra Strength Tablets	Acetaminophen 500mg	**Adults & Peds: ≥12 yrs:** 2 tabs q6h. **Max:** 8 tabs q24h.
Feverall Childrens' Suppositories	Acetaminophen 120mg	**Peds: 3-6 yrs:** 1-2 supp. q4-6h. **Max:** 6 supp q24h.
Feverall Infants' Suppositories	Acetaminophen 80mg	**Peds: 3-11 months:** 1 supp q6h. **12-36 months:** 1 supp q4h. **Max:** 6 supp q24h.
Feverall Jr. Strength Suppositories	Acetaminophen 325mg	**Peds: 6-12 yrs:** 1 supp q4-6h. **Max:** 6 supp q24h.
Tylenol 8 Hour Caplets	Acetaminophen 650mg	**Adults & Peds: ≥12 yrs:** 2 tabs q8h prn. **Max:** 6 tabs q24h.
Tylenol 8 Hour Geltabs	Acetaminophen 650mg	**Adults & Peds: ≥12 yrs:** 2 tabs q8h prn. **Max:** 6 tabs q24h.
Tylenol Arthritis Caplets	Acetaminophen 650mg	**Adults:** 2 tabs q8h prn. **Max:** 6 tabs q24h.
Tylenol Arthritis Geltabs	Acetaminophen 650mg	**Adults:** 2 tabs q8h prn. **Max:** 6 tabs q24h.
Tylenol Children's Meltaways Tablets	Acetaminophen 80mg	**Peds: 2-3 yrs (24-35 lbs):** 2 tabs. **4-5 yrs (36-47 lbs):** 3 tabs. **6-8 yrs (48-59 lbs):** 4 tabs. **9-10 yrs (60-71 lbs):** 5 tabs. **11 yrs (72-95 lbs):** 6 tabs. May repeat q4h. **Max:** 5 doses q24h.
Tylenol Children's Suspension	Acetaminophen 160mg/5mL	**Peds: 2-3 yrs (24-35 lbs):** 1 tsp (5mL). **4-5 yrs (36-47 lbs):** 1.5 tsp (7.5mL). **6-8 yrs (48-59 lbs):** 2 tsp (10mL). **9-10 yrs (60-71 lbs):** 2.5 tsp (12.5mL). **11 yrs (72-95 lbs):** 3 tsp (15mL). May repeat q4h. **Max:** 5 doses q24h.
Tylenol Extra Strength Caplets	Acetaminophen 500mg	**Adults & Peds: ≥12 yrs:** 2 tabs q4-6h prn. **Max:** 8 tabs q24h.
Tylenol Extra Strength Cool Caplets	Acetaminophen 500mg	**Adults & Peds: ≥12 yrs:** 2 tabs q4-6h prn. **Max:** 8 tabs q24h.
Tylenol Extra Strength Gelcaps	Acetaminophen 500mg	**Adults & Peds: ≥12 yrs:** 2 caps q4-6h prn. **Max:** 8 caps q24h.
Tylenol Extra Strength Geltabs	Acetaminophen 500mg	**Adults & Peds: ≥12 yrs:** 2 tabs q4-6h prn. **Max:** 8 tabs q24h.
Tylenol Extra Strength Liquid	Acetaminophen 1000mg/30mL	**Adults & Peds: ≥12 yrs:** 2 tbl (30mL) q4-6h prn. **Max:** 8 tbl (120mL) q24h.
Tylenol Extra Strength Tablets	Acetaminophen 500mg	**Adults & Peds: ≥12 yrs:** 2 tabs q4-6h prn. **Max:** 8 tabs q24h.
Tylenol Infants' Suspension	Acetaminophen 80mg/0.8mL	**Peds: 2-3 yrs (24-35 lbs):** 1.6 mL q4h prn. **Max:** 5 doses (8mL) q24h.
Tylenol Junior Meltaways Tablets	Acetaminophen 160mg	**Peds: 6-8 yrs (48-59 lbs):** 2 tabs. **9-10 yrs (60-71 lbs):** 2.5 tabs. **11 yrs (72-95 lbs):** 3 tabs. **12 yrs (≥96 lbs):** 4 tabs. May repeat q4h. **Max:** 5 doses q24h.
Tylenol Regular Strength Tablets	Acetaminophen 325mg	**Adults & Peds: ≥12 yrs:** 2 tabs q4-6h prn. **Max:** 12 tabs q24h. **Peds: 6-11 yrs:** 1 tab q4-6h. **Max:** 5 tabs q24h.

Table 8. ANTIPYRETIC PRODUCTS (cont.)

BRAND	INGREDIENT/STRENGTH	DOSE
NONSTEROIDAL ANTI-INFLAMMATORY DRUGS (NSAIDs)		
Advil Children's Chewable Tablets	Ibuprofen 50mg	**Peds: 2-3 yrs (24-35 lbs):** 2 tabs q6-8h. **4-5 yrs (36-47 lbs):** 3 tabs q6-8h. **6-8 yrs (48-59 lbs):** 4 tabs q6-8h. **9-10 yrs (60-71 lbs):** 5 tabs q6-8h. **11 yrs (72-95 lbs):** 6 tabs q6-8h. **Max:** 4 doses q24h
Advil Children's Suspension	Ibuprofen 100mg/5mL	**Peds: 2-3 yrs (24-35 lbs):** 1 tsp (5mL). **4-5 yrs (36-47 lbs):** 1.5 tsp (7.5mL). **6-8 yrs (48-59 lbs):** 2 tsp (10mL). **9-10 yrs (60-71 lbs):** 2.5 tsp (12.5mL). **11 yrs (72-95 lbs):** 3 tsp (15mL). May repeat q6-8h. **Max:** 4 doses q24h.
Advil Gel Caplets	Ibuprofen 200mg	**Adults & Peds: ≥12 yrs:** 1-2 caps q4-6h. **Max:** 6 caps q24h.
Advil Infants' Concentrated Drops	Ibuprofen 50mg/1.25mL	**Peds: 6-11 months (12-17 lbs):** 1.25mL. **12-23 months (18-23 lbs):** 1.875mL. May repeat q6-8h. **Max:** 4 doses q24h.
Advil Junior Strength Chewable Tablets	Ibuprofen 100mg	**Peds: 6-8 yrs (48-59 lbs):** 2 tabs. **9-10 yrs (60-71 lbs):** 2.5 tabs. **11 yrs (72-95 lbs):** 3 tabs. May repeat q6-8h. **Max:** 4 doses q24h.
Advil Junior Strength Swallow Tablets	Ibuprofen 100mg	**Peds: 6-10 yrs (48-71 lbs):** 2 tabs **11 yrs (72-95 lbs):** 3 tabs. May repeat q6-8h. **Max:** 4 doses q24h.
Advil Liqui-Gels	Ibuprofen 200mg	**Adults & Peds: ≥12 yrs:** 1-2 caps q4-6h. **Max:** 6 caps q24h.
Advil Tablets	Ibuprofen 200mg	**Adults & Peds: ≥12 yrs:** 1-2 tabs q4-6h. **Max:** 6 tabs q24h.
Aleve Caplets	Naproxen Sodium 220mg	**Adults & Peds: ≥12 yrs:** 1 tab q8-12h. May take 1 additional tab within 1 hour of first dose. **Max:** 3 tabs q24h.
Aleve Liquid Gels	Naproxen Sodium 220mg	**Adults & Peds: ≥12 yrs:** 1 cap q8-12h. May take 1 additional tab within 1 hour of first dose. **Max:** 3 caps q24h.
Aleve Smooth Gels	Naproxen Sodium 220mg	**Adults & Peds: ≥12 yrs:** 1 cap q8-12h. May take 1 additional tab within 1 hour of first dose. **Max:** 3 caps q24h.
Aleve Tablets	Naproxen Sodium 220mg	**Adults & Peds: ≥12 yrs:** 1 tab q8-12h. May take 1 additional tab within 1 hour of first dose. **Max:** 3 caps q24h.
Motrin Children's Suspension	Ibuprofen 100mg/5mL	**Peds: 2-3 yrs (24-35 lbs):** 1 tsp (5mL). **4-5 yrs (36-47 lbs):** 1.5 tsp (7.5mL). **6-8 yrs (48-59 lbs):** 2 tsp (10mL). **9-10 yrs (60-71 lbs):** 2.5 tsp (12.5mL). **11 yrs (72-95 lbs):** 3 tsp (15mL). May repeat q6-8h. **Max:** 4 doses q24h.
Motrin IB Caplets	Ibuprofen 200mg	**Adults & Peds: ≥12 yrs:** 1-2 tabs q4-6h. **Max:** 6 tabs q24h.
Motrin IB Tablets	Ibuprofen 200mg	**Adults & Peds: ≥12 yrs:** 1-2 tabs q4-6h. **Max:** 6 tabs q24h.
Motrin Infants' drops	Ibuprofen 50mg/1.25mL	**Peds: 6-11 months (12-17 lbs):** 1.25mL. **12-23 months (18-23 lbs):** 1.875mL. May repeat q6-8h. **Max:** 4 doses q24h.

Table 8. ANTIPYRETIC PRODUCTS (cont.)

BRAND	INGREDIENT/STRENGTH	DOSE
Motrin Junior Strength Caplets	Ibuprofen 100mg	**Peds: 6-8 yrs (48-59 lbs):** 2 tabs. **9-10 yrs (60-71 lbs):** 2.5 tabs. **11 yrs (72-95 lbs):** 3 tabs. May repeat q6-8h. **Max:** 4 doses q24h.
Motrin Junior Strength Chewable Tablets	Ibuprofen 100mg	**Peds: 6-8 yrs (48-59 lbs):** 2 tabs. **9-10 yrs (60-71 lbs):** 2.5 tabs. **11 yrs (72-95 lbs):** 3 tabs. May repeat q6-8h. **Max:** 4 doses q24h.
SALICYLATES		
Anacin 81 Tablets	Aspirin 81mg	**Adults & Peds: ≥12 yrs:** 2 tabs q6h. **Max:** 8 tabs q24h.
Aspergum Chewable Tablets	Aspirin 227mg	**Adults & Peds: ≥12 yrs:** 2 tabs q4h. **Max:** 16 tabs q24h.
Bayer Aspirin Extra Strength Caplets	Aspirin 500mg	**Adults & Peds: ≥12 yrs:** 1-2 tabs q4-6h. **Max:** 8 tabs q24h.
Bayer Genuine Aspirin Caplets	Aspirin 325mg	**Adults & Peds: ≥12 yrs:** 1-2 tabs q4h or 3 tabs q6h. **Max:** 12 tabs q24h.
Bayer Aspirin Safety Coated Caplets	Aspirin 325mg	**Adults & Peds: ≥12 yrs:** 1-2 tabs q4h or 3 tabs q6h. **Max:** 12 tabs q24h.
Bayer Children's Aspirin Chewable Tablets	Aspirin 81mg	**Adults & Peds: ≥12 yrs:** 4-8 tabs q4h. **Max:** 48 tabs q24h.
Bayer Low Dose Aspirin Tablets	Aspirin 81mg	**Adults & Peds: ≥12 yrs:** 4-8 tabs q4h. **Max:** 48 tabs q24h.
Ecotrin Low Strength Tablets	Aspirin 81mg	**Adults:** 4-8 tabs q4h. **Max:** 48 tabs q24h
Ecotrin Enteric Regular Strength Tablets	Aspirin 325mg	**Adults & Peds: ≥12 yrs:** 1-2 tabs q4h. **Max:** 12 tabs q24h.
Ecotrin Maximum Strength Tablets	Aspirin 500mg	**Adults & Peds: ≥12 yrs:** 2 tabs q6h. **Max:** 8 tabs q24h.
Halfprin 162mg Tablets	Aspirin 162mg	**Adults & Peds: ≥12 yrs:** 2-4 tabs q4h. **Max:** 24 tabs q24h.
Halfprin 81mg Tablets	Aspirin 81mg	**Adults & Peds: ≥12 yrs:** 4-8 tabs q4h. **Max:** 48 tabs q24h.
St. Joseph Aspirin Chewable Tablets	Aspirin 81mg	**Adults & Peds: ≥12 yrs:** 4-8 tabs q4h. **Max:** 48 tabs q24h.
St. Joseph Enteric Safety-Coated Tablets	Aspirin 81mg	**Adults & Peds: ≥12 yrs:** 4-8 tabs q4h. **Max:** 48 tabs q24h.
SALICYLATES, BUFFERED		
Bayer Extra Strength Plus Caplets	Aspirin Buffered with Calcium Carbonate 500mg	**Adults & Peds: ≥12 yrs:** 1-2 tabs q4-6h. **Max:** 8 tabs q24h.
Bufferin Extra Strength Tablets	Aspirin Buffered with Calcium Carbonate/Magnesium Oxide/Magnesium Carbonate 500mg	**Adults & Peds: ≥12 yrs:** 2 tabs q6h. **Max:** 8 tabs q24h.
Bufferin Tablets	Aspirin Buffered with Calcium Carbonate/Magnesium Oxide/Magnesium Carbonate 325mg	**Adults & Peds: ≥12 yrs:** 2 tabs q4h. **Max:** 12 tabs q24h.

Table 9. ANTISEBORRHEAL PRODUCTS

Brand Name	Ingredient/Strength	Dose
COAL TAR		
DHS Tar Dermatological Hair & Scalp Shampoo	Coal Tar 0.5%	**Adults & Peds:** Use biw.
DHS Tar Shampoo	Coal Tar 0.5%	**Adults & Peds:** Use at least biw.
Neutrogena T/Gel Shampoo Original Formula	Coal Tar 0.5%	**Adults & Peds:** Use at least biw.
Neutrogena T/Gel Stubborn Itch Shampoo	Coal Tar 0.5%	**Adults & Peds:** Use at least biw.
Polytar Shampoo	Coal Tar 0.5%	**Adults & Peds:** Use at least biw.
Polytar Soap	Coal Tar 0.5%	**Adults & Peds:** Use prn.
Psoriasin Liquid Dab-on	Coal Tar 0.66%	**Adults:** Apply to affected area qd-qid.
Ionil-T Shampoo	Coal Tar 1%	**Adults & Peds:** Use at least biw.
Neutrogena T/Gel Shampoo Extra Strength	Coal Tar 1%	**Adults & Peds:** Use at least biw.
Psoriasin Gel	Coal Tar 1.25%	**Adults:** Apply to affected area qd-qid.
Ionil-T Plus Shampoo	Coal Tar 2%	**Adults & Peds:** Use at least biw.
MG217 Ointment	Coal Tar 2%	**Adults & Peds:** Apply to affected area qd-qid.
Denorex Therapeutic Protection 2-in-1 Shampoo	Coal Tar 2.5%	**Adults & Peds:** Use at least biw.
Denorex Therapeutic Protection Shampoo	Coal Tar 2.5%	**Adults & Peds:** Use at least biw.
MG217 Tar Shampoo	Coal Tar 3%	**Adults & Peds:** Use at least biw.
Ionil T Therapeutic Coal Tar Shampoo	Coal Tar 5%	**Adults & Peds:** Use biw.
CORTICOSTEROIDS		
Aveeno Hydrocortisone 1% Anti-Itch Cream	Hydrocortisone 1%	**Adults & Peds: ≥2 yrs:** Apply to affected area tid-qid.
Cortaid Advanced 12-Hour Anti-Itch Cream	Hydrocortisone 1%	**Adults & Peds: ≥2 yrs:** Apply to affected area tid-qid.
Cortaid Intensive Therapy Cooling Spray	Hydrocortisone 1%	**Adults & Peds: ≥2 yrs:** Apply to affected area tid-qid.
Cortaid Intensive Therapy Moisturizing Cream	Hydrocortisone 1%	**Adults & Peds: ≥2 yrs:** Apply to affected area tid-qid.
Cortaid Maximum Strength Cream	Hydrocortisone 1%	**Adults & Peds: ≥2 yrs:** Apply to affected area tid-qid.
Cortaid Maximum Strength Ointment	Hydrocortisone 1%	**Adults & Peds: ≥2 yrs:** Apply to affected area tid-qid.
Cortizone-10 Cream	Hydrocortisone 1%	**Adults & Peds: ≥2 yrs:** Apply to affected area tid-qid.
Cortizone-10 Maximum Strength Anti-Itch Ointment	Hydrocortisone 1%	**Adults & Peds: ≥2 yrs:** Apply to affected area tid-qid.
Cortizone-10 Ointment	Hydrocortisone 1%	**Adults & Peds: ≥2 yrs:** Apply to affected area tid-qid.
Cortizone-10 Intensive Healing Formula	Hydrocortisone 1%	**Adults & Peds: ≥2 yrs:** Apply to affected area tid-qid.
PYRITHIONE ZINC		
Denorex Dandruff Shampoo, Daily Protection	Pyrithione Zinc 2%	**Adults & Peds:** Use biw.
Garnier Fructis Fortifying Shampoo, Anti-Dandruff	Pyrithione Zinc 1%	**Adults & Peds:** Use biw.
Head & Shoulders Dry Scalp Care Dandruff Shampoo Plus Conditioner, Shampoo; Conditioner	Pyrithione Zinc 1%	**Adults & Peds:** Use biw.
Head & Shoulders Smooth & Silky Dandruff Shampoo Plus Conditioner; Shampoo; Conditioner	Pyrithione Zinc 1%	**Adults & Peds:** Use biw.

Table 9. ANTISEBORRHEAL PRODUCTS (cont.)

Brand Name	Ingredient/Strength	Dose
Head & Shoulders Citrus Breeze Dandruff Shampoo Plus Conditioner; Shampoo	Pyrithione Zinc 1%	**Adults & Peds:** Use biw.
Head & Shoulders Classic Clean Dandruff Shampoo Plus Conditioner; Shampoo; Conditioner	Pyrithione Zinc 1%	**Adults & Peds:** Use biw.
Head & Shoulders Extra Volume Dandruff Shampoo	Pyrithione Zinc 1%	**Adults & Peds:** Use biw.
Head & Shoulders Ocean Lift Dandruff Shampoo Plus Conditioner; Shampoo	Pyrithione Zinc 1%	**Adults & Peds:** Use biw.
Head & Shoulders Dandruff Refresh Shampoo Plus Conditioner; Shampoo	Pyrithione Zinc 1%	**Adults & Peds:** Use biw.
Head & Shoulders Restoring Shine Dandruff Shampoo Plus Conditioner; Shampoo	Pyrithione Zinc 1%	**Adults & Peds:** Use biw.
Head & Shoulders Sensitive Care Dandruff Shampoo Plus Conditioner; Shampoo	Pyrithione Zinc 1%	**Adults & Peds:** Use biw.
Head & Shoulders Intensive Solutions Dandruff Shampoo and Conditioner; Shampoo	Pyrithione Zinc 1%	**Adults & Peds:** Use biw.
L'Oreal VIVE Pro Anti-Dandruff for Men Shampoo	Pyrithione Zinc 1%	**Adults & Peds:** Use biw.
Neutrogena T-Gel Daily Control Dandruff Shampoo	Pyrithione Zinc 1%	**Adults & Peds:** Use biw.
Pantene Pro-V Shampoo + Conditioner, Anti-Dandruff	Pyrithione Zinc 1%	**Adults & Peds:** Use biw.
Pert Plus Shampoo Plus Conditioner, Dandruff Control	Pyrithione Zinc 0.45%	**Adults & Peds:** Use biw.
Selsun Salon 2-in-1 Pyrithione Zinc Shampoo	Pyrithione Zinc 1%	**Adults & Peds:** Use biw.
Suave for Men 2 in 1 Shampoo/ Conditioner, Dandruff	Pyrithione Zinc 0.5%	**Adults & Peds:** Use biw.
SALICYLIC ACID		
Neutrogena T/Gel Conditioner	Salicylic Acid 2%	**Adults & Peds:** Use at least tiw.
Psoriasin Therapeutic Shampoo and Body Wash	Salicylic Acid 3%	**Adults & Peds:** Use biw.
Neutrogena T/Sal Shampoo, Scalp Build-up Control	Salicylic Acid 3%	**Adults & Peds:** Use biw.
Scalpicin Anti-Itch Liquid Scalp Treatment (Combe)	Salicylic Acid 3%	**Adults:** Apply to affected area qd-qid.
SELENIUM SULFIDE		
Head & Shoulders Dandruff Shampoo, Intensive Treatment	Selenium Sulfide 1%	**Adults & Peds:** Use biw.
Selsun Blue Dandruff Shampoo, Medicated Treatment	Selenium Sulfide 1%	**Adults & Peds:** Use biw.
Selsun Blue Dandruff Shampoo Plus Conditioner	Selenium Sulfide 1%	**Adults & Peds:** Use biw.
Selsun Blue Dandruff Shampoo	Selenium Sulfide 1%	**Adults & Peds:** Use biw.
Selsun Blue Dandruff Shampoo, Moisturizing Treatment	Selenium Sulfide 1%	**Adults & Peds:** Use biw.
SULFUR/SALICYLIC ACID		
Sebulex Medicated Dandruff Shampoo	Sulfur/Salicylic Acid 2%-2%	**Adults & Peds:** Use qd.

Table 10. ARTIFICIAL TEAR PRODUCTS

Brand Name	Ingredient/Strength	Dose
Akwa Tears Lubricant Eye Drops	Polyvinyl Alcohol 1.4%	**Adults:** Instill 1-2 drops to affected eye prn.
Akwa Tears Lubricant Ophthalmic Ointment	White Petrolatum/Mineral Oil/ Lanolin 83%-15%-21%	**Adults:** Place ¼ in oint inside eyelid qd.
Allergan Optive Lubricant Eye Drops	Carboxymethylcellulose/ Sodium Glycerin 0.5%-0.9%	**Adults:** Instill 1-2 drops to affected eye prn.
Allergan Lacri-Lube S.O.P. Lubricant Eye Ointment	Mineral Oil/White Petrolatum 42.5%-56.8%	**Adults:** Place ¼ in oint inside eyelid qd.
Allergan Refresh Celluvisc Lubricant Eye Drops	Carboxymethylcellulose Sodium 1%	**Adults:** Instill 1-2 drops to affected eye prn.
Allergan Refresh Dry Eye Therapy Eye Drops	Glycerin/Polysorbate 80. 1%-1%	**Adults:** Instill 1-2 drops to affected eye prn.
Allergan Refresh Liquigel Lubricant Eye Drops	Carboxymethylcellulose Sodium 1%	**Adults:** Instill 1-2 drops to affected eye prn.
Allergan Refresh Lubricant Eye Drops	Polyvinyl Alcohol/Povidone 1.4%-0.6%	**Adults:** Instill 1-2 drops to affected eye prn.
Allergan Refresh Plus Lubricant Eye Drops	Carboxymethylcellulose Sodium 0.5%	**Adults:** Instill 1-2 drops to affected eye prn.
Allergan Refresh PM Lubricant Eye Ointment	White Petrolatum/Mineral Oil 57.3%-42.5%	**Adults:** Place ¼ in oint inside eyelid.
Allergan Refresh Tears Lubricant Eye Drops	Carboxymethylcellulose Sodium 0.5%	**Adults:** Instill 1-2 drops to affected eye prn.
AMO Blink Tears Lubricating Eye Drops for Mild-Moderate Dry Eyes	Polyethylene Glycol 400 0.25%	**Adults:** Instill 1-2 drops to affected eye prn.
Bausch & Lomb Advanced Eye Relief Dry Eye Environmental Lubricant Eye Drops	Propylene Glycol/Glycerin 1.0%-0.3%	**Adults:** Instill 1 or 2 drops in the affected eye as needed.
Bausch & Lomb Advanced Eye Relief Preservative Free Dry Eye Rejuvenation Lubricant Eye Drops	Propylene Glycol 0.95%	**Adults:** Instill 1 or 2 drops in the affected eye as needed.
Bausch & Lomb Advanced Eye Relief Night Time Lubricant Eye Ointment (Preservative Free)	Mineral Oil/White Petrolatum 20%-80%	**Adults:** Apply a small amount (¼ inch) of ointment to the inside of lower eyelid one or more times daily.
Bion Tears Lubricant Eye Drops	Dextran 70/Hydroxypropyl Methylcellulose 2910 0.01%-0.3%	**Adults:** Instill 1-2 drops to affected eye prn.
Clear Eyes Eye Drops for Dry Eyes	Carboxymethylcellulose Sodium/ Glycerine 1.0%-0.25%	**Adults:** Instill 1-2 drops to affected eye prn.
GenTeal Mild Dry Eyes Drops	Hypromellose 0.2%	**Adults:** Instill 1-2 drops to affected eye prn.
GenTeal Moderate Dry Eyes Drops	Hypromellose 0.3%	**Adults:** Instill 1-2 drops to affected eye prn.
GenTeal PM Ointment	Mineral Oil/White Petrolatum 15%-85%	**Adults:** Apply a small amount (¼ inch) of ointment to the inside of lower eyelid one or more times daily.
GenTeal Lubricant Eye Drops for Moderate to Severe Dry Eye Relief, Gel Drops.	Carboxymethylcellulose Sodium/ Hypromellose 0.25%-0.3%	**Adults:** Instill 1-2 drops to affected eye prn.
GenTeal PF Dry Eye Drops	Hydroxypropylmethylcellulose 0.3%	**Adults:** Instill 1-2 drops to affected eye prn.
Murine Tears Lubricant Eye Drops	Polyvinyl Alcohol/Povidone 0.5%-0.6%	**Adults:** Instill 1-2 drops to affected eye prn.
Optics Laboratory Minidrops Eye Therapy	Polyvinylpyrrolidone/ Polyvinyl Alcohol 6mg-14mg	**Adults:** Instill 1-2 drops to affected eye prn.
Rohto Zi For Eyes Lubricant Eye Drops	Povidone 1.8%	**Adults:** Instill 1-2 drops to affected eye prn.
Soothe XP Emollient Lubricant Eye Drops	Light Mineral Oil/Mineral Oil 1%-4.5%	**Adults:** Instill 1-2 drops in the affected eye as needed, or as directed by your doctor.
Soothe Lubricant Eye Drops	Glycerin/Propylene Glycol 0.6%-0.6%	**Adults:** Instill 1-2 drops in the affected eye as needed, or as directed by your doctor.

Table 10. ARTIFICIAL TEAR PRODUCTS (cont.)

Brand Name	Ingredient/Strength	Dose
Systane Lubricant Eye Drops	Polyethylene Glycol 400/ Propylene Glycol 0.4%-0.3%	**Adults:** Instill 1-2 drops to affected eye prn.
Tears Naturale Forte Lubricant Eye Drops	Dextran 70 0.1%, Glycerin 0.2% Hypromellose 0.3%	**Adults:** Instill 1-2 drops to affected eye prn.
Tears Naturale Free Lubricant Eye Drops	Dextran 70/Hydroxypropyl Methylcellulose 2910 0.1%-0.3%	**Adults:** Instill 1-2 drops to affected eye prn.
Tears Naturale II Polyquad Lubricant Eye Drops	Dextran 70/Hydroxypropyl Methylcellulose 2910 0.1%-0.3%	**Adults:** Instill 1-2 drops tq affected eye prn.
Tears Naturale P.M. Lubricant Eye Ointment	White Petrolatum/Mineral Oil 94%-3%	**Adults:** Place ¼ inch oint inside eyelid qd.
TheraTears Liquid Gel Lubricant Eye Gel	Sodium Carboxymethylcellulose 1%	**Adults:** Instill 1-2 drops to affected eye prn.
TheraTears Lubricant Eye Drops	Sodium Carboxymethylcellulose 0.25%	**Adults:** Instil 1-2 drops to affected eye prn.
Visine Pure Tears Lubricant Eye Drops	Glycerin/Hypromellose/Polyethylene Glycol 400 0.2%-0.2%-1%	**Adults and Peds: >6 yrs:** Instill 1-2 drops to affected eye prn.
Viva-Drops Lubricant Eye Drops	Polysorbate 80	**Adults:** Instill 1-2 drops to affected eye prn.

Table 11. CANKER AND COLD SORE PRODUCTS

Brand	Ingredient/Strength	Dose
Abreva Cold Sore/Fever Blister Treatment	Docosanol 10%	**Adults & Peds:** ≥12 yrs: Use 5 times a day until healed. **Max:** 10 days
Abreva Pump Cold Sore/Fever Blister Treatment	Docosanol 10%	**Adults & Peds:** ≥12 yrs: Use 5 times a day until healed. **Max:** 10 days
Anbesol Cold Sore Therapy Ointment	Allantoin/Benzocaine/Camphor/White Petrolatum 1%-20%-3%-64.9%	**Adults & Peds:** ≥2 yrs: Apply to affected area tid-qid.
Anbesol Jr. Gel	Benzocaine 10%	**Adults & Peds:** ≥2 yrs: Apply to affected area qid.
Anbesol Maximum Strength Gel Core Sore Treatment	Benzocaine/Camphor 20%-3%	**Adults & Peds:** ≥2 yrs: Apply to affected area qid.
Anbesol Regular Strength Gel	Benzocaine 10%	**Adults & Peds:** ≥2 yrs: Apply to affected area qid.
Anbesol Regular Strength Liquid	Benzocaine 10%	**Adults & Peds:** ≥2 yrs: Apply to affected area qid.
Campho-Phenique Cold Sore Gel	Camphor/Phenol 10.8%-4.7%	**Adults & Peds:** ≥2 yrs: Apply to affected area qd-tid.
Carmex Cold Sore Reliever and Lip Moisturizer	Menthol/Camphor/Phenol 0.4%-1.7%-0.4%	**Adults & Peds:** ≥12 yrs: Apply to affected area prn.
ChapStick Cold Sore Therapy	Allantoin/Benzocaine/Camphor/White Petrolatum 1%-20%-3%-64.9%	**Adults & Peds:** ≥2 yrs: Apply to affected area tid-qid.
Chloraseptic Mouth Pain Spray	Phenol 1.4%	**Peds:** ≥2 yrs: Apply to affected area for 15 seconds, then spit. Use prn.
Herpecin-L Lip Balm Stick, SPF 30	Dimethicone/Methyl Anthranilate/Octyl Methoxycinnamate/Octyl Salicylate/Oxybenzone 1%-5%-7.5%-5%- 6%	**Adults & Peds:** ≥12 yrs: Apply prn.
Kank-A Soft Brush Mouth Pain Gel	Benzocaine 20%	**Adults & Peds:** ≥2 yrs: Apply to affected area qid.
Kanka-A Mouth Pain Liquid	Benzocaine 20%	**Adults & Peds:** ≥2 yrs: Apply to affected area qid.
Novitra Cold Sore Maximum Strength Cream	Zincum Oxydatum 2X HPUS	**Adults & Peds:** ≥2 yrs: Apply to affected area q2-3h, 6 to 8 times daily.
Orabase Medicated Cold Sore Swabs	Benzocaine 20%	**Adults & Peds:** ≥2 yrs: Apply to affected area qid.
Orajel Ultra Mouth Sore Medicine Film-Forming Gel	Benzocaine/Menthol 15%-2%	**Adults & Peds:** ≥2 yrs: Apply to affected area qid.
Orajel Mouth Sore Gel	Benzocaine/Benzalkonium Chloride/Zinc Chloride 20%-0.02%-0.1%	**Adults & Peds:** ≥2 yrs: Apply to affected area qid.
Orajel Mouth Sore Swabs	Benzocaine 20%	**Adults & Peds:** ≥2 yrs: Apply to affected area qid.
Orajel Multi-Action Cold Sore Medicine Gel	Allantoin/Benzocaine/Camphor/Dimethicone/White Petrolatum 0.5%-20%-3%-2%-65%	**Adults & Peds:** ≥2 yrs: Apply to affected area tid-qid.
Orajel Protective Mouth Sore Discs	Benzocaine 15%	**Adults & Peds:** ≥2 yrs: Apply to affected area qiq 2h prn.
Releev 1-Day Cold Sore Treatment	Benzalkonium Chloride 0.13%	**Adults & Peds:** ≥2 yrs: Apply to clean dry affected area tid-qid.
Swabplus Mouth Sore Relief Swabs	Benzocaine 20%	**Adults & Peds:** ≥2 yrs: Apply to affected area qid.
Tanac Liquid	Benzalkonium Chloride/Benzocaine 0.12%-10%	**Adults & Peds:** ≥2 yrs: Apply to affected area tid-qid.
Zilactin Cold Sore Gel	Benzyl Alcohol 10%	**Adults & Peds:** ≥2 yrs: Apply to affected area qid.

Table 12. CONTACT DERMATITIS PRODUCTS

BRAND	INGREDIENT/STRENGTH	DOSE
ANTIHISTAMINE		
Benadryl Extra Strength Gel	Diphenhydramine HCl 2%	**Adults & Peds ≥2 yrs:** Apply to affected area tid-qid.
ANTIHISTAMINE COMBINATION		
Benadryl Extra Strength Itch-Stopping Cream	Diphenhydramine HCl/Zinc Acetate 2%-0.1%	**Adults & Peds ≥2 yrs:** Apply to affected area tid-qid.
Benadryl Extra Strength Spray	Diphenhydramine HCl/Zinc Acetate 2%-0.1%	**Adults & Peds ≥12 yrs:** Apply to affected area tid-qid.
Benadryl Itch Relief Spray	Diphenhydramine HCl/Zinc Acetate 2%-0.1%	**Adults & Peds ≥2 yrs:** Apply to affected area tid-qid.
Benadryl Itch Relief Stick	Diphenhydramine HCl/Zinc Acetate 2%-0.1%	**Adults & Peds ≥2 yrs:** Apply to affected area tid-qid.
Benadryl Original Cream	Diphenhydramine HCl/Zinc Acetate 1%-0.1%	**Adults & Peds ≥2 yrs:** Apply to affected area tid-qid.
CalaGel Anti-Itch Gel	Diphenhydramine HCl/Zinc Acetate/Benzenthonium Chloride 2%-0.215%-0.15%	**Adults & Peds ≥2 yrs:** Apply to affected area tid-qid.
Ivarest Anti-Itch Cream	Diphenhydramine HCl/Calamine 2%-14%	**Adults & Peds ≥2 yrs:** Apply to affected area tid-qid.
ASTRINGENT		
Domeboro Powder Packets	Aluminum Acetate/Aluminum Sulfate	**Adults & Peds:** Dissolve 1-2 packets and apply to affected area for 15-30 min tid.
Ivy-Dry Super Lotion Extra Strength	Zinc Acetate/Benzyl Alcohol/Camphor/Menthol 2%-10%-0.5%-0.25%	**Adults & Peds: ≥6 yrs:** Apply to affected area qd-tid.
ASTRINGENT COMBINATION		
Aveeno Calamine and Pramoxine HCl Anti-Itch Cream	Calamine/Pramoxine HCl 3%-1%	**Adults & Peds ≥2 yrs:** Apply to affected area tid-qid.
Aveeno Anti-Itch Concentrated Lotion	Calamine/Pramoxine HCl/Camphor 3%-1%-0.47%	**Adults & Peds ≥2 yrs:** Apply to affected area qid.
Caladryl Clear Lotion	Zinc Acetate/Pramoxine HCl 0.1%-1%	**Adults & Peds ≥2 yrs:** Apply to affected area tid-qid.
Caladryl Lotion	Calamine/Pramoxine HCl 8%-1%	**Adults & Peds ≥2 yrs:** Apply to affected area tid-qid.
Calamine Lotion (generic)	Calamine/Zinc Oxide	**Adults & Peds:** Apply to affected area prn.
CLEANSER		
Ivy-Dry Scrub	Polyethylene, sodium lauryl sulfoacetate, cetearyl alcohol, nonoxynol-9, camellia sinensis oil, phenoxyethanol, methylparaben, propylparaben, triethanolamine, carbomer, erythorbic acid, aloe barbadensis extract, tocopheryl acetate extract, tetrasodium EDTA	**Adults & Peds:** Wash affected area prn.
Cortaid Poison Ivy Care Toxin Removal Cloths	Water, lauroyl sarcosinate, glycerin, DMDM, hydantoin, methylparaben, tetrasodium EDTA, Aloe barnadenis leaf extract, citric acid	**Adults & Peds:** Wash affected area prn.
CORTICOSTEROID		
Aveeno 1% Hydrocortisone Anti-Itch Cream	Hydrocortisone 1%	**Adults & Peds ≥2 yrs:** Apply to affected area tid-qid.
Cortaid Advanced 12-Hour Anti-Itch Cream	Hydrocortisone 1%	**Adults & Peds ≥2 yrs:** Apply to affected area tid-qid.
Cortaid Intensive Therapy Cooling Spray	Hydrocortisone 1%	**Adults & Peds ≥2 yrs:** Apply to affected area tid-qid.

Table 12. CONTACT DERMATITIS PRODUCTS (cont.)

BRAND	INGREDIENT/STRENGTH	DOSE
Cortaid Intensive Therapy Moisturizing Cream	Hydrocortisone 1%	**Adults & Peds ≥2 yrs:** Apply to affected area tid-qid.
Cortaid Maximum Strength Cream	Hydrocortisone 1%	**Adults & Peds ≥2 yrs:** Apply to affected area tid-qid.
Cortaid Maximum Strength Ointment	Hydrocortisone 1%	**Adults & Peds ≥2 yrs:** Apply to affected area tid-qid.
Cortizone-10 Cream	Hydrocortisone 1%	**Adults & Peds ≥2 yrs:** Apply to affected area tid-qid.
Cortizone-10 Maximum Strength Anti-Itch Ointment	Hydrocortisone 1%	**Adults & Peds ≥2 yrs:** Apply to affected area tid-qid.
Cortizone-10 Ointment	Hydrocortisone 1%	**Adults & Peds ≥2 yrs:** Apply to affected area tid-qid.
Cortizone-10 Plus Intensive Healing Formula	Hydrocortisone 1%	**Adults & Peds ≥2 yrs:** Apply to affected area tid-qid.
IvyStat!	Hydrocortisone 1%	**Adults & Peds ≥2 yrs:** Apply to affected area tid-qid.
Dermarest Eczema Lotion	Hydrocortisone 1%	**Adults & Peds ≥2 yrs:** Apply to affected area tid-qid.
COUNTERIRRITANT		
Gold Bond First Aid Quick Spray	Menthol/Benzethonium Chloride 1%-0.13%	**Adults & Peds ≥2 yrs:** Apply to affected area tid-qid.
Gold Bond Medicated Maximum Strength Anti-Itch Cream	Menthol/Pramoxine HCl 1%-1%	**Adults & Peds ≥2 yrs:** Apply to affected area tid-qid.
Ivy Block Lotion	Bentoquatam 5%	**Adults & Peds ≥2 yrs:** Apply q4h for continued protection.
LOCAL ANESTHETIC		
Solarcaine Aloe Extra Burn Relief Gel	Lidocaine HCl 0.5%	**Adults & Peds ≥2 yrs:** Apply to affected area tid-qid.
Solarcaine Aloe Extra Spray	Lidocaine HCl 0.5%	**Adults & Peds ≥2 yrs:** Apply to affected area tid-qid.
Solarcaine First Aid Medicated Spray	Benzocaine/Triclosan 20%-0.13%	**Adults & Peds ≥2 yrs:** Apply to affected area qd-tid.
LOCAL ANESTHETIC COMBINATION		
Bactine First Aid Liquid	Lidocaine HCl/Benzalkonium Chloride 2.5%-0.13%	**Adults & Peds ≥2 yrs:** Apply to affected area qd-tid.
Lanacane Maximum Strength Cream	Benzocaine/Benzethonium Chloride 20%-0.2%	**Adults & Peds ≥2 yrs:** Apply to affected area qd-tid.
Lanacane Maximum Strength Spray	Benzocaine/Benzethonium Chloride 20%-0.2%	**Adults & Peds ≥2 yrs:** Apply to affected area qd-tid.
Lanacane Original Formula Cream	Benzocaine/Benzethonium Chloride 6%-0.2%	**Adults & Peds ≥2 yrs:** Apply to affected area qd-tid.
SKIN PROTECTANT		
Aveeno Skin Relief Moisturizing Cream	Dimethicone 2.5%	**Adults & Peds ≥2 yrs:** Apply to affected area tid-qid.
SKIN PROTECTANT COMBINATION		
Aveeno Itch Relief Lotion	Dimethicone/Menthol	**Adults & Peds ≥2 yrs:** Apply to affected area tid-qid.
Gold Bond Extra Strength Medicated Body Lotion Triple Action Relief	Dimethicone/Menthol 5%-0.5%	**Adults & Peds:** Apply to affected area tid-qid.
Gold Bond Medicated Body Lotion	Dimethicone/Menthol 5%-0.15%	**Adults & Peds:** Apply to affected area prn.

Table 12. CONTACT DERMATITIS PRODUCTS (cont.)

BRAND	INGREDIENT/STRENGTH	DOSE
Gold Bond Medicated Extra Strength Powder	Zinc Oxide/Menthol 0.5%-0.8%	**Adults & Peds ≥2 yrs:** Apply to affected area tid-qid.
Vaseline Intensive Care Lotion Advanced Healing	Dimethicone 1%-White Petrolatum	**Adults & Peds:** Apply to affected area prn.

Table 13. COUGH-COLD-FLU PRODUCTS

Brand Name	Analgesic	Antihistamine	Decongestant	Cough Suppressant	Expectorant	Dose
ANTIHISTAMINE + DECONGESTANT						
Actifed Cold & Allergy Tablets		Chlorpheniramine Maleate 4mg	Phenylephrine HCl 10mg			**Adults: ≥12 yrs:** 1 tab q4-6h. **Max:** 6 doses q24h. **Peds: 6-12 yrs:** ½ tab q4-6h. **Max:** 2 tabs q24h.
Benadryl Children's Allergy & Cold Fastmelt Tablets		Diphenhydramine HCl 19mg	Pseudoephedrine HCl 30mg			**Adults: ≥12 yrs:** 2 tabs q4h. **Max:** 8 tabs q24h. **Peds: 6-12 yrs:** 1 tab q4h. **Max:** 4 tabs q24h.
Benadryl-D Allergy/Sinus Tablets		Diphenhydramine HCl 25mg	Phenylephrine HCl 10mg			**Adults & Peds: ≥12 yrs:** 1 tab q4h. **Max:** 6 tab q24h.
Children's Benadryl-D Allergy & Sinus Liquid		Diphenhydramine HCl 12.5mg/5mL	Phenylephrine HCl 5mg/5mL			**Adults: ≥12 yrs:** 2 tsp (10mL) q4h. **Peds: 6-12 yrs:** 1 tsp (5mL) q4h. **Max:** 6 doses q24h.
Dimetapp Children's Cold & Allergy Elixir		Brompheniramine Maleate 1mg/5mL	Phenylephrine HCl 2.5mg/5mL			**Adults & Peds: ≥12 yrs:** 2 tabs q4h. **Max:** 8 tabs q24h. **Peds: 6-12 yrs:** 1 tab q4hr. **Max:** 6 doses q24h.
Dimetapp Children's Cold & Allergy Chewable Tablets		Brompheniramine Maleate 1mg	Phenylephrine HCl 2.5mg			**Peds: 6-12 yrs:** 2 tabs q4h. **Max:** 6 doses q24h.
Pedicare Children's NightRest Multi-Symptom Cold Liquid		Diphenhydramine HCl 12.5mg/5mL	Phenylephrine HCl 5mg/5mL			**Peds: 6-12 yrs:** 1 tsp (5mL) q4h. **Max:** 6 doses q24h.
Robitussin Night Time Cough & Cold Liquid		Diphenhydramine HCl 6.25mg/5mL	Phenylephrine HCl 2.5mg/5mL			**Adults & Peds: ≥12 yrs:** 4 tsp (20mL) q4h. **Peds: 6-12 yrs:** 2 tsp (10mL) q4h. **Max:** 6 doses q24h.
Robitussin Pediatric Night Time Cough & Cold Liquid		Diphenhydramine HCl 6.25mg/5mL	Phenylephrine HCl 2.5mg/5mL			**Adults & Peds: ≥12 yrs:** 4 tsp (20mL) q4h. **Peds: 6-12 yrs:** 2 tsp (10mL) q4h. **Max:** 6 doses q24h.
Sudafed Sinus & Allergy Tablets		Chlorpheniramine Maleate 4mg	Pseudoephedrine HCl 60mg			**Adults: ≥12 yrs:** 1 tab q4-6h. **Peds: 6-12 yrs:** ½ tab q4-6h. **Max:** 4 doses q24h.
Sudafed Sinus Nighttime Tablets		Triprolidine HCl 2.5mg	Pseudoephedrine HCl 60mg			**Adults: & Peds: ≥12 yrs:** 1 tab q4-6h. **Peds: 6-12 yrs:** ½ tab q4-6h. **Max:** 4 doses q24h.
Theraflu Nighttime Cold & Cough Thin Strips		Diphenhydramine HCl 25mg/strips	Phenylephrine HCl 10mg/strip			**Adults: ≥12 yrs:** 1 strip q4h. **Max:** 6 strips q24h.
Triaminic Cold & Allergy Liquid		Chlorpheniramine Maleate 1mg/5mL	Phenylephrine HCl 2.5mg/5mL			**Peds: 6-12 yrs:** 2 tsp (10mL) q4h. **Max:** 6 doses q24h.
Triaminic Nighttime Cough & Cold Liquid		Diphenhydramine HCl 6.25mg/5mL	Phenylephrine HCl 2.5mg/5mL			**Peds: 6-12 yrs:** 2 tsp (10mL) q4h. **Max:** 6 doses q24h.
Triaminic Nighttime Cough & Cold Thin Strips		Diphenhydramine HCl 12.5mg/strip	Phenylephrine HCl 5mg/strip			**Peds: 6-12 yrs:** 1 strip q4h. **Max:** 6 strips q24h.

Table 13. COUGH-COLD-FLU PRODUCTS (cont.)

ANTIHISTAMINE + DECONGESTANT + ANALGESIC

Brand Name	Analgesic	Antihistamine	Decongestant	Cough Suppressant	Expectorant	Dose
Actifed Cold & Sinus Caplets	Acetaminophen 500mg	Chlorpheniramine Maleate 2mg	Pseudoephedrine HCl 30mg			**Adults & Peds:** ≥**12 yrs:** 2 tabs q6h. **Max:** 8 tabs q24h.
Advil Multi-Symptom Cold Caplets	Ibuprofen 200mg	Chlorpheniramine Maleate 2mg	Pseudoephedrine HCl 30mg			**Adults & Peds:** ≥**12 yrs:** 1 tab q4-6h. **Max:** 6 tabs q24h.
Advil Allergy Sinus Caplets	Ibuprofen 200mg	Chlorpheniramine Maleate 2mg	Pseudoephedrine HCl 30mg			**Adults & Peds:** ≥**12 yrs:** 1 tab q4-6h. **Max:** 6 tabs q24h.
Advil Allergy Sinus Children's Liquid	Ibuprofen 100mg	Chlorpheniramine Maleate 1mg	Pseudoephedrine HCl 15mg			**Peds: 6-11 yrs (48-95 lbs):** 2 tsp q6h. **Max:** 8 tsp q24h.
Alka-Seltzer Plus Cold Effervescent Tablets	Acetaminophen 325mg	Chlorpheniramine Maleate 2mg	Phenylephrine HCl 5mg			**Adults & Peds:** ≥**12 yrs:** 2 tabs q4h. **Max:** 8 tabs q24h.
Alka-Seltzer Plus Cold Cherry Burst Formula Effervescent Tablets	Acetaminophen 250mg	Chlorpheniramine Maleate 2mg	Phenylephrine HCl 5mg			**Adults & Peds:** ≥**12 yrs:** 2 tabs q4h. **Max:** 8 tabs q24h.
Alka-Seltzer Plus Cold Orange Zest Formula Effervescent Tablets	Acetaminophen 250mg	Chlorpheniramine Maleate 2mg	Phenylephrine HCl 5mg			**Adults & Peds:** ≥**12 yrs:** 2 tabs q4h. **Max:** 8 tabs q24h.
Alka-Seltzer Plus Regular Seltzer Multi-Symptom Cold Relief Effervescent Tablets	Acetaminophen 250mg	Chlorpheniramine Maleate 2mg	Phenylephrine HCl 5mg			**Adults & Peds:** ≥**12 yrs:** 2 tabs q4h. **Max:** 8 tabs q24h.
Benadryl Allergy & Cold Caplets	Acetaminophen 325mg	Diphenhydramine HCl 12.5mg	Phenylephrine HCl 5mg			**Adults & Peds:** ≥**12 yrs:** 2 tabs q4h. **Max:** 12 tabs q24h. **Peds: 6-12 yrs:** 1 tab q4h. **Max:** 5 tabs q24h.
Benadryl Allergy & Sinus Headache Caplets	Acetaminophen 325mg	Diphenhydramine HCl 12.5mg	Phenylephrine HCl 5mg			**Adults & Peds:** ≥**12 yrs:** 2 tabs q4h. **Max:** 12 tabs q24h. **Peds: 6-12 yrs:** 1 tab q4h. **Max:** 5 tabs q24h.
Benadryl Severe Allergy & Sinus Headache Caplets	Acetaminophen 325mg	Diphenhydramine HCl 25mg	Phenylephrine HCl 5mg			**Adults & Peds:** ≥**12 yrs:** 2 tabs q4h. **Max:** 12 tabs q24h.
Comtrex Day & Night Severe Cold & Sinus Caplets	Acetaminophen 325mg	Chlorpheniramine Maleate 2mg (nighttime dose only)	Phenylephrine HCl 5mg			**Adults & Peds:** ≥**12 yrs:** *Daytime:* 2 daytime tabs q4h. **Max:** 8 daytime tabs q24h. *Nighttime:* 2 nighttime tabs q4h. **Max:** 4 nighttime tabs q24h.
Contac Cold & Flu Maximum Strength Caplets	Acetaminophen 500mg	Chlorpheniramine Maleate 2mg	Phenylephrine HCl 5mg			**Adults & Peds:** ≥**12 yrs:** 2 tabs q4-6h **Max:** 8 tabs q24h.
Dristan Cold Multi-Symptom Tablets	Acetaminophen 325mg	Chlorpheniramine Maleate 2mg	Phenylephrine HCl 5mg			**Adults & Peds:** ≥**12 yrs:** 2 tabs q4h. **Max:** 12 tabs q24h.
Robitussin Cold & Congestion Tablets	Acetaminophen 325mg	Chlorpheniramine Maleate 2mg	Phenylephrine HCl 5mg			**Adults & Peds:** ≥**12 yrs:** 2 tabs q4h. **Max:** 12 tabs q24h.
Sudafed Sinus PE Nighttime Cold Caplets	Acetaminophen 325mg	Diphenhydramine HCl 25mg	Phenylephrine HCl 5mg			**Adults & Peds:** ≥**12 yrs:** 2 tabs q4h. **Max:** 12 tabs q24h.
Sudafed PE Nighttime Cold Caplets	Acetaminophen 325mg	Diphenhydramine HCl 12.5mg	Phenylephrine HCl 5mg			**Adults & Peds:** ≥**12 yrs:** 2 tabs q4h. **Max:** 12 tabs q24h. **Peds: 6-12 yrs:** 1 tab q4h. **Max:** 5 tabs q24h.

Table 13: COUGH-COLD-FLU PRODUCTS (cont.)

Brand Name	Analgesic	Antihistamine	Decongestant	Cough Suppressant	Expectorant	Dose
Sudafed PE Severe Cold Caplets	Acetaminophen 325mg	Diphenhydramine HCl 12.5mg	Phenylephrine HCl 5mg			**Adults & Peds: ≥12 yrs:** 2 tabs q4h. **Max:** 12 tabs q24h. **Peds: 6-12 yrs:** 1 tab q4h. **Max:** 5 tabs q24h.
Theraflu Cold & Sore Throat Hot Liquid	Acetaminophen 325mg/packet	Pheniramine Maleate 20mg/packet	Phenylephrine HCl 10mg/packet			**Adults & Peds: ≥12 yrs:** 1 packet q4h. **Max:** 6 packets q24h.
Theraflu Nighttime Severe Hot Liquid	Acetaminophen 650mg/packet	Pheniramine Maleate 20mg/packet	Phenylephrine HCl 10mg/packet			**Adults & Peds: ≥12 yrs:** 1 packet q4h. **Max:** 6 packets q24h.
Theraflu Flu & Sore Throat Liquid	Acetaminophen 650mg/packet	Pheniramine Maleate 20mg/packet	Phenylephrine HCl 10mg/packet			**Adults & Peds: ≥12 yrs:** 1 packet q4h. **Max:** 6 packets q24h.
Theraflu Nighttime Warming Relief Syrup	Acetaminophen 325mg/15mL	Diphenhydramine HCl 12.5mg/15mL	Phenylephrine HCl 5mg/15mL			**Adults & Peds: ≥12 yrs:** 2 tbl (30mL) q4h. **Max:** 6 doses (12 tbl) q24h.
Theraflu Flu & Sore Throat Relief Syrup	Acetaminophen 325mg/15mL	Diphenhydramine HCl 12.5mg/15mL	Phenylephrine HCl 5mg/15mL			**Adults & Peds: ≥12 yrs:** 2 tbl (30mL) q4h. **Max:** 6 doses (12 tbl) q24h.
Tylenol Children's Plus Cold Liquid	Acetaminophen 160mg/5mL	Chlorpheniramine Maleate 1mg/5mL	Phenylephrine HCl 2.5mg/5mL			**Peds: 6-11 yrs (48-95 lbs):** 2 tsp (10mL) q4h. **Max:** 5 doses q24h.
Tylenol Children's Plus Cold & Allergy Liquid	Acetaminophen 160mg/5mL	Diphenhydramine HCl 12.5mg/5mL	Phenylephrine HCl 2.5mg/5mL			**Peds: 6-11 yrs (48-95 lbs):** 2 tsp (10mL) q4-6h. **Max:** 4 doses q24h.
Tylenol Children's Plus Cold & Allergy Liquid	Acetaminophen 160mg/5mL	Diphenhydramine HCl 12.5mg/5mL	Pseudoephedrine HCl 15mg/5mL			**Peds: 6-11 yrs (48-95 lbs):** 2 tsp (10mL) q4-6h. **Max:** 4 doses q24h.
Tylenol Sinus Congestion & Pain Nighttime Caplets	Acetaminophen 325mg	Chlorpheniramine Maleate 2mg	Phenylephrine HCl 5mg			**Adults & Peds: ≥12 yrs:** 2 tabs q4h. **Max:** 12 tabs q24h.
Tylenol Allergy Multi-Symptom Caplets	Acetaminophen 325mg	Chlorpheniramine Maleate 2mg	Phenylephrine HCl 5mg			**Adults & Peds: ≥12 yrs:** 2 tabs q4h. **Max:** 12 tabs q24h.
Tylenol Allergy Multi-Symptom Nighttime Caplets	Acetaminophen 325mg	Diphenhydramine HCL 25mg	Phenylephrine HCl 5mg			**Adults & Peds: ≥12 yrs:** 2 tabs q4h. **Max:** 12 tabs q24h.
Vicks NyQuil Sinus Liquicaps	Acetaminophen 325mg	Doxylamine Succinate 6.25 mg	Phenylephrine HCl 5mg			**Adults & Peds: ≥12 yrs:** 2 tabs q4h. **Max:** 6 doses q24h.
COUGH SUPPRESSANT						
Delsym 12 Hour Cough Relief Liquid				Dextromethorphan Polistrex 30mg/5mL		**Adults: ≥12 yrs:** 2 tsp (10mL) q12h. **Max:** 4 doses q24h. **Peds: 6-12 yrs:** 1 tsp (5mL) q12h. **Max:** 2 doses q24h. **2-6 yrs:** ½ tsp (2.5mL) q12h. **Max:** 1 dose q24h.
PediaCare Long-Acting Cough Liquid				Dextromethorphan HBr 7.5mg/5mL		**Peds: 6-12 yrs:** 2 tsp q6-8h. **2-6 yrs:** 1 tsp q6-8h. **Max:** 4 doses q24h.
Robitussin Cough Long-Acting Liquid				Dextromethorphan HBr 15mg/5mL		**Adults & Peds: ≥12 yrs:** 2 tsp (10mL) q6-8h. **Max:** 8 tsp (40mL) q24h.
Robitussin CoughGels Liqui-gels				Dextromethorphan HBr 15mg		**Adults & Peds: ≥12 yrs:** 2 caps q6-8h. **Max:** 8 caps q24h.
Robitussin Pediatric Cough Liquid				Dextromethorphan HBr 7.5mg/5mL		**Adults: ≥12 yrs (≥96 lbs):** 4 tsp (20mL) q6-8h. **Peds: 6-12 yrs (48-95 lbs):** 2 tsp (10mL) q6-8h. **2-6 yrs:** 1 tsp (5mL) q6-8h. **Max:** 4 doses q24h.

Table 13. COUGH-COLD-FLU PRODUCTS (cont.)

Brand Name	Analgesic	Antihistamine	Decongestant	Cough Suppressant	Expectorant	Dose
Triaminic Long Acting Cough Liquid				Dextromethorphan HBr 7.5mg/5mL		**Peds: 6-12 yrs:** 2 tsp (10mL) q6-8h. **2-6 yrs:** 1 tsp (5mL) q6-8h. **Max:** 4 doses q24h.
Triaminic Long Acting Cough Thin Strips				Dextromethorphan 5.5mg/strip		**Peds: 6-12 yrs:** 2 strips q6-8h. **Max:** 8 strips q24h.
Vicks DayQuil Cough Liquid				Dextromethorphan HBr 15mg/15mL		**Adults & Peds: ≥12 yrs:** 2 tbl (30mL) q6-8h. **Peds: 6-12 yrs:** 1 tbl (15mL) q6-8h. **Max:** 4 doses q24h.
Vicks 44 Liquid				Dextromethorphan HBr 30mg/15mL		**Adults & Peds: ≥12 yrs:** 1 tbl (15mL) q6-8h. **Peds: 6-12 yrs:** 1.5 tsp (7.5mL) q6-8h. **Max:** 4 doses q24h.
Vicks BabyRub				Eucalyptus, petrolatum, fragrance, aloe extract, eucalyptus oil, lavender oil, rosemary oil		**Peds:** Gently massage on the chest, neck, and back to help soothe and comfort.
Vicks Casero Cough Suppressant/Topical Analgesic				Camphor 4.7%, Menthol 2.6%, Eucalyptus 1.2%		**Adults & Peds: ≥2 yrs:** Apply 3 times q24h.
Vicks Cough Drops Cherry Flavor				Menthol 1.7mg		**Adults & Peds: ≥5 yrs:** 3 drops q1-2h.
Vicks Cough Drops Original Flavor				Menthol 3.3mg		**Adults & Peds: ≥5 yrs:** 2 drops q1-2h.
Vicks VapoRub Cream				Camphor 5.2%, Menthol 2.8%, Eucalyptus 1.2%		**Adults & Peds: ≥2 yrs:** Apply q8h.
Vicks VapoRub Ointment				Camphor 4.8%, Menthol 2.6%, Eucalyptus 1.2%		**Adults & Peds: ≥2 yrs:** Apply q8h.
Vicks VapoSteam				Camphor 6.2%		**Adults & Peds: ≥2 yrs:** 1 tbl/quart q8h.
COUGH SUPPRESSANT + ANTIHISTAMINE						
Coricidin HBP Cough & Cold Tablets		Chlorpheniramine Maleate 4mg		Dextromethorphan HBr 30mg		**Adults & Peds: ≥12 yrs:** 1 tab q6h. **Max:** 4 tabs q24h.
Dimetapp Long-Acting Cold Plus Cough Elixir		Chlorpheniramine Maleate 1mg/5mL		Dextromethorphan HBr 7.5mg/5mL		**Peds: ≥12 yrs:** 4 tsp (20mL) q6h. **6-12 yrs:** 2 tsp (10 mL) q6h. **Max:** 4 doses q24h.
Robitussin Cough & Cold Long-Acting Liquid		Chlorpheniramine Maleate 2mg/5mL		Dextromethorphan HBr 15mg/5mL		**Adults & Peds: ≥12 yrs:** 2 tsp (10mL) q6h. **Max:** 4 doses q24h.
Robitussin Pediatric Cough & Cold Long-Acting Liquid		Chlorpheniramine Maleate 1mg/5mL		Dextromethorphan HBr 7.5mg/5mL		**Adults & Peds: ≥12 yrs:** 4 tsp (20mL) q6h. **Peds: 6-12 yrs:** 2 tsp (10mL) q6h. **Max:** 4 doses q24h.

Table 13. COUGH-COLD-FLU PRODUCTS (cont.)

Brand Name	Analgesic	Antihistamine	Decongestant	Cough Suppressant	Expectorant	Dose
Triaminic Softchews Cough & Runny Nose		Chlorpheniramine Maleate 1mg		Dextromethorphan HBr 5mg		**Peds: 6-12 yrs:** 2 tabs q4-6h. **Max:** 6 doses q24h.
Vicks Children's NyQuil Liquid		Chlorpheniramine Maleate 2mg/15mL		Dextromethorphan HBr 15mg/15mL		**Adults: ≥12 yrs:** 2 tbl (30mL) q6h. **Peds: 6-11 yrs:** 1 tbl (15mL) q6h. **Max:** 4 doses q24h.
Vicks NyQuil Cough Liquid		Doxylamine Succinate 6.25mg/15mL		Dextromethorphan HBr 15mg/15mL		**Adults & Peds: ≥12 yrs:** 2 tbl (30mL) q6h. **Max:** 8 tbl (120mL) q24h.
Vicks Pediatric Formula 44M Cough & Cold Relief		Chlorpheniramine Maleate 2mg/15mL		Dextromethorphan HBr 15mg/15mL		**Adults & Peds: ≥12 yrs:** 2 tbl (30mL) q6h. **Peds: 6-12 yrs:** 1 tbl (15mL) q6h. **Max:** 4 doses q24h.
COUGH SUPPRESSANT + ANALGESIC						
Triaminic Cough & Sore Throat Liquid	Acetaminophen 160mg/5mL			Dextromethorphan HBr 5mg/5mL		**Peds: 6-12 yrs:** 2 tsp (10mL) q4h. **2-6 yrs:** 1 tsp (5mL) q4h. **Max:** 5 doses q24h.
Triaminic Softchews Cough & Sore Throat Tablets	Acetaminophen 160mg			Dextromethorphan HBr 5mg		**Peds: 6-12 yrs:** 2 tabs q4h. **2-6 yrs:** 1 tab q4h. **Max:** 5 doses q24h.
Tylenol Children's Plus Cough & Sore Throat Liquid	Acetaminophen 160mg/5mL			Dextromethorphan HBr 5mg/5mL		**Peds: 6-11 yrs: (48-95 lbs):** 2 tsp (10mL) q4h. **2-5 yrs (24-47 lbs):** 1 tsp (5mL) q4h. **Max:** 5 doses q24h.
Tylenol Cough & Sore Throat Daytime Liquid	Acetaminophen 1000mg/30mL			Dextromethorphan HBr 30mg/30mL		**Adults & Peds: ≥12 yrs:** 2 tbl (30mL) q6h. **Max:** 8 tbl q24h.
COUGH SUPPRESSANT + ANTIHISTAMINE + ANALGESIC						
Alka-Seltzer Plus Flu Effervescent Tablets	Aspirin 500mg	Chlorpheniramine Maleate 2mg		Dextromethorphan HBr 15mg		**Adults & Peds: ≥12 yrs:** 2 tabs q6h. **Max:** 8 tabs q24h.
Alka-Seltzer Plus Nighttime Liquid Gels	Acetaminophen 325mg	Doxylamine Succinate 6.25mg		Dextromethorphan HBr 15mg		**Adults & Peds: ≥12 yrs:** 2 tabs q6h. **Max:** 12 tabs q24h.
Tylenol Children's Plus Cough & Runny Nose Liquid	Acetaminophen 160mg/5mL	Chlorpheniramine Maleate 1mg/5mL		Dextromethorphan HBr 5mg/5mL		**Peds: 6-11 yrs: (48-95 lbs):** 2 tsp (10mL) q4h. **Max:** 5 doses q24h.
Coricidin HBP Maximum Strength Flu Tablets	Acetaminophen 500mg	Chlorpheniramine Maleate 2mg		Dextromethorphan HBr 15mg		**Adults & Peds: ≥12 yrs:** 2 tabs q6h. **Max:** 8 tabs q24h.
Triaminic Flu Cough & Fever Liquid	Acetaminophen 160mg/5mL	Chlorpheniramine Maleate 1mg/5mL		Dextromethorphan HBr 7.5mg/5mL		**Peds: 6-12 yrs:** 2 tsp (10mL) q6h. **Max:** 4 doses (20mL) q24h.
Tylenol Nighttime Cough & Sore Throat Cool Burst Liquid	Acetaminophen 1000mg/30mL	Doxylamine 12.5mg/30mL		Dextromethorphan HBr 30mg/30mL		**Adults & Peds: ≥12 yrs:** 2 tbl (30mL) q6h. **Max:** 8 tbl (120mL) q24h.
Vicks 44M Liquid	Acetaminophen 162.5mg/5mL	Chlorpheniramine Maleate 1mg/5mL		Dextromethorphan HBr 7.5mg/5mL		**Adults & Peds: ≥12 yrs:** 4 tsp (20mL) q6h. **Max:** 16 tsp (80mL) q24h.
Vicks NyQuil Liquicaps	Acetaminophen 325mg	Doxylamine Succinate 6.25mg		Dextromethorphan HBr 15mg		**Adults & Peds: ≥12 yrs:** 2 caps q6h. **Max:** 8 caps q24h.
Vicks NyQuil Liquid	Acetaminophen 500mg/15mL	Doxylamine Succinate 6.25mg/15mL		Dextromethorphan HBr 15mg/15mL		**Adults & Peds: ≥12 yrs:** 2 tbl (30mL) q6h. **Max:** 8 tbl (120mL) q24h.

Table 13. COUGH-COLD-FLU PRODUCTS (cont.)

COUGH SUPPRESSANT + ANTIHISTAMINE + ANALGESIC + DECONGESTANT

Brand Name	Analgesic	Antihistamine	Decongestant	Cough Suppressant	Expectorant	Dose
Alka-Seltzer Plus Cough & Cold Liquid Gels	Acetaminophen 325mg	Chlorpheniramine Maleate 2mg	Phenylephrine HCl 5mg	Dextromethorphan HBr 10mg		**Adults & Peds:** ≥12 yrs: 2 caps q4h. **Max:** 12 caps q24h.
Alka-Seltzer Plus Effervescent Tablets	Acetaminophen 250mg	Doxlamine Succinate 6.25mg	Phenylephrine HCl 5mg	Dextromethorphan HBr 10mg		**Adults & Peds:** ≥12 yrs: 2 tabs q4h. **Max:** 8 tabs q24h.
Alka-Seltzer Plus Cough & Cold Effervescent Tablets	Acetaminophen 250mg	Chlorpheniramine Maleate 2mg	Phenylephrine HCl 5mg	Dextromethorphan HBr 10mg		**Adults & Peds:** ≥12 yrs: 2 tabs q4h. **Max:** 8 tabs q24h.
Alka-Seltzer Plus Cough & Cold Liquid	Acetaminophen 162.5mg/5mL	Chlorpheniramine Maleate 1mg/5mL	Phenylephrine HCl 2.5mg/5mL	Dextromethorphan HBr 5mg/5mL		**Adults & Peds:** ≥12 yrs: 4 tsp q4h. **Max:** 24 tsp q24h.
Alka-Seltzer Plus Night Cold Liquid	Acetaminophen 162.5mg/5mL	Doxylamine Succinate 3.125/5mL	Phenylephrine HCl 2.5mg/5mL	Dextromethorphan HBr 5mg/5mL		**Adults & Peds:** ≥12 yrs: 4 tsp q4h. **Max:** 24 tsp q24h.
Comtrex Nighttime Cold & Cough Caplets	Acetaminophen 325mg	Chlorpheniramine Maleate 2mg	Phenylephrine HCl 5mg	Dextromethorphan HBr 10mg		**Adults & Peds:** ≥12 yrs: 2 tabs q6h. **Max:** 8 tabs q24h.
Dimetapp Children's Nighttime Flu Liquid	Acetaminophen 160mg/5mL	Chlorpheniramine Maleate 1mg/5mL	Phenylephrine HCl 2.5mg/5mL	Dextromethorphan HBr 5mg/5mL		**Adults:** ≥12 yrs: 4 tsp (20mL) q4h. **Peds:** 6-12 yrs: 2 tsp (10mL) q4h. **Max:** 5 doses q24h.
Robitussin Nighttime Cold Cough & Flu Liquid	Acetaminophen 160mg/5mL	Chlorpheniramine Maleate 1mg/5mL	Phenylephrine HCl 2.5mg/5mL	Dextromethorphan HBr 5mg/5mL		**Adults:** ≥12 yrs: 4 tsp (20mL) q4h. **Peds:** 6-12 yrs: 2 tsp (10mL) q4h. **Max:** 5 doses q24h.
Theraflu Nighttime Severe Cold Caplets	Acetaminophen 325mg	Chlorpheniramine Maleate 2mg	Phenylephrine HCl 5mg	Dextromethorphan HBr 10mg		**Adults & Peds:** ≥12 yrs: 2 tabs q6h. **Max:** 8 tabs q24h.
Tylenol Children's Plus Multisymptom Cold Liquid	Acetaminophen 160mg/5mL	Chlorpheniramine Maleate 1mg/5mL	Phenylephrine HCl 2.5mg/5mL	Dextromethorphan HBr 5mg/5mL		**Peds:** 6-11 yrs (48-95 lbs): 2 tsp (10mL) q4h. **Max:** 5 doses q24h.
Tylenol Children's Plus Flu Liquid	Acetaminophen 160mg/5mL	Chlorpheniramine Maleate 1mg/5mL	Phenylephrine HCl 2.5mg/5mL	Dextromethorphan HBr 5mg/5mL		**Peds:** 6-11 yrs (48-95 lbs): 2 tsp (10mL) q6-8h. **Max:** 4 doses q24h.
Tylenol Children's Plus Flu Liquid	Acetaminophen 160mg/5mL	Chlorpheniramine Maleate 1mg/5mL	Pseudoephedrine HCl 15mg/5mL	Dextromethorphan HBr 7.5mg/5mL		**Peds:** 6-11 yrs (48-95 lbs): 2 tsp (10mL) q6-8h. **Max:** 4 doses q24h.
Tylenol Cold Head Congestion Nighttime Caplets	Acetaminophen 325mg	Chlorpheniramine Maleate 2mg	Phenylephrine HCl 5mg	Dextromethorphan HBr 10mg		**Adults & Peds:** ≥12 yrs: 2 tabs q4h. **Max:** 12 tabs q24h.
Tylenol Cold Multi-Symptom Nighttime Caplets	Acetaminophen 325mg	Chlorpheniramine Maleate 2mg	Phenylephrine HCl 5mg	Dextromethorphan HBr 10mg		**Adults & Peds:** ≥12 yrs: 2 tabs q4h. **Max:** 12 tabs q24h.
Tylenol Cold Multi-Symptom Nighttime Liquid	Acetaminophen 325mg/15mL	Doxylamine 6.25mg/30mL	Phenylephedrine HCl 5mg/15mL	Dextromethorphan HBr 10mg/15mL		**Adults & Peds:** ≥12 yrs: 2 tbl (30mL) q4h. **Max:** 12 tbl (180mL) q24h.
Vicks NyQuil D Liquid	Acetaminophen 500mg/15mL	Doxylamine 6.25mg/15mL	Phenylephedrine HCl 30mg/15mL	Dextromethorphan HBr 15mg/15mL		**Adults & Peds:** ≥12 yrs: 2 tbl (30mL) q6h. **Max:** 4 doses q24h.

COUGH SUPPRESSANT + ANTIHISTAMINE + DECONGESTANT

Brand Name	Analgesic	Antihistamine	Decongestant	Cough Suppressant	Expectorant	Dose
Dimetapp DM Children's Cold & Cough Elixir		Brompheniramine Maleate 1mg/5mL	Phenylephrine HCl 2.5mg/5mL	Dextromethorphan HBr 5mg/5mL		**Adults:** ≥12 yrs: 4 tsp (20mL) q4h. **Peds:** 6-12 yrs: 2 tsp (10mL) q4h. **Max:** 6 doses q24h.
Robitussin Allergy & Cough Liquid		Chlorpheniramine Maleate 2mg/5mL	Phenylephrine HCl 5mg/5mL	Dextromethorphan HBr 10mg/5mL		**Adults:** ≥12 yrs: 2 tsp (10mL) q4h. **Peds:** 6-12 yrs: 1 tsp (5mL) q4h. **Max:** 6 doses q24h.

Table 13. COUGH-COLD-FLU PRODUCTS (cont.)

Brand Name	Analgesic	Antihistamine	Decongestant	Cough Suppressant	Expectorant	Dose
Theraflu Cold & Cough Hot Liquid		Pheniramine Maleate 20mg/packet	Phenylephrine HCl 10mg/packet	Dextromethorphan HBr 20mg/packet		**Adults & Peds: ≥12 yrs:** 1 packet q4h. **Max:** 6 packets q24h.
COUGH SUPPRESSANT + DECONGESTANT						
Dimetapp Toddler's Decongestant Plus Cough Drops			Phenylephrine HCl 1.25mg/0.8mL	Dextromethorphan HBr 2.5mg/0.8mL		**Peds: 2-6 yrs:** 1.6mL q4h. **Max:** 6 doses q24h.
PediaCare Children's Multi-Symptom Cold Liquid			Phenylephrine HCl 2.5mg/5mL	Dextromethorphan HBr 5mg/5mL		**Peds: 6-12 yrs:** 2 tsp (10mL) q4h. **2-6 yrs:** 1 tsp (5mL) q4h. **Max:** 6 doses q24h.
Sudafed Children's Cold & Cough Liquid			Pseudoephedrine HCl 15mg/5mL	Dextromethorphan HBr 5mg/5mL		**Adults & Peds: ≥12 yrs:** 4 tsp (20mL) q4h. **Peds: 6-12 yrs:** 2 tsp (10mL) q4h. **2-6 yrs:** 1 tsp (5mL) q4h. **Max:** 4 doses q24h.
Theraflu Daytime Cold & Cough Thin Strips			Phenylephrine HCl 10mg/strip	Dextromethorphan HBr 20mg/strip		**Adults & Peds: ≥12 yrs:** 1 strip q4h. **Max:** 6 strips q24h.
Triaminic Daytime Cold & Cough Liquid			Phenylephrine HCl 2.5mg/5mL	Dextromethorphan HBr 5mg/5mL		**Peds: 6-12 yrs:** 2 tsp (10mL) q4h. **2-6 yrs:** 1 tsp (5mL) q4h. **Max:** 6 doses q24h.
Triaminic Daytime Cold & Cough Thin Strips			Phenylephrine HCl 2.5mg/strip	Dextromethorphan HBr 3.67mg/strip		**Peds: 6-12 yrs:** 2 strips q4h. **2-6 yrs:** 1 strip q4h. **Max:** 6 doses q24h.
Vicks 44D Cough & Congestion Relief Liquid			Phenylephrine HCl 10mg/15mL	Dextromethorphan HBr 20mg/15mL		**Adults: ≥12 yrs:** 1 tbl (15mL) q4h. **Peds: 6-12 yrs:** 1.5 tsp (7.5mL) q4h. **Max:** 6 doses q24h.
COUGH SUPPRESSANT + DECONGESTANT + ANALGESIC						
Alka-Seltzer Plus Day Cold Liquid Gels	Acetaminophen 325mg		Phenylephrine HCl 5mg	Dextromethorphan HBr 10mg		**Adults & Peds: ≥12 yrs:** 2 caps q4h. **Max:** 12 caps q24h.
Alka-Seltzer Plus Day & Night Liquid Gels	Acetaminophen 325mg		Phenylephrine HCl 5mg	Dextromethorphan HBr 10mg		**Adults & Peds: ≥12 yrs:** 2 caps q4h. **Max:** 12 caps q24h.
Alka-Seltzer Plus Day & Night Effervescent Tablets	Acetaminophen 250mg		Phenylephrine HCl 5mg	Dextromethorphan HBr 10mg		**Adults & Peds: ≥12 yrs:** 2 tabs q4h. **Max:** 8 tabs q24h.
Alka-Seltzer Plus Day Cold Liquid	Acetaminophen 162.5mg/5mL		Phenylephrine HCl 2.5mg/5mL	Dextromethorphan HBr 5mg/5mL		**Adults & Peds: ≥12 yrs:** 4 tsps q4h. **Max:** 6 doses q24h.
Comtrex Cold & Cough Caplets	Acetaminophen 325mg		Phenylephrine HCl 5mg	Dextromethorphan HBr 10mg		**Adults & Peds: ≥12 yrs:** 2 tabs q4h. **Max:** 12 tabs q24h.
Theraflu Daytime Warming Relief Syrup	Acetaminophen 325mg/15mL		Phenylephrine HCl 5mg/15mL	Dextromethorphan HBr 10mg/15mL		**Adults & Peds: ≥12 yrs:** 2 tbl (30mL) q4h. **Max:** 6 doses (12 tbl) q24h.
Theraflu Daytime Severe Cold Caplets	Acetaminophen 325mg		Phenylephrine HCl 5mg	Dextromethorphan HBr 15mg		**Adults & Peds: ≥12 yrs:** 2 tabs q6h. **Max:** 8 tabs q24h.
Tylenol Cold Head Congestion Daytime Capsules	Acetaminophen 325mg		Phenylephephrine HCl 5mg	Dextromethorphan HBr 10mg		**Adults & Peds: ≥12 yrs:** 2 caps q4h. **Max:** 12 caps q24h.
Tylenol Cold Head Congestion Day/Night Pack	Acetaminophen 325mg		Phenylephedrine HCl 5mg	Dextromethorphan HBr 10mg		**Adults & Peds: ≥12 yrs:** 2 tabs q4h. **Max:** 12 tabs q24h.

Table 13: COUGH-COLD-FLU PRODUCTS (cont.)

Brand Name	Analgesic	Antihistamine	Decongestant	Cough Suppressant	Expectorant	Dose
Tylenol Cold Multi-Symptom Daytime Capsules	Acetaminophen 325mg		Phenylephrine HCl 5mg	Dextromethorphan HBr 10mg		**Adults & Peds: ≥12 yrs:** 2 caps q4h. **Max:** 12 caps q24h.
Tylenol Cold Multi-Symptom Daytime Cool Burst Liquid	Acetaminophen 325mg/15mL		Phenylephrine HCl 5mg/15mL	Dextromethorphan HBr 10mg/15mL		**Adults & Peds: ≥12 yrs:** 2 tbl (30mL) q4h. **Max:** 6 doses (12 tbl) q24h.
Tylenol Cold Multi-Symptom Day/Night Pack	Acetaminophen 325mg		Phenylephrine HCl 5mg	Dextromethorphan HBr 10mg		**Adults & Peds: ≥12 yrs:** 2 caps q4h. **Max:** 12 caps q24h.
Tylenol Flu Daytime Gelcaps	Acetaminophen 500mg		Pseudoephedrine HCl 30mg	Dextromethorphan HBr 15mg		**Adults & Peds: ≥12 yrs:** 2 caps q6h. **Max:** 8 caps q24h.
Vicks DayQuil Liquicaps	Acetaminophen 325mg		Phenylephrine HCl 5mg	Dextromethorphan HBr 10mg		**Adults & Peds: ≥12 yrs:** 2 caps q4h. **Max:** 6 caps q24h.
Vicks DayQuil Liquid	Acetaminophen 325mg/15mL		Phenylephrine HCl 5mg/15mL	Dextromethorphan HBr 10mg/15mL		**Adults & Peds: ≥12 yrs:** 2 tbl (30mL) q4h. **Max:** 12 tbl (120mL) q24h.
COUGH SUPPRESSANT + DECONGESTANT + EXPECTORANT						
Robitussin CF Liquid			Phenylephrine HCl 5mg/5mL	Dextromethorphan HBr 10mg/5mL	Guaifenesin 100mg/5mL	**Adults: ≥12 yrs:** 2 tsp (10mL) q4h. **Peds: 6-12 yrs:** 1 tsp (5mL) q4h. **2-6 yrs:** ½ tsp (2.5mL) q4h. **Max:** 6 doses q24h.
COUGH SUPPRESSANT + DECONGESTANT + EXPECTORANT + ANALGESIC						
Sudafed Cold & Cough Capsules	Acetaminophen 250mg		Pseudoephedrine HCl 30mg	Dextromethorphan HBr 10mg	Guaifenesin 100mg	**Adults & Peds: ≥12 yrs:** 2 caps q4h. **Max:** 8 caps q24h.
Sudafed PE Cold & Cough Caplets	Acetaminophen 325mg		Phenylephrine HCl 5mg	Dextromethorphan HBr 10mg	Guaifenesin 100mg	**Adults & Peds: ≥12 yrs:** 2 tabs q4h. **Max:** 12 tabs q24h.
Tylenol Cold Multi-Symptom Severe Liquid	Acetaminophen 325mg/15mL		Phenylephrine HCl 5mg/15mL	Dextromethorphan HBr 10mg/15mL	Guaifenesin 200mg/15mL	**Adults & Peds: ≥12 yrs:** 2 tbs q4h. **Max:** 12 tbs q24h.
Tylenol Cold Multi-Symptom Severe Caplets	Acetaminophen 325mg		Phenylephrine HCl 5mg	Dextromethorphan HBr 10mg	Guaifenesin 200mg	**Adults & Peds: ≥12 yrs:** 2 tabs q4h. **Max:** 12 tabs q24h.
Tylenol Cold Head Congestion Severe Caplets	Acetaminophen 325mg		Phenylephrine HCl 5mg	Dextromethorphan HBr 10mg	Guaifenesin 200mg	**Adults & Peds: ≥12 yrs:** 2 tabs q4h. **Max:** 12 tabs q24h.
Tylenol Cold Severe Congestion Daytime Caplets	Acetaminophen 325mg		Pseudoephedrine HCl 30mg	Dextromethorphan HBr 15mg	Guaifenesin 200mg	**Adults & Peds: ≥12 yrs:** 2 tabs q6h. **Max:** 8 tabs q24h.
COUGH SUPPRESSANT + EXPECTORANT						
Alka-Seltzer Plus Mucus & Congestion Effervescent Tablets				Dextromethorphan HBr 10mg	Guaifenesin 200mg	**Adults & Peds: ≥12 yrs:** 2 tabs q4h. **Max:** 8 tabs q24h.
Coricidin HBP Chest Congestion & Cough Softgels				Dextromethorphan HBr 10mg	Guaifenesin 200mg	**Adults & Peds: ≥12 yrs:** 1-2 caps q4h. **Max:** 12 caps q24h.
Mucinex DM Extended-Release Tablets				Dextromethorphan HBr 30mg	Guaifenesin 600mg	**Adults & Peds: ≥12 yrs:** 1-2 tabs q12h. **Max:** 4 tabs q24h.
Mucinex Liquid Cherry				Dextromethorphan HBr 5mg	Guaifenesin 100mg	**Peds: 6-12 yrs:** 1-2 tsp q4h. **2-6 yrs:** ½-1 tsp q4h. **Max:** 6 doses q24h.

Table 13. COUGH-COLD-FLU PRODUCTS (cont.)

Brand Name	Analgesic	Antihistamine	Cough Suppressant	Decongestant	Expectorant	Dose
Robitussin Cough & Congestion Liquid			Dextromethorphan HBr 10mg/5mL		Guaifenesin 200mg/5mL	**Adults: ≥12 yrs:** 2 tsp (10mL) q4h. **Peds: 6-12 yrs:** 1 tsp (5mL) q4h. **2-6 yrs:** ½ tsp (2.5mL) q4h. **Max:** 6 doses q24h.
Robitussin DM Liquid			Dextromethorphan HBr 10mg/5mL		Guaifenesin 100mg/5mL	**Adults: ≥12 yrs:** 2 tsp (10mL) q4h. **Peds: 6-12 yrs:** 1 tsp (5mL) q4h. **2-6 yrs:** ½ tsp (2.5mL) q4h. **Max:** 6 doses q24h.
Robitussin Sugar-Free Cough Liquid			Dextromethorphan HBr 10mg/5mL		Guaifenesin 100mg/5mL	**Adults: ≥12 yrs:** 2 tsp (10mL) q4h. **Peds: 6-12 yrs:** 1 tsp (5mL) q4h. **2-6 yrs:** ½ tsp (2.5mL) q4h. **Max:** 6 doses q24h.
Vicks 44E Liquid			Dextromethorphan HBr 20mg/15mL		Guaifenesin 200mg/15mL	**Adults: ≥12 yrs:** 1 tbl (15mL) q4h. **Peds: 6-12 yrs:** 1.5 tsp (7.5mL) q4h. **Max:** 6 doses q24h.
Vicks 44E Pediatric Liquid			Dextromethorphan HBr 10mg/15mL		Guaifenesin 100mg/15mL	**Adults: ≥12 yrs:** 2 tbl (30mL) q4h. **Peds: 6-12 yrs:** 1 tbl (15mL) q4h. **2-5 yrs:** ½ tbl (7.5mL) q4h. **Max:** 6 doses q24h.
DECONGESTANT						
Contac-D Cold Decongestant Tablets				Phenylephrine HCl 10mg		**Adults & Peds: ≥12 yrs:** 1 tabs q4h. **Max:** 6 tabs q24h.
Dimetapp Toddler's Drops Decongestant				Phenylephrine HCl 1.25mg/0.8mL		**Peds: 2-6 yrs:** 1.6mL q4h. **Max:** 6 doses q24h.
PediaCare Children's Decongestant Liquid				Phenylephrine HCl 2.5mg/5mL		**Peds: 6-12 yrs:** 2 tsp (10mL) q4h. **2-6 yrs:** 1 tsp (5mL) q4h. **Max:** 6 doses q24h.
Sudafed 12-Hour Tablets				Pseudoephedrine HCl 120mg		**Adults & Peds: ≥12 yrs:** 1 tab q12h. **Max:** 2 tabs q24h.
Sudafed 24-Hour Tablets				Pseudoephedrine HCl 240mg		**Adults & Peds: ≥12 yrs:** 1 tab q24h. **Max:** 1 tab q24h.
Sudafed Children's Chewable Tablets				Pseudoephedrine HCl 15mg		**Adults & Peds: ≥12 yrs:** 4 tabs q4-6h. **Peds: 6-12 yrs:** 2 tabs q4-6h. **2-6 yrs:** 1 tab q4-6h. **Max:** 4 doses q24h.
Sudafed Children's Liquid				Pseudoephedrine HCl 15mg/5mL		**Adults & Peds: ≥12 yrs:** 4 tsp (20mL) q4-6h. **Peds: 6-12 yrs:** 2 tsp (10mL) q4-6h. **2-6 yrs:** 1 tsp (5mL) q4-6h. **Max:** 4 doses q24h.
Sudafed PE Tablets				Phenylephrine HCl 10mg		**Adults & Peds: ≥12 yrs:** 1 tab q4h. **Max:** 6 tabs q24h.
Sudafed PE Quick Dissolve Strips				Phenylephrine HCl 10mg		**Adults & Peds: ≥12 yrs:** 1 film q4h. **Max:** 6 films q24h.

Table 13. COUGH-COLD-FLU PRODUCTS (cont.)

Brand Name	Analgesic	Antihistamine	Decongestant	Cough Suppressant	Expectorant	Dose
Sudafed Nasal Decongestant Tablets			Pseudoephedrine HCl 30mg			**Adults: ≥12 yrs:** 2 tabs q4-6h. **Peds: 6-12 yrs:** 1 tab q4-6h. **Max:** 4 doses q24h.
Triaminic Cold with Stuffy Nose Thin Strips			Phenylephrine HCl 2.5mg/strip			**Peds: 6-12 yrs:** 2 strips q4h. **2-6 yrs:** 1 strip q4h. **Max:** 6 doses q24h.
Vicks Sinex 12-Hour Nasal Spray			Oxymetazoline HCl 0.05%			**Adults & Peds: ≥6 yrs:** 2-3 sprays q10-12h. **Max:** 2 doses q24h.
Vicks Sinex Nasal Spray			Phenylephrine HCl 0.5%			**Adults & Peds: ≥12 yrs:** 2-3 sprays q4h. **Max:** 18 sprays q24h.
Vicks Sinex UltraFine Mist			Phenylephrine HCl 0.5%			**Adults & Peds: ≥12 yrs:** 2-3 sprays q4h. **Max:** 18 sprays q24h.
Vicks Sinex 12-Hour UltraFine Mist			Oxymetazoline HCl 0.05%			**Adults & Peds: ≥6 yrs:** 2-3 sprays q10-12h. **Max:** 2 doses q24h
Vicks Vapor Inhaler			Levmetamfetamine 50mg			**Adults & Peds: ≥12 yrs:** 2 inhalations q2h. **Max:** 24 inhalations q24h **Peds: 6-12 yrs:** 1 inhalation q2h. **Max:** 12 inhalations q24h.

DECONGESTANT + ANALGESIC

Brand Name	Analgesic	Antihistamine	Decongestant	Cough Suppressant	Expectorant	Dose
Advil Children's Cold Liquid	Ibuprofen 100mg/5mL		Pseudoephedrine HCl 15mg/5mL			**Peds: 6-11 yrs (48-95 lbs):** 2 tsp (10mL) q6h. **2-5 yrs (24-47 lbs):** 1 tsp (5mL) q6h. **Max:** 4 doses q24h
Advil Cold & Sinus Caplets	Ibuprofen 200mg		Pseudoephedrine HCl 30mg			**Adults & Peds: ≥12 yrs:** 1-2 tabs q4-6h. **Max:** 6 tabs q24h.
Advil Cold & Sinus Liqui-gels	Ibuprofen 200mg		Pseudoephedrine HCl 30mg			**Adults & Peds: ≥12 yrs:** 1-2 caps q4-6h. **Max:** 6 caps q24h.
Alka-Seltzer Plus Cold & Sinus Tablets	Acetaminophen 250mg		Phenylephrine HCl 5mg			**Adults & Peds: ≥12 yrs:** 2 tabs q4h. **Max:** 8 tab q24h.
Alka-Seltzer Plus Sinus Effervescent Tablets	Acetaminophen 250mg		Phenylephrine HCl 5mg			**Adults & Peds: ≥12 yrs:** 2 tabs q4h. **Max:** 8 tab q24h.
Contac Cold & Flu Day & Night Caplets	Acetaminophen 500mg		Phenylephrine HCl 5mg			**Adults & Peds: ≥12 yrs:** 2 tabs q4-6h. **Max:** 8 tabs q24h.
Contac Cold & Flu Non-Drowsy Maximum Strength Caplets	Acetaminophen 500mg		Phenylephrine HCl 5mg			**Adults & Peds: ≥12 yrs:** 2 tabs q4-6h. **Max:** 8 tabs q24h.
Motrin Children's Cold Suspension	Ibuprofen 100mg/5mL		Pseudoephedrine HCl 15mg/5mL			**Peds: 6-12 yrs (48-95 lbs):** 2 tsp (10mL) q6h. **2-6 yrs (24-47 lbs):** 1 tsp (5mL) q6h. **Max:** 4 doses q24h
Sinutab Sinus Tablets	Acetaminophen 500mg		Phenylephrine HCl 5mg			**Adults & Peds: ≥12 yrs:** 2 tabs q6h. **Max:** 8 tabs q24h.
Sudafed PE Sinus Headache Caplets	Acetaminophen 325mg		Phenylephrine HCl 5mg			**Adults & Peds: ≥12 yrs:** 2 tabs q4h. **Max:** 12 tabs q24h.
Sudafed Sinus & Cold Liquid Capsules	Acetaminophen 325mg		Pseudoephedrine HCl 30mg			**Adults & Peds: ≥12 yrs:** 2 caps q4-6h. **Max:** 8 caps q24h.

Table 13. COUGH-COLD-FLU PRODUCTS (cont.)

Brand Name	Analgesic	Antihistamine	Decongestant	Cough Suppressant	Expectorant	Dose
Theraflu Daytime Severe Cold Hot Liquid	Acetaminophen 650mg		Phenylephrine HCl 10mg			**Adults & Peds: ≥12 yrs:** 1 packet q4h. **Max:** 6 packets q24h.
Tylenol Sinus Congestion & Pain Daytime Caplets	Acetaminophen 325 mg		Phenylephrine HCl 5mg			**Adults & Peds: ≥12 yrs:** 2 tabs q4h. **Max:** 12 tabs q24h.
Tylenol Sinus Congestion & Pain Daytime Gelcaps	Acetaminophen 325 mg		Phenylephrine HCl 5mg			**Adults & Peds: ≥12 yrs:** 2 caps q4h. **Max:** 12 caps q24h.
Tylenol Sinus Congestion & Pain Daytime Rapid Release Gelcaps	Acetaminophen 325 mg		Phenylephrine HCl 5mg			**Adults & Peds: ≥12 yrs:** 2 caps q4h. **Max:** 12 caps q24h.
Vicks DayQuil Sinus Liquicaps	Acetaminophen 325 mg		Phenylephrine HCl 5mg			**Adults & Peds: ≥12 yrs:** 2 caps q4h. **Max:** 6 caps q24h.
DECONGESTANT + EXPECTORANT						
Dimetapp Children's Cold & Chest Congestion Syrup			Phenylephrine HCl 5mg/5mL		Guaifenesin 100mg/5mL	**Adults: ≥12 yrs:** 2 tsp (10mL) q4h. **Peds: 6-12 yrs:** 1 tsp (5mL) q4h. 2-6 yrs: ½ tsp (2.5mL) 14 h. **Max:** 6 doses q24h.
Mucinex D Extended-Release Tablets			Pseudoephedrine HCl 60mg		Guaifenesin 600mg	**Adults & Peds: ≥12 yrs:** 2 tabs q12h. **Max:** 4 tabs q24h.
Robitussin PE Head & Chest Liquid			Phenylephrine HCl 5mg/5mL		Guaifenesin 100mg/5mL	**Adults: ≥12 yrs:** 2 tsp (10mL) q4h. **Peds: 6-12 yrs:** 1 tsp (5mL) q4h. **Max:** 6 doses q24h.
Sudafed Non-Drying Sinus Liquid Caps			Pseudoephedrine HCl 30mg		Guaifenesin 200mg	**Adults & Peds: ≥12 yrs:** 2 caps q4h. **Max:** 8 caps q24h.
Sudafed PE Non-Drying Sinus Caplets			Phenylephrine HCl 5mg		Guaifenesin 200mg	**Adults & Peds: ≥12 yrs:** 2 tabs q4h. **Max:** 12 tabs q24h.
Triaminic Chest & Nasal Liquid		2.5mg/5mL	Phenylephrine HCl	50mg/5mL	Guaifenesin **Max:** 6 doses q24h.	**Adults & Peds: ≥12 yrs:** 1 tsp q 4h. **Peds: 6-12 yrs:** 2 tsp (10mL). **2-6 yrs:** 1 tsp (5mL).
DECONGESTANT + EXPECTORANT + ANALGESIC						
Tylenol Sinus Congestion & Severe Pain Caplets	Acetaminophen 325 mg		Phenylephrine HCl 5mg		Guaifenesin 200mg	**Adults & Peds: ≥12 yrs:** 2 tabs q4h. **Max:** 12 tabs q24h.
EXPECTORANT						
Mucinex Extended-Release Tablets					Guaifenesin 600mg	**Adults & Peds: ≥12 yrs:** 1-2 tabs q12h. **Max:** 4 tabs q24h.
Mucinex Liquid Grape					Guaifenesin 100mg/5mL	**Peds: 6-12 yrs:** 1-2 tsp q4h. **2-6 yrs:** ½-1 tsp q4h. **Max:** 6 doses 24h.
Mucinex Mini-Melts Bubble Gum Packets					Guaifenesin 100mg	**Adults & Peds: ≥12 yrs:** 2-4 packets q4h. **Peds: 6-12 yrs:** 1-2 packets q4h. **2-6 yrs:** 1 packet q4h. **Max:** 6 doses q24h.
Mucinex Mini-Melts Grape Packets					Guaifenesin 50mg	**Peds: 6-12 yrs:** 2-4 packets q4h. **2-6 yrs:** 1-2 packets q4h. **Max:** 6 doses 24h.

Table 13. COUGH-COLD-FLU PRODUCTS (cont.)

Brand Name	Analgesic	Antihistamine	Decongestant	Cough Suppressant	Expectorant	Dose
Robitussin Chest Congestion Liquid					Guaifenesin 100mg/5mL	**Adults: ≥12 yrs:** 2-4 tsp (10-20mL) q4h. **Peds: 6-12 yrs:** 1-2 tsp (5-10mL) q4h. **2-6 yrs:** ½-1 tsp (2.5-5mL) q4h. **Max:** 6 doses q24h.
Vicks Casero Chest Congestion Relief Liquid					Guaifenesin 100mg/ 6.25mL	**Adults & Peds: ≥12 yrs:** 2.5 tsp (12.5mL) q4h. **Peds: 6-12 yrs:** 1.25 tsp (6.25mL) q4h. **2-6 yrs:** 3.12mL q4h. **Max:** 6 doses q24h.
EXPECTORANT + ANALGESIC						
Comtrex Deep Chest Cold Caplets	Acetaminophen 325mg				Guaifenesin 200mg	**Adults & Peds: ≥12 yrs:** 2 tabs q4-6h. **Max:** 12 tabs q24h.
Tylenol Chest Congestion Caplets	Acetaminophen 325mg				Guaifenesin 200mg	**Adults & Peds: ≥12 yrs:** 2 tabs q4-6h. **Max:** 12 tabs q24h.
Tylenol Chest Congestion Liquid	Acetaminophen 500mg/15mL				Guaifenesin 200mg/ 15mL	**Adults & Peds: ≥12 yrs:** 2 tbl (30mL) q4-6h. **Max:** 8 tbl (120mL) q24h.
Theraflu Flu & Chest Liquid	Acetaminophen 1000mg/packet				Guaifenesin 400mg/ packet	**Adults & Peds: ≥12 yrs:** 1 packet q6h. **Max:** 4 packets q24h.
EXPECTORANT + DECONGESTANT + COUGH SUPPRESSANT						
Robitussin Cold & Cough CF Liquid			Phenylephrine HCl 5mg/5mL	Dextromethorphan HBr 10mg/5mL	Guaifenesin 100mg/5mL	**Adults & Peds: ≥12 yrs:** 2 tsp (10mL) q4h. **Peds: 6-12 yrs:** 1 tsp (5mL) q4h. **2-6 yrs:** ½ tsp (2.5mL) q4h. **Max:** 6 doses q24h.
Robitussin Pediatric Cold & Cough CF Liquid			Phenylephrine HCl 2.5mg/5mL	Dextromethorphan HBr 5mg/2.5mL	Guaifenesin 100mg/ 2.5mL	**Peds: 2-6 yrs:** 2.5mL q4h. **Max:** 6 doses q24h.
EXPECTORANT + DECONGESTANT + ANALGESIC						
Tylenol Sinus Congestion & Severe Pain Caplets	Acetaminophen 325mg		Phenylephrine HCl 5mg		Guaifenesin 200mg	**Adults & Peds: ≥12 yrs:** 2 tabs q4h. **Max:** 12 tabs q24h.
Tylenol Sinus Severe Congestion Daytime Caplets	Acetaminophen 325mg		Pseudoephedrine HCl 30mg		Guaifenesin 200mg	**Adults & Peds: ≥12 yrs:** 2 tabs q6h. **Max:** 8 tabs q24h.
ANTIHISTAMINE + ANALGESIC						
Coricidin Cold & Flu Tablets	Acetaminophen 325mg	Chlorpheniramine Maleate 2mg				**Adults & Peds: ≥12 yrs:** 2 tabs q4-6h. **Max:** 12 tabs q24h.
Tylenol Sore Throat Nighttime Liquid	Acetaminophen 1000mg/30mL	Diphenhydramine HCl 50mg/30mL				**Adults & Peds: ≥12 yrs:** 2 tbl (120mL) q4-6h. **Max:** 8 tbl (120mL) q24h.

Table 14. DANDRUFF PRODUCTS

BRAND NAME	INGREDIENT/STRENGTH	DOSE
COAL TAR		
Denorex Therapeutic Protection 2-in-1 Shampoo	Coal Tar 2.5%	**Adults & Peds:** Use biw.
DHS Tar Dermatological Hair & Scalp Shampoo	Coal Tar 0.5%	**Adults & Peds:** Use biw.
Ionil T Shampoo	Coal Tar 1%	**Adults & Peds:** Use biw.
Ionil T Plus Shampoo	Coal Tar 2%	**Adults & Peds:** Use biw.
Neutrogena T-Gel Shampoo Original Formula	Coal Tar 0.5%	**Adults & Peds:** Use biw.
Neutrogena T-Gel Shampoo, Extra Strength	Coal Tar 1%	**Adults & Peds:** Use biw.
Neutrogena T-Gel Stubborn Itch Shampoo	Coal Tar 0.5%	**Adults & Peds:** Use biw.
KETOCONAZOLE		
Nizoral Anti-Dandruff Shampoo	Ketoconazole 1%	**Adults & Peds ≥12:** Use q3-4d prn.
PYRITHIONE ZINC		
Denorex Dandruff Shampoo, Daily Protection	Pyrithione Zinc 2%	**Adults & Peds:** Use biw.
Garnier Fructis Fortifying Shampoo, Anti-Dandruff	Pyrithione Zinc 1%	**Adults & Peds:** Use biw.
Head & Shoulders Dry Scalp Care Dandruff Shampoo Plus Conditioner; Shampoo; Conditioner	Pyrithione Zinc 0.5%	**Adults & Peds:** Use biw.
Head & Shoulders Smooth & Silky Dandruff Shampoo Plus Conditioner; Shampoo; Conditioner	Pyrithione Zinc 1%	**Adults & Peds:** Use biw.
Head & Shoulders Citrus Breeze Dandruff Shampoo Plus Conditioner; Shampoo	Pyrithione Zinc 1%	**Adults & Peds:** Use biw.
Head & Shoulders Classic Clean Dandruff Shampoo Plus Conditioner; Shampoo; Conditioner	Pyrithione Zinc 1%	**Adults & Peds:** Use biw.
Head & Shoulders Extra Volume Dandruff Shampoo	Pyrithione Zinc 1%	**Adults & Peds:** Use biw.
Head & Shoulders Ocean Lift Dandruff Shampoo Plus Conditioner; Shampoo	Pyrithione Zinc 1%	**Adults & Peds:** Use biw.
Head & Shoulders Dandruff Refresh Shampoo Plus Conditioner; Shampoo	Pyrithione Zinc 1%	**Adults & Peds:** Use biw.
Head & Shoulders Restoring Shine Dandruff Shampoo Plus Conditioner; Shampoo	Pyrithione Zinc 1%	**Adults & Peds:** Use biw.
Head & Shoulders Sensitive Care Dandruff Shampoo Plus Conditioner; Shampoo	Pyrithione Zinc 1%	**Adults & Peds:** Use biw.
Head & Shoulders Intensive Solutions Dandruff Shampoo and Conditioner; Shampoo	Pyrithione Zinc 2%	**Adults & Peds:** Use biw.
L'Oreal VIVE Pro Anti-Dandruff for Men Shampoo	Pyrithione Zinc 1%	**Adults & Peds:** Use biw.
Neutrogena T-Gel Daily Control Dandruff Shampoo	Pyrithione Zinc 1%	**Adults & Peds:** Use biw.
Pantene Pro-V Shampoo + Conditioner, Anti-Dandruff	Pyrithione Zinc 1%	**Adults & Peds:** Use biw.

Table 14. DANDRUFF PRODUCTS (cont.)

BRAND NAME	INGREDIENT/STRENGTH	DOSE
Pert Plus Shampoo Plus Conditioner, Dandruff Control	Pyrithione Zinc 0.45%	**Adults & Peds:** Use biw.
Selsun Salon 2-in-1 Pyrithione Zinc Shampoo	Pyrithione Zinc 1%	**Adults & Peds:** Use biw.
Suave for Men 2 in 1 Shampoo/ Conditioner, Dandruff	Pyrithione Zinc 0.5%	**Adults & Peds:** Use biw.
SALICYLIC ACID		
Denorex Dandruff Shampoo, Extra Strength	Salicylic Acid 3%	**Adults & Peds:** Use biw.
Neutrogena T/Sal Shampoo, Scalp Build-up Control	Salicylic Acid 3%	**Adults & Peds:** Use biw.
Scalpicin Anti-Itch Liquid Scalp Treatment	Salicylic Acid 3%	**Adults & Peds:** Apply to affected area qd-qid.
SELENIUM SULFIDE		
Head & Shoulders Dandruff Shampoo, Intensive Treatment	Selenium Sulfide 1%	**Adults & Peds:** Use biw.
Selsun Blue Dandruff Shampoo, Medicated Treatment	Selenium Sulfide 1%	**Adults & Peds:** Use biw.
Selsun Blue Dandruff Shampoo Plus Conditioner	Selenium Sulfide 1%	**Adults & Peds:** Use biw.
Selsun Blue Dandruff Shampoo	Selenium Sulfide 1%	**Adults & Peds:** Use biw.
Selsun Blue Dandruff Shampoo, Moisturizing Treatment	Selenium Sulfide 1%	**Adults & Peds:** Use biw.
SULFUR/SALICYLIC ACID		
Sebulex Medicated Dandruff Shampoo	Sulfur/Salicylic Acid 2%-2%	**Adults & Peds ≥12yrs:** Use qd.

Table 15. HEADACHE/MIGRAINE PRODUCTS

Brand Name	Ingredient/Strength	Dose
ACETAMINOPHEN		
Anacin Extra Strength Aspirin Free Tablets	Acetaminophen 500mg	**Adults & Peds: ≥12 yrs:** 2 tabs q6h. **Max:** 8 tabs q24h.
Tylenol 8 Hour Caplets	Acetaminophen 650mg	**Adults & Peds: ≥12 yrs:** 2 tabs q8h prn. **Max:** 6 tabs q24h.
Tylenol 8 Hour Geltabs	Acetaminophen 650mg	**Adults & Peds: ≥12 yrs:** 2 tabs q8h prn. **Max:** 6 tabs q24h.
Tylenol Arthritis Caplets	Acetaminophen 650mg	**Adults:** 2 tabs q8h prn. **Max:** 6 tabs q24h.
Tylenol Arthritis Geltabs	Acetaminophen 650mg	**Adults:** 2 tabs q8h prn. **Max:** 6 tabs q24h.
Tylenol Children's Meltaway Tablets	Acetaminophen 80mg	**Peds: 2-3 yrs (24-35 lbs):** 2 tabs **4-5 yrs (36-47 lbs):** 3 tabs. **6-8 yrs (48-59 lbs):** 4 tabs. **9-10 yrs (60-71 lbs):** 5 tabs. **11 yrs (72-95 lbs):** 6 tabs. May repeat q4h. **Max:** 5 doses q24h.
Tylenol Children's Suspension	Acetaminophen 160mg/5mL	**Peds: 2-3 yrs (24-35 lbs):** 1 tsp (5mL). **4-5 yrs (36-47 lbs):** 1.5tsp (7.5mL). **6-8 yrs (48-59 lbs):** 2 tsp (10mL). **9-10 yrs (60-71 lbs):** 2.5 tsp (12.5mL). **11 yrs (72-95 lbs):** 3 tsp (15mL). May repeat q4h. **Max:** 5 doses q24h.
Tylenol Extra Strength Caplets	Acetaminophen 500mg	**Adults & Peds: ≥12 yrs:** 2 tabs q4-6h prn. **Max:** 8 tabs q24h.
Tylenol Extra Strength Cool Caplets	Acetaminophen 500mg	**Adults & Peds: ≥12 yrs:** 2 tabs q4-6h prn. **Max:** 8 tabs q24h.
Tylenol Extra Strength Rapid Release Gels	Acetaminophen 500mg	**Adults & Peds: ≥12 yrs:** 2 caps q4-6h prn. **Max:** 8 caps q24h.
Tylenol Extra Strength Rapid Blast Liquid	Acetaminophen 1000mg/30mL	**Adults & Peds: ≥12 yrs:** 2 tbl (30mL) q4-6h prn. **Max:** 8 tbl (120mL) q24h.
Tylenol Extra Strength EZ Tabs	Acetaminophen 500mg	**Adults & Peds: ≥12 yrs:** 2 tabs q4-6h prn. **Max:** 8 tabs q24h.
Tylenol Extra Strength Go Tabs	Acetaminophen 500mg	**Adults & Peds: ≥12 yrs:** 2 tabs q4-6h prn. **Max:** 8 tabs q24h.
Tylenol Infants' Suspension	Acetaminophen 80mg/0.8mL	**Peds: 2-3 yrs (24-35 lbs):** 1.6 mL q4h prn. **Max:** 5 doses (8mL) q24h.
Tylenol Junior Meltaways Tablets	Acetaminophen 160mg	**Peds: 6-8 yrs (48-59 lbs):** 2 tabs. **9-10 yrs (60-71 lbs):** 2.5 tabs. **11 yrs (72-95 lbs):** 3 tabs. **12 yrs (≥96 lbs):** 4 tabs. May repeat q4h. **Max:** 5 doses q24h.
Tylenol Regular Strength Tablets	Acetaminophen 325mg	**Adults & Peds: ≥12 yrs:** 2 tabs q4-6h prn. **Max:** 12 tabs q24h. **Peds: 6-11 yrs:** 1 tab q4-6h. **Max:** 5 tabs q24h.
ACETAMINOPHEN COMBINATIONS		
Excedrin Extra Strength Caplets	Acetaminophen/Aspirin/Caffeine 250mg-250mg-65mg	**Adults & Peds: ≥12 yrs:** 2 tabs q6h. **Max:** 8 tabs q24h.
Excedrin Extra Strength Geltabs	Acetaminophen/Aspirin/Caffeine 250mg-250mg-65mg	**Adults & Peds: ≥12 yrs:** 2 tabs q6h. **Max:** 8 tabs q24h.
Excedrin Extra Strength Tablets	Acetaminophen/Aspirin/Caffeine 250mg-250mg-65mg	**Adults & Peds: ≥12 yrs:** 2 tabs q6h. **Max:** 8 tabs q24h.
Excedrin Migraine Caplets	Acetaminophen/Aspirin/Caffeine 250mg-250mg-65mg	**Adults:** 2 tabs prn. **Max:** 2 tabs q24h.
Excedrin Migraine Geltabs	Acetaminophen/Aspirin/Caffeine 250mg-250mg-65mg	**Adults:** 2 tabs prn. **Max:** 2 tabs q24h.
Excedrin Migraine Tablets	Acetaminophen/Aspirin/Caffeine 250mg-250mg-65mg	**Adults:** 2 tabs prn. **Max:** 2 tabs q24h.

Table 15. HEADACHE/MIGRAINE PRODUCTS (cont.)

Brand Name	Ingredient/Strength	Dose
Excedrin Sinus Headache Caplets	Acetaminophen/Phenylephrine HCl 325mg-5mg	**Adults & Peds:** ≥12 yrs: 2 tabs q4h. **Max:** 12 tabs q24h.
Excedrin Sinus Headache Tablets	Acetaminophen/Phenylephrine HCl 325mg-5mg	**Adults & Peds:** ≥12 yrs: 2 tabs q4h. **Max:** 12 tabs q24h.
Excedrin Tension Headache Caplets	Acetaminophen/Caffeine 500mg-65mg	**Adults & Peds:** ≥12 yrs: 2 tabs q6h. **Max:** 8 tabs q24h.
Excedrin Tension Headache Geltabs	Acetaminophen/Caffeine 500mg-65mg	**Adults & Peds:** ≥12 yrs: 2 tabs q6h. **Max:** 8 tabs q24h.
Excedrin Tension Headache Tablets	Acetaminophen/Caffeine 500mg-65mg	**Adults & Peds:** ≥12 yrs: 2 tabs q6h. **Max:** 8 tabs q24h.
Goody's Extra Strength Headache Powders	Acetaminophen/Aspirin/Caffeine 260mg-520mg-32.5mg	**Adults & Peds:** ≥12 yrs: 1 powder q4-6h. **Max:** 4 powders q24h.
Sudafed PE Sinus Headache Coated Caplets	Acetaminophen/Phenylephrine HCl 325mg-5mg	**Adults & Peds:** ≥12 yrs: 2 tabs q4h. **Max:** 12 tabs q24h.
Tylenol Sinus Congestion & Pain Daytime Gelcaps	Acetaminophen/Phenylephrine HCl 325mg-5mg	**Adults & Peds:** ≥12 yrs: 2 caps q4h. **Max:** 12 caps q24h.
Tylenol Sinus Congestion & Pain Daytime Rapid Release Gelcaps	Acetaminophen/Phenylephrine HCl 325mg-5mg	**Adults & Peds:** ≥12 yrs: 2 caps q4h. **Max:** 12 caps q24h.
Vanquish Caplets	Acetaminophen/Aspirin/Caffeine 194mg-227mg-33mg	**Adults & Peds:** ≥12 yrs: 2 tabs q6h. **Max:** 8 tabs q24h.
ACETAMINOPHEN/SLEEP AIDS		
Excedrin PM Caplets	Acetaminophen/Diphenhydramine 500mg-38mg	**Adults & Peds:** ≥12 yrs: 2 tabs qhs.
Excedrin PM Geltabs	Acetaminophen/Diphenhydramine citrate 500mg-38 mg	**Adults & Peds:** ≥12 yrs:2 tabs qhs.
Excedrin PM Tablets	Acetaminophen/Diphenhydramine citrate 500mg-38 mg	**Adults & Peds:** ≥12 yrs:2 tabs qhs.
Goody's PM Powder	Acetaminophen/Diphenhydramine 1000mg-76mg/dose	**Adults & Peds:** ≥12 yrs: 1 packet (2 powders) qhs.
Tylenol PM Caplets	Acetaminophen/Diphenhydramine 500mg-25mg	**Adults & Peds:** ≥12 yrs: 2 tabs qhs.
Tylenol PM Rapid Release Gels	Acetaminophen/Diphenhydramine 500mg-25mg	**Adults & Peds:** ≥12 yrs: 2 caps qhs.
Tylenol PM Geltabs	Acetaminophen/Diphenhydramine 500mg-25mg	**Adults & Peds:** ≥12 yrs: 2 tabs qhs.
Tylenol Sinus Night Time Caplets	Acetaminophen/Pseudoephedrine HCl/ Doxylamine Succinate 500mg-30mg-6.25mg	**Adults & Peds:** ≥12 yrs: 2 tbl (30mL) qhs. **Max:** 8 tbl (120mL)q24h.
NONSTEROIDAL ANTI-INFLAMMATORY DRUGS (NSAIDS)		
Advil Caplets	Ibuprofen 200mg	**Adults & Peds:** ≥12 yrs: 1-2 tabs q4-6h. **Max:** 6 tabs q24h.
Advil Children's Chewable Tablets	Ibuprofen 50mg	**Peds: 2-3 yr (24-35 lbs):** 2 tabs q6-8h. **4-5 yr (36-47 lbs):** 3 tabs q6-8h. **6-8 yr (48-59 lbs):** 4 tabs q6-8h. **9-10 yr (60-71 lbs):** 5 tabs q6-8h. **11 yr (72-95 lbs):** 6 tabs q6-8h. **Max:** 4 doses q24h
Advil Children's Suspension	Ibuprofen 100mg/5mL	**Peds: 2-3 yrs (24-35 lbs):** 1 tsp (5mL). **4-5 yrs (36-47 lbs):** 1.5 tsp (7.5mL). **6-8 yrs (48-59 lbs):** 2 tsp (10mL). **11 yrs 9-10 yrs (60-71 lbs):** 2.5 tsp (12.5mL). **(72-95 lbs):** 3 tsp (15mL). May repeat q6-8h. **Max:** 4 doses q24h.
Advil Gel Caplets	Ibuprofen 200mg	**Adults & Peds:** ≥12 yrs: 1-2 caps q4-6h. **Max:** 6 caps q24h.

Table 15. HEADACHE/MIGRAINE PRODUCTS (cont.)

BRAND NAME	INGREDIENT/STRENGTH	DOSE
Advil Infants' Concentrated Drops	Ibuprofen 50mg/1.25mL	**Peds: 6-11 months (12-17 lbs):** 1.25mL. **12-23 months (18-23 lbs):** 1.875mL. May repeat q6-8h. **Max:** 4 doses q24h.
Advil Junior Strength Swallow Tablets	Ibuprofen 100mg	**Peds: 6-10 yrs (48-71 lbs):** 2 tabs. **11 yrs (72-95 lbs):** 3 tabs. May repeat q6-8h. **Max:** 4 doses q24h.
Advil Junior Strength Chewable Tablets	Ibuprofen 100mg	
Advil Liqui-Gels	Ibuprofen 200mg	**Adults & Peds: ≥12 yrs:** 1-2 caps q4-6h. **Max:** 6 caps q24h.
Advil Migraine Capsules	Ibuprofen 200mg	**Adults:** 2 caps prn. **Max:** 2 caps q24h.
Advil Tablets	Ibuprofen 200mg	**Adults & Peds: ≥12 yrs:** 1-2 tabs q4-6h. **Max:** 6 tabs q24h.
Aleve Caplets	Naproxen Sodium 220mg	**Adults & Peds: ≥12 yrs:** 1 tab q8-12h. May take 1 additional tab within 1 hour of first dose. **Max:** 3 tabs q24h.
Aleve Gelcaps	Naproxen Sodium 220mg	**Adults & Peds: ≥12 yrs:** 1 cap q8-12h. May take 1 additional tab within 1 hour of first dose. **Max:** 3 caps q24h.
Aleve Tablets	Naproxen Sodium 220mg	**Adults & Peds: ≥12 yrs:** 1 tab q8-12h. May take 1 additional tab within 1 hour of first dose. **Max:** 3 q24h.
Motrin Children's Suspension	Ibuprofen 100mg/5mL	**Peds: 2-3 yrs (24-35 lbs):** 1 tsp (5mL). **4-5 yrs (36-47 lbs):** 1.5tsp (7.5mL). **6-8 yrs (48-59 lbs):** 2 tsp (10mL). **9-10 yrs (60-71 lbs):** 2.5 tsp (12.5mL). **11 yrs (72-95 lbs):** 3 tsp (15mL). May repeat q6-8h. **Max:** 4 doses q24h.
Motrin IB Caplets	Ibuprofen 200mg	**Adults & Peds: ≥12 yrs:** 1-2 tabs q4-6h. **Max:** 6 tabs q24h.
Motrin IB Tablets	Ibuprofen 200mg	**Adults & Peds: ≥12 yrs:** 1-2 tabs q4-6h. **Max:** 6 tabs q24h.
Motrin Infants' Drops	Ibuprofen 50mg/1.25mL	**Peds: 6-11 months (12-17 lbs):** 1.25mL. **12-23 months (18-23 lbs):** 1.875mL. May repeat q6-8h. **Max:** 4 doses q24h.
Motrin Junior Strength Chewable Tablets	Ibuprofen 100mg	**Peds: 6-8 yrs (48-59 lbs):** 2 tabs. **9-10 yrs (60-71 lbs):** 2.5 tabs. **11 yrs (72-95 lbs):** 3 tabs. May repeat q6-8h. **Max:** 4 doses q24h.
NSAID COMBINATIONS		
Aleve Sinus & Headache Caplets	Naproxen Sodium/Pseudoephedrine HCl 220 mg-120 mg	**Adults & Peds: ≥12 yrs:** 1 tab q12h. **Max:** 2 tabs q24h.
SALICYLATES		
Anacin 81 Tablets	Aspirin 81mg	**Adults & Peds: ≥12 yrs:** 2 tabs q6h. **Max:** 8 tabs q24h.
Aspergum Chewable Tablets	Aspirin 227mg	**Adults & Peds: ≥12 yrs:** 2 tabs q4h. **Max:** 16 tabs q24h.
Bayer Aspirin Extra Strength Caplets	Aspirin 500mg	**Adults & Peds: ≥12 yrs:** 1-2 tabs q4-6h. **Max:** 8 tabs q24h.
Bayer Genuine Aspirin Tablets	Aspirin 325mg	**Adults & Peds: ≥12 yrs:** 1-2 tabs q4h or 3 tabs q6h. **Max:** 12 tabs q24h.
Bayer Genuine Aspirin Caplets	Aspirin 325mg	**Adults & Peds: ≥12 yrs:** 1-2 tabs q4h or 3 tabs q6h. **Max:** 12 tabs q24h.
Bayer Aspirin Chewable Tablets	Aspirin 81mg	**Adults & Peds: ≥12 yrs:** 4-8 tabs q4h. **Max:** 48 tabs q24h.

Table 15. HEADACHE/MIGRAINE PRODUCTS (cont.)

Brand Name	Ingredient/Strength	Dose
Bayer Low Dose Aspirin Tablets	Aspirin 81mg	**Adults & Peds: ≥12 yrs:** 4-8 tabs q4h. **Max:** 48 tabs q24h.
Doan's Extra Strength Caplets	Magnesium Salicylate Tetrahydrate 580mg	**Adults & Peds: ≥12 yrs:** 2 tabs q6h. **Max:** 8 tabs q24h.
Ecotrin Low Strength Tablets	Aspirin 81mg	**Adults:** 4-8 tabs q4h. **Max:** 48 tabs q24h.
Ecotrin Regular Strength Tablets	Aspirin 325mg	**Adults & Peds: ≥12 yrs:** 1-2 tabs q4h. **Max:** 12 tabs q24h.
Ecotrin Maximum Strength Tablets	Aspirin 500mg	**Adults & Peds: ≥12 yrs:** 2 tabs q6h. **Max:** 8 tabs q24h.
Halfprin 162mg Tablets	Aspirin 162mg	**Adults & Peds: ≥12 yrs:** 2-4 tabs q4h. **Max:** 24 tabs q24h.
Halfprin 81mg Tablets	Aspirin 81mg	**Adults & Peds: ≥12 yrs:** 4-8 tabs q4h. **Max:** 48 tabs q24h.
St. Joseph Chewable	Aspirin 81mg	**Adults & Peds: ≥12 yrs:** 4-8 tabs q4h.
St. Joseph Enteric	Aspirin 81mg	**Adults & Peds: ≥12 yrs:** 4-8 tabs q4h.
SALICYLATES, BUFFERED		
Alka-Seltzer Original Effervescent Tablets	Aspirin/Citric Acid/Sodium Bicarbonate 325mg-1000mg-1916mg	**Adults & Peds: ≥12 yrs:** 2 tabs q4h. **Max:** 8 tabs q24h. **≥60 yrs: Max:** 4 tabs q24h.
Alka-Seltzer Extra Strength Effervescent Tablets	Aspirin/Citric Acid/Sodium Bicarbonate 500mg-1000mg-1985mg	**Adults & Peds: ≥12 yrs:** 2 tabs q6h. **Max:** 7 tabs q24h. **≥60 yrs: Max:** 3 tabs q24h.
Ascriptin Maximum Strength Tablets	Aspirin Buffered with Maalox/Calcium Carbonate 500mg	**Adults & Peds: ≥12 yrs:** 2 tabs q4h. **Max:** 8 tabs q24h.
Ascriptin Regular Strength Tablets	Aspirin Buffered with Maalox/Calcium Carbonate 325mg	**Adults & Peds: ≥12 yrs:** 2 tabs q4h. **Max:** 12 tabs q24h.
Bayer Extra Strength Plus Caplets	Aspirin Buffered with Calcium Carbonate 500mg	**Adults & Peds: ≥12 yrs:** 1-2 tabs q4-6h. **Max:** 8 tabs q24h.
Bufferin Extra Strength Tablets	Aspirin Buffered with Calcium Carbonate/ Magnesium Oxide/Magnesium Carbonate 500mg	**Adults & Peds: ≥12 yrs:** 2 tabs q6h. **Max:** 8 tabs q24h.
Bufferin Tablets	Aspirin Buffered with Benzoic Acid/ Citric Acid 325	**Adults & Peds: ≥12 yrs:** 2 tabs q4h. **Max:** 12 tabs q24h.
SALICYLATE COMBINATIONS		
Alka-Seltzer Morning Relief Effervescent Tablets	Aspirin/Caffeine 500mg-65mg	**Adults & Peds: ≥12 yrs:** 2 tabs q6h. **Max:** 8 tabs q24h. **≥60 yrs: Max:** 4 tabs q24h.
Anacin Max Strength Tablets	Aspirin/Caffeine 500mg-32mg	**Adults & Peds: ≥12 yrs:** 2 tabs q6h. **Max:** 8 tabs q24h.
Anacin Tablets	Aspirin/Caffeine 400mg-32mg	**Adults & Peds: ≥12 yrs:** 2 tabs q6h. **Max:** 8 tabs q24h.
Bayer Back & Body Pain Caplets	Aspirin/Caffeine 500mg-32.5mg	**Adults & Peds: ≥12 yrs:** 2 tabs q6h. **Max:** 8 tabs q24h.
BC Arthritis Strength Powders	Aspirin/Caffeine/Salicylamide 742mg-38mg-222mg	**Adults & Peds: ≥12 yrs:** 1 powder q3-4h. **Max:** 4 powders q24h.
BC Original Formula Powders	Aspirin/Caffeine/Salicylamide 650mg-33.3mg-195mg	**Adults & Peds: ≥12 yrs:** 1 powder q3-4h. **Max:** 4 powders q24h.
SALICYLATE/SLEEP AIDS		
Alka-Seltzer PM Pain Reliever & Sleep Aid Effervescent Tablets	Aspirin/Diphenhydramine Citrate 325mg-38 mg	**Adults & Peds: ≥12 yrs:** 2 tabs qpm.
Bayer PM Relief Caplets	Aspirin/Diphenhydramine 500mg-38.3mg	**Adults & Peds: ≥12 yrs:** 2 tabs qhs.
Doan's Extra Strength PM Caplets	Magnesium Salicylate Tetrahydrate/ Diphenhydramine 580mg-25mg	**Adults & Peds: ≥12 yrs:** 2 tabs qhs.

Table 16. HEMORRHOIDAL PRODUCTS

BRAND NAME	INGREDIENT/STRENGTH	DOSE
ANESTHETICS/ANESTHETIC COMBINATIONS		
Tucks Hemorrhoidal Ointment	Pramoxine HCl/Zinc Oxide/ Mineral Oil 1%-12.5% - 46.6%	**Adults: ≥12 yrs:** Apply to affected area prn. **Max:** 5 times q24h.
Fleet Pain Relief Pre-Moistened Anorectal Pads	Pramoxine HCl/Glycerin 1%-12%	**Adults & Peds: ≥12 yrs:** Apply to affected area prn. **Max:** 5 times q24h.
Hemorid Maximum Strength Hemorrhoidal Creme with Aloe	Petrolatum/Mineral Oil/Pramoxine HCl/ Phenylephrine HCl 30%-20%-1%-0.25%	**Adults & Peds: ≥12 yrs:** Apply to affected area qid.
Nupercainal Ointment	Dibucaine 1%	**Adults & Peds: ≥12 yrs:** Apply to affected area qid.
Preparation H Hemorrhoidal Cream, Maximum Strength Pain Relief	Glycerin/Phenylephrine HCl/Pramoxine HCl/ White Petrolatum 14.4%-0.25%-1%-15%	**Adults & Peds: ≥12 yrs:** Apply to affected area qid.
Tronolane Anesthetic Hemorrhoid Cream	Pramoxine HCl/Zinc Oxide 1%-5%	**Adults:** Apply to affected area prn. **Max:** 5 times q24h.
BULK-FORMING LAXATIVES		
Citrucel Caplets	Methylcellulose 500mg	**Adults: ≥12 yrs:** 2 caps qd prn. **Max:** 12 tabs q24h. **Peds: 6-12 yrs:** 1 cap qd prn. **Max:** 6 tabs q24h.
Citrucel Powder	Methylcellulose 2g/tbl	**Adults: ≥12 yrs:** 1 tbl (11.5g) qd-tid. **Peds: 6-12 yrs:** ½ tbl (5.75g) qd.
Equalactin Chewable Tablet	Calcium Polycarbophil 625mg	**Adults & Peds: ≥12 yrs:** 2 tabs qd. **Max:** 8 tabs qd. **Peds: 6-12 yrs:** 1 tab qd. **Max:** 4 tabs qd. **2 to <6 yrs:** 1 tab qd. **Max:** 2 tabs qd.
Fibercon Caplets	Calcium Polycarbophil 625mg	**Adults & Peds: ≥12 yrs:** 2 caps qd. **Max:** 8 caps qd. **Peds: <12 yrs:** Ask doctor.
Konsyl Easy Mix Powder	Psyllium 6g/tsp	**Adults & Peds: ≥12 yrs:** 1 tsp qd-tid. **Max:** ½ tsp qd-tid.
Konsyl Fiber Caplets	Calcium Polycarbophil 625mg	**Adults & Peds: ≥2 yrs:** 2 caps qd. **Max:** 8 caps qd.
Konsyl Orange Powder	Psyllium 3.4g	**Adults & Peds: ≥12 yrs:** 1 tsp qd-tid. **Max:** ½ tsp qd-tid.
Konsyl Original Powder	Psyllium 6g/tsp	**Adults ≥12 yrs:** 1 tsp qd-tid. **Peds: 6-12 yrs:** ½ tsp qd-tid.
Konsyl-D Powder	Psyllium 3.4g/tsp	**Adults ≥12 yrs:** 1 tsp qd-tid. **Peds: 6-12 yrs:** ½ tsp qd-tid.
Metamucil Capsules	Psyllium 0.52g	**Adults & Peds: ≥12 yrs:** 5 caps qd-tid.
Metamucil Original	Psyllium 3.4g/tbs Texture Powder	**Adults ≥12 yrs:** 1 tbs qd-tid. **Peds: 6-12 yrs:** ½ tsp qd-tid.
Metamucil Smooth Texture Powder	Psyllium 3.4g/tbs	**Adults ≥12 yrs:** 1 tbs qd-tid. **Peds: 6-12 yrs:** ½ tsp qd-tid.
Metamucil Wafers	Psyllium 3.4g/dose	**Adults ≥12 yrs:** 2 wafers qd-tid. **Peds: 6-12 yrs:** 1 wafer qd-tid.
HYDROCORTISONE		
Tucks Anti-Itch Ointment	Hydrocortisone Acetate 1.12%	**Adults & Peds: ≥12 yrs:** Apply to affected area ud. **Max:** Apply to affected area tid-qid q24h.
Preparation H Anti-Itch Cream	Hydrocortisone 1.0%	**Adults & Peds: ≥12 yrs:** Apply to affected area tid-qid.
STOOL SOFTENER		
Colace Capsules	Docusate Sodium 100mg	**Adults: ≥12 yrs:** 1-3 caps qd. **Peds: 2-12 yrs:** 1 cap qd.
Colace Capsules	Docusate Sodium 50mg	**Adults: ≥12 yrs:** 1-6 caps qd. **Peds: 2-12 yrs:** 1-3 caps qd.
Colace Liquid	Docusate Sodium 10mg/mL	**Adults: ≥12 yrs:** 5-15mL qd-bid. **Peds: 2-12 yrs:** 5-15mL qd.
Colace Syrup	Docusate Sodium 60mg/15mL	**Adults: ≥12 yrs:** 15-90mL qd. **Peds: 2-12 yrs:** 5-37.5mL qd.

Table 16. HEMORRHOIDAL PRODUCTS (cont.)

Brand Name	Ingredient/Strength	Dose
Correctol Stool Softener Laxative Soft-Gels	Docusate Sodium 100mg	**Adults: ≥12 yrs:** Take 2 caps qd. **Peds: 2-12 yrs:** Take 1 cap qd.
Docusol Constipation Relief, Mini Enemas	Docusate Sodium 283mg	**Adults: ≥12 yrs:** Take 1-3 units qd. **Peds: 6-12 yrs:** Take 1 unit qd.
Dulcolax Stool Softener Capsules	Docusate Sodium 100mg	**Adults: ≥12 yrs:** 1-3 caps qd. **Peds: 6-12 yrs:** 1 cap qd.
Ex-Lax Stool Softener Tablets	Docusate Sodium 100mg	**Adults: ≥12 yrs:** 1-3 caps qd. **Peds: 2-12 yrs:** 1 cap qd.
Kaopectate Liqui-Gels	Docusate Calcium 240mg	**Adults & Peds: ≥12 yrs:** 1 cap qd until normal bowel movement.
Phillips Stool Softener Capsules	Docusate Sodium 100mg	**Adults: ≥12 yrs:** 1-3 caps qd. **Peds: 6-12 yrs:** 1 cap qd.
WITCH HAZEL/WITCH HAZEL COMBINATIONS		
Hemspray Hemorrhoid Relief Spray	Witch Hazel/Glycerin/Phenylephrine HCl/ Camphor 50%-20%-0.25%-0.15%	**Adults & Peds: ≥12 yrs:** Apply to affected area prn. **Max:** 5 times q24h.
Preparation H Hemorrhoidal Cooling Gel	Phenylephrine HCl/Witch Hazel 0.25%-50.0%	**Adults & Peds: ≥12 yrs:** Apply to affected area qid.
Preparation H Medicated Wipes	Witch Hazel 50%	**Adults & Peds: ≥12 yrs:** Apply to affected area prn. **Max:** 6 times q24h.
T.N. Dickinson's Witch Hazel Hemorrhoidal Pads	Witch Hazel 50%	**Adults & Peds: ≥12 yrs:** Apply to affected area prn. **Max:** 6 times q24h.
Tucks Hemorrhoidal Pads with Witch Hazel	Witch Hazel 50%	**Adults & Peds: ≥12 yrs:** Apply to affected area prn. **Max:** 6 times q24h.
Tucks Hemorrhoidal Towelettes with Witch Hazel	Witch Hazel 50%	**Adults & Peds: ≥12 yrs:** Apply to affected area prn. **Max:** 6 times q24h.
MISCELLANEOUS		
Preparation H Hemorrhoidal Ointment	Mineral Oil/Petrolatum/Phenylephrine HCl/ Shark Liver Oil 14%-71.9%-0.25%-3.0%	**Adults & Peds: ≥12 yrs:** Apply to affected area qid.
Preparation H Hemorrhoidal Suppositories	Cocoa Butter/Phenylephrine HCl/ Shark Liver Oil 85.5%-0.25%-3.0%	**Adults & Peds: ≥12 yrs:** Insert 1 supp qid.
Rectal Medicone Suppositories	Phenylephrine HCl 0.25%	**Adults & Peds: ≥12 yrs:** Insert 1 supp tid-qid.
Tronolane Suppositories	Hard Fat/Phenylephrine HCl 88.7%-0.25%	**Adults & Peds: ≥12 yrs:** Insert 1 supp prn. **Max:** 4 times q24h.
Tucks Topical Starch Hemorrhoidal Suppositories	Topical Starch 51%	**Adults & Peds: ≥12 yrs:** Insert 1 supp prn. **Max:** 6 times q24h.

Table 17. INSOMNIA PRODUCTS

Brand Name	Ingredient/Strength	Dose
DIPHENHYDRAMINE		
Nytol Quick Caps Caplets	Diphenhydramine 25mg	**Adults & Peds: ≥12 yrs:** 2 tabs qpm.
Nytol Quick Gels Capsules	Diphenhydramine 50mg	**Adults & Peds: ≥12 yrs:** 1 tab qpm.
Simply Sleep Nighttime Sleep Aid Caplets	Diphenhydramine 25mg	**Adults & Peds: ≥12 yrs:** 2 tabs qpm.
Sominex Original Formula	Diphenhydramine 25mg	**Adults & Peds: ≥12 yrs:** 2 tabs qpm.
Sominex Maximum Strength Formula	Diphenhydramine 50mg	**Adults & Peds: ≥12 yrs:** 1 tab qpm.
Unisom Nighttime Sleep-Aid Sleep Gels	Diphenhydramine 50mg	**Adults & Peds: ≥12 yrs:** 1 tab qpm.
DIPHENHYDRAMINE COMBINATION		
Alka-Seltzer PM	Aspirin/Diphenhydramine Citrate 325mg-38mg	**Adults & Peds: ≥12 yrs:** 2 tabs qpm.
Bayer PM Relief Caplets	Aspirin/Diphenhydramine 500mg-38.3mg	**Adults & Peds: ≥12 yrs:** 2 tabs qhs.
Doan's Extra Strength PM Caplets	Magnesium Salicylate Tetrahydrate/ Diphenhydramine 580mg-25mg	**Adults & Peds: ≥12 yrs:** 2 tabs qhs.
Excedrin PM Caplets	Acetaminophen/Diphenhydramine 500mg-38mg	**Adults & Peds: ≥12 yrs:** 2 tabs qhs.
Excedrin PM Geltabs	Acetaminophen/Diphenhydramine 500mg-38mg	**Adults & Peds: ≥12 yrs:** 2 tabs qhs.
Excedrin PM Tablets	Acetaminophen/Diphenhydramine 500mg-38mg	**Adults & Peds: ≥12 yrs:** 2 tabs qhs.
Goody's PM Powders	Acetaminophen/Diphenhydramine 1000mg-76mg/dose	**Adults & Peds: ≥12 yrs:** 1 packet (2 powders) qhs.
Tylenol PM Caplets	Acetaminophen/Diphenhydramine 500mg-25mg	**Adults & Peds: ≥12 yrs:** 2 tabs qhs.
Tylenol PM Rapid Release Gelcaps	Acetaminophen/Diphenhydramine 500mg-25mg	**Adults & Peds: ≥12 yrs:** 2 caps qhs.
Tylenol PM Geltabs	Acetaminophen/Diphenhydramine 500mg-25mg	**Adults & Peds: ≥12 yrs:** 2 tabs qhs.
Tylenol PM Liquid	Acetaminophen/Diphenhydramine 1000g-50mg/30mL	**Adults & Peds: ≥12 yrs:** 2 tbl (30mL) qhs. **Max:** 8 tbl (120mL) q24h.
DOXYLAMINE		
Unisom Nighttime Sleep-Aid Sleep Tabs	Doxylamine Succinate 25mg	**Adults & Peds: ≥12 yrs:** 1 tab 30 min before hs.

Table 18. IS IT A COLD, THE FLU, OR AN ALLERGY?

	COLD	FLU	AIRBORNE ALLERGY
SYMPTOMS			
Chest discomfort	Mild to moderate	Common; can become severe	Sometimes
Cough	Common (hacking cough)	Sometimes	Sometimes
Duration	3-14 days	Days to weeks	Weeks (eg, 6 weeks for ragweed or grass pollen seasons)
Extreme exhaustion	Never	Early and prominent	Never
Fatigue, weakness	Sometimes	Can last up to 2-3 weeks	Sometimes
Fever	Rare	Characteristic, high (100-102°F); lasts 3-4 days	Never
General aches, pains	Slight	Usual; often severe	Never
Headache	Rare	Prominent	Sometimes
Itchy eyes	Rare or never	Rare or never	Common
Runny nose	Common		Common
Sneezing	Usual	Sometimes	Usual
Sore throat	Common	Sometimes	Sometimes
Stuffy nose	Common	Sometimes	Common
TREATMENT*			
	Antihistamines	Amantadine	Antihistamines
	Decongestants	Rimantadine	Nasal steroids
	Nonsteroidal anti-inflammatories	Oseltamivir	Decongestants
		Zanamavir	
PREVENTION			
	Wash your hands often; avoid close contact with anyone with a cold	Annual vaccination Amantadine Rimantadine Oseltamivir	Avoid allergens such as pollen, house flies, dust mites, mold, pet dander, cockroaches
COMPLICATIONS			
	Sinus infection	Bronchitis	Sinus infection
	Middle ear infection	Pneumonia	Asthma
	Asthma	Can be life-threatening	

Adapted from the National Institute of Allergy and Infectious Diseases, September 2005.

*Used only for temporary relief of cold symptoms.

Table 19. LAXATIVE PRODUCTS

BRAND NAME	INGREDIENT/STRENGTH	DOSE
BULK-FORMING		
Citrucel Caplets	Methylcellulose 500mg	**Adults: ≥12 yrs:** 2 caps qd prn. **Max:** 12 tabs q24h. **Peds: 6-12 yrs:** 1 cap qd prn. **Max:** 6 tabs q24h.
Citrucel Powder	Methylcellulose 2g/tbl	**Adults: ≥12 yrs:** 1 tbl (11.5g) qd tid. **Peds: 6-12 yrs:** ½ tbl (5.75g) qd.
Equalactin Chewable Tablet	Calcium Polycarbophil 625mg	**Adults & Peds: ≥12 yrs:** 2 tabs qd. **Max:** 8 tabs qd. **Peds: 6-12 yrs:** 1 tab qd. **Max:** 2 tabs qd. **2 to <6 yrs:** 1 tab qd. **Max:** 2 tabs qd.
Fibercon Caplets	Calcium Polycarbophil 625mg	**Adults & Peds: ≥12 yrs:** 2 tabs qd. **Max:** 8 tabs qd. **Peds: 6-12 yrs:** 1 tab qd. **Max:** 4 tabs qd. **2 to <6 yrs:** 1 tab qd. **Max:** 2 tabs qd.
Konsyl Easy Mix Powder	Psyllium 6g/tsp	**Adults: ≥12 yrs:** 1 tsp qd-tid. **Peds: 6-12 yrs:** ½ tsp qd-tid.
Konsyl Fiber Caplets	Calcium Polycarbophil 625mg	**Adults & Peds: ≥12 yrs:** 2 tabs qd. **Max:** 8 tabs qd.
Konsyl Orange Powder	Psyllium 3.4g	**Adults: ≥12 yrs:** 1 tsp qd-tid. **Peds: 6-12 yrs:** ½ tsp qd-tid.
Konsyl Original Powder	Psyllium 6g/tsp	**Adults: ≥12 yrs:** 1 tsp qd-tid. **Peds: 6-12 yrs:** ½ tsp qd-tid.
Konsyl-D Powder	Psyllium 3.4g/tsp	**Adults: ≥12 yrs:** 1 tsp qd-tid. **Peds: 6-12 yrs:** ½ tsp qd-tid.
Metamucil Capsules	Psyllium 0.52g	**Adults & Peds: ≥12 yrs:** 5 caps qd-tid.
Metamucil Original Texture Powder	Psyllium 3.4g/tbs	**Adults: ≥12 yrs:** 1 tbs qd-tid. **Peds: 6-12 yrs:** ½ tsp qd-tid.
Metamucil Smooth Texture Powder	Psyllium 3.4g/tbs	**Adults: ≥12 yrs:** 1 tbs qd-tid. **Peds: 6-12 yrs:** ½ tsp qd-tid.
Metamucil Wafers	Psyllium 3.4 g/dose	**Adults: ≥12 yrs:** 2 wafers qd-tid. **Peds: 6-12 yrs:** 1 wafer qd-tid.
HYPEROSMOTICS		
Fleet Children's Babylax Suppositories	Glycerin 2.3g	**Peds: 2-5 yrs:** 1 supp. ud.
Fleet Glycerin Suppositories	Glycerin 2g	**Adults & Peds: ≥6 yrs:** 1 supp ud.
Fleet Liquid Glycerin Suppositories	Glycerin 5.6g	**Adults & Peds: ≥6 yrs:** 1 supp ud.
Fleet Mineral Oil Enema	Mineral Oil 133mL	**Adults: ≥12 yrs:** 1 bottle (133mL). **Peds: 2-12 yrs:** ½ bottle (66.5mL)
HYPEROSMOTIC COMBINATION		
Fleet Pain Relief Pre-Moistened Anorectal Pads	Glycerin/Pramoxine HCl 12%-1%	**Adults & Peds: ≥12 yrs:** Apply to affected area up to five times daily.
OSMOTIC		
MiraLAX	Polyethylene Glycol 3350	**Adults & Peds: ≥17 yrs:** Stir and dissolve 17g in 4-8 oz of beverage and drink qd. Use no more than 7 days.
SALINES		
Ex-Lax Milk of Magnesia Liquid	Magnesium Hydroxide 400mg/5mL	**Adults & Peds: ≥12 yrs:** Take 2-4 tbs hs. **Peds: 6-11 yrs:** 1-2 tbs hs. **2-5 yrs:** 1-3 tbs hs.
Fleet Children's Enema	Monobasic Sodium Phosphate/Dibasic Sodium Phosphate 9.5g-3.5g/66mL	**Peds: 5-11 yrs:** 1 bottle (66mL). **2-5 yrs:** ½ bottle (33mL).
Fleet Enema	Monobasic Sodium Phosphate/Dibasic Sodium Phosphate 19g-7g/133mL	**Adults & Peds: ≥12 yrs:** 1 bottle (133mL).
Fleet Phospho-Soda	Monobasic Sodium Phosphate/Dibasic Sodium Phosphate 2.4g-0.9g/5mL	**Adults: ≥12 yrs:** 1 tbl in 8 oz of water. **Max:** 3 tbl. **Peds: 10-11 yrs:** 1 tbl in 8 oz of water. **Max:** 1 tbl. **5-9 yrs:** ½ tbl in 8 oz of water. **Max:** ½ tbl.
Magnesium Citrate Solution	Magnesium Citrate 1.75gm/30mL	**Adults: ≥12 yrs:** 300mL. **Peds: 6-12 yrs:** 90-210mL. **2-6 yrs:** 60-90mL.

Table 19. LAXATIVE PRODUCTS (cont.)

BRAND NAME	INGREDIENT/STRENGTH	DOSE
Phillips Antacid/Laxative Chewable Tablets	Magnesium Hydroxide 311mg	**Adults: ≥12 yrs:** 6-8 tabs qd. **Peds: 6-11 yrs:** 3-4 tabs qd. **2-5 yrs:** 1-2 tabs qd.
Phillips Soft Chews, Laxative	Magnesium/Sodium 500mg-10 mg	**Adults & Peds: ≥12 yrs:** Take 2-4 tab qd. **Max:** 4 tab q24h.
Phillips Cramp-Free Laxative Caplets	Magnesium 500 mg	**Adults & Peds: ≥12 yrs:** Take 2-4 tabs qd. **Max:** 4 tabs q24h.
Phillips Milk of Magnesia Concentrated Liquid	Magnesium Hydroxide 800mg/5mL	**Adults: ≥12 yrs:** 15-30mL qd. **Peds: 6-11 yrs:** 7.5-15mL qd. **2-5 yrs:** 2.5-7.5mL qd.
Phillips Milk of Magnesia Liquid	Magnesium Hydroxide 400mg/5mL	**Adults: ≥12 yrs:** 30-60mL qd. **Peds: 6-11 yrs:** 15-30mL qd. **2-5 yrs:** 5-15mL qd.
SALINE COMBINATION		
Phillips M-O Liquid	Magnesium Hydroxide/Mineral Oil 300mg-1.25mL/5mL	**Adults: ≥12 yrs:** 30-60mL qd. **Peds: 6-11 yrs:** 5-15mL qd.
STIMULANTS		
Alophen Enteric Coated Stimulant Laxative Pills	Bisacodyl 5mg	**Adults: ≥12 yrs:** Take 1-3 tabs qd. **Peds: 6-12 yrs:** Take 1 tab qd.
Carter's Laxative, Sodium Free Pills	Bisacodyl 5mg	**Adults:** qd.**12 yrs:** Take 1-3 tabs (usually 2 tabs) qd. **Peds: 6-12 yrs:** Take 1 tab qd.
Castor Oil	Castor Oil	**Adults: ≥12 yrs:** 15-60mL. **Peds: 2-12 yrs:** 5-15mL.
Correctol Stimulant Laxative Tablets For Women	Bisacodyl 5mg	**Adults: ≥12 yrs:** Take 1-3 tabs qd. **Peds: 6-12 yrs:** Take 1 tab qd.
Doxidan Capsules	Bisacodyl 5mg	**Adults: ≥12 yrs:** 1-3 caps (usually 2) qd. **Peds: 6-12 yrs:** 1 cap qd.
Dulcolax Overnight Relief Laxative Tablets	Bisacodyl 5mg	**Adults: ≥12 yrs:** 1-3 tabs (usually 2) qd. **Peds: 6-12 yo:** 1 tab qd.
Dulcolax Suppository	Bisacodyl 10mg	**Adults: ≥12 yrs:** 1 supp qd. **Peds: 6-12 yrs:** ½ supp qd.
Dulcolax Tablets	Bisacodyl 5mg	**Adults: ≥12 yrs:** 1-3 tabs (usually 2) qd. **Peds: 6-12 yrs:** 1 tab qd.
Ex-Lax Maximum Strength Tablets	Sennosides 25mg	**Adults: ≥12 yrs:** 2 tabs qd-bid. **Peds: 6-12 yrs:** 1 tab qd-bid.
Ex-Lax Tablets	Sennosides 15mg	**Adults: ≥12 yrs:** 2 tabs qd-bid. **Peds: 6-12 yrs:** 1 tab qd-bid.
Ex-Lax Ultra Stimulant Laxative Tablets	Bisacodyl 5mg	**Adults: ≥12 yrs:** 1-3 tabs qd. **Peds: 6-12 yrs:** 1 tab qd.
Fleet Bisacodyl Suppositories	Bisacodyl 10mg	**Adults: ≥12 yrs:** 1 supp. qd. **Peds: 6-12 yrs:** ½ supp. qd.
Fleet Stimulant Laxative Tablets	Bisacodyl 5mg	**Adults: ≥12 yrs:** 1-3 tabs (usually 2) qd. **Peds: 6-12 yrs:** 1 tab qd.
Nature's Remedy Caplets	Aloe/Cascara Sagrada 100mg-150mg	**Adults: ≥12 yrs:** 2 tabs qd-bid. **Max:** 4 tabs bid. **Peds: 6-12 yrs:** 1 tab qd-bid. **Max:** 2 tabs bid. **2-6 yrs:** ½ tab qd-bid. **Max:** 1 tab bid.
Perdiem Overnight Relief Tablets	Sennosides 15mg	**Adults: ≥12 yrs:** 2 tabs qd-bid. **Peds: 6-12 yrs:** 1 tab qd-bid.
Senokot Tablets	Sennosides 8.6mg	**Adults: ≥12 yrs:** 2 tabs qd. **Max** 4 tabs bid. **Peds: 6-12 yrs:** 1 tab qd. **Max:** 2 tabs bid. **2-6 yrs:** ½ tab qd. **Max:** 1 tab bid.
STIMULANT COMBINATIONS		
Peri-Colace Tablets	Sennosides/Docusate 8.6mg-50mg	**Adults: ≥12 yrs:** 2-4 tabs qd. **Peds: 6-12 yrs:** 1-2 tabs qd. **2-6 yrs:** 1 tab qd.
Senokot S Tablets	Sennosides/Docusate 8.6mg-50mg	**Adults: ≥12 yrs:** 2 tabs qd. **Max:** 4 tabs bid. **Peds: 6-12 yrs:** 1 tab qd. **Max:** 2 tabs bid. **2-6 yrs:** ½ tab qd. **Max:** 1 tab bid.

Table 19. LAXATIVE PRODUCTS (cont.)

BRAND NAME	INGREDIENT/STRENGTH	DOSE
SURFACTANTS (STOOL SOFTENERS)		
Colace Capsules	Docusate Sodium 100mg	**Adults: ≥12 yrs:** 1-3 caps qd. **Peds: 2-12 yrs:** 1 cap qd.
Colace Capsules	Docusate Sodium 50mg	**Adults: ≥12 yrs:** 1-6 caps qd. **Peds: 2-12 yrs:** 1-3 caps qd.
Colace Liquid	Docusate Sodium 10mg/mL	**Adults: ≥12 yrs:** 5-15mL qd-bid. **Peds: 2-12 yrs:** 5-15mL qd.
Colace Syrup	Docusate Sodium 60mg/15mL	**Adults: ≥12 yrs:** 15-90mL qd. **Peds: 2-12 yrs:** 5-37.5mL qd.
Correctol Stool Softener Laxative Soft-Gels	Docusate Sodium 100mg	**Adults: ≥12 yrs:** Take 2 caps qd. **Peds: 2-12 yrs:** Take 1 cap qd
Docusol Constipation Relief, Mini Enemas	Docusate Sodium 283mg	**Adults: ≥12 yrs:** Take 1-3 units qd. **Peds: 6-12 yrs:** Take 1 unit qd
Dulcolax Stool Softener Capsules	Docusate Sodium 100mg	**Adults: ≥12 yrs:** 1-3 caps qd. **Peds: 2-12 yrs:** 1 cap qd.
Ex-Lax Stool Softener Tablets	Docusate Sodium 100mg	**Adults: ≥12 yrs:** 1-3 caps qd. **Peds: 2-12 yrs:** 1 cap qd.
Kaopectate Liqui-Gels	Docusate Calcium 240mg	**Adults & Peds: ≥12 yrs:** 1 cap qd until normal bowel movement.
Phillips Stool Softener Capsules	Docusate Sodium 100mg	**Adults: ≥12 yrs:** 1-3 caps qd. **Peds: 6-12 yrs:** 1 cap qd.
Kaopectate Liqui-Gels	Docusate Calcium 240mg	**Adults & Peds: ≥12 yrs:** 1 cap qd until normal bowel movement.
Phillips Stool Softener Capsules	Docusate Sodium 100mg	**Adults: ≥12 yrs:** 1-3 caps qd. **Peds: 2-12 yrs:** 1 cap qd.

Table 20. NASAL DECONGESTANT/MOISTURIZING PRODUCTS

BRAND NAME	INGREDIENT/STRENGTH	DOSE
PSEUDOEPHEDRINE		
Sudafed 12 Hour Tablets	Pseudoephedrine HCl 120mg	**Adults & Peds: ≥12 yrs:** 1 tab q12h. **Max:** 2 tabs/day.
Sudafed 24 Hour Tablets	Pseudoephedrine HCl 240mg	**Adults & Peds: ≥12 yrs:** 1 tab q24h. **Max:** 1 tab/day.
Sudafed Children's Nasal Decongestant Chewable Tablets	Pseudoephedrine HCl 15mg	**Peds: 6-12 yrs:** 2 tabs q4-6h. **Max:** 4 doses/day.
Sudafed Children's Nasal Decongestant Liquid	Pseudoephedrine HCl 15mg/5mL	**Adults: ≥12 yrs:** 4 tsp (20mL) q4-6h. **Peds: 6-12 yrs:** 2 tsp (10mL) q4h. **2-6 yrs:** 1 tsp (5mL) q4-6h. **Max:** 4 doses/day.
Sudafed Nasal Decongestant Tablets	Pseudoephedrine HCl 30mg	**Adults: ≥12 yrs:** 2 tabs q4-6h. **Peds: 6-12 yrs:** 1 tab q4-6h. **Max:** 4 doses/day.
PHENYLEPHRINE		
Pediacare Children's Decongestant Liquid	Phenylephrine 2.5/5mL	**Peds: 6-12 yrs:** 2 tsp (10mL) q4h. **2-6 yrs:** 1 tsp (5mL) q4-6h. **Max:** 4 doses/day.
Sudafed PE	Phenylephrine 10mg	**Adults & Peds: ≥12 yrs:** 1 tablet every 4 hours. **Max:** 6 tabs per day.
Sudafed PE Quick Dissolve Strips	Phenylephrine 10mg	**Adults & Peds: ≥12 yrs:** Dissolve 1 strip on tongue every 4 hours. **Max:** 6 doses per day.
TOPICAL NASAL DECONGESTANTS		
4-Way Fast Acting Nasal Decongestant Spray	Phenylephrine HCl 1%	**Adults & Peds: ≥12 yrs:** Instill 2-3 sprays per nostril q4h.
4-Way Mentholated Nasal Decongestant Spray	Phenylephrine HCl 1%	**Adults & Peds: ≥12 yrs:** Instill 2-3 sprays per nostril q4h.
4-Way No Drip Nasal Decongestant Spray	Oxymetazoline HCl 0.05%	**Adults & Peds: ≥6 yrs:** Instill 2-3 sprays per nostril q10-12h.
Afrin No Drip Extra Moisturizing Nasal Spray	Oxymetazoline HCl 0.05%	**Adults & Peds: ≥6 yrs:** Instill 2-3 sprays per nostril q10-12h. **Max:** 2 doses q24h.
Afrin No Drip Sinus Nasal Spray	Oxymetazoline HCl 0.05%	**Adults & Peds: ≥6 yrs:** Instill 2-3 sprays per nostril q10-12h.
Afrin Original Nasal Spray	Oxymetazoline HCl 0.05%	**Adults & Peds: ≥6 yrs:** Instill 2-3 sprays per nostril q10-12h.
Afrin No-Drip Original Pump Mist Nasal Spray	Oxymetazoline HCl 0.05%	**Adults & Peds: ≥6 yrs:** Instill 2-3 sprays per nostril q10-12h.
Afrin No Drip Severe Congestion Nasal Spray	Oxymetazoline HCl 0.05%	**Adults & Peds: ≥6 yrs:** Instill 2-3 sprays per nostril q10-12h.
Afrin No Drip All Night 12 Hour Pump Mist	Oxymetazoline HCl 0.05%	**Adults & Peds: ≥6 yrs:** Instill 2-3 sprays per nostril q10-12h.
Benzedrex Inhaler	Propylhexedrine 250 mg	**Adults & Peds: ≥6 yrs:** Inhale 2 sprays per nostril q2h.
Dristan 12 Hour Nasal Spray	Oxymetazoline HCl 0.05%	**Adults & Peds: ≥6 yrs:** Instill 2-3 sprays per nostril q10-12h. **Max:** 2 doses q24h.
Neo-Synephrine 12 Hour Extra Moisturizing Nasal Spray	Oxymetazoline HCl 0.05%	**Adults & Peds: ≥6 yrs:** Instill 2-3 sprays per nostril q10-12h. **Max:** 2 doses q24h.
Neo-Synephrine 12 Hour Nasal Decongestant Spray	Oxymetazoline HCl 0.05%	**Adults & Peds: ≥6 yrs:** Instill 2-3 sprays per nostril q10-12h.
Neo-Synephrine Extra Strength Nasal Decongestant Drops	Phenylephrine HCl 1%	**Adults & Peds: ≥12 yrs:** Instill 2-3 drops per nostril q4h.

Table 20. NASAL DECONGESTANT/MOISTURIZING PRODUCTS (cont.)

BRAND NAME	INGREDIENT/STRENGTH	DOSE
Neo-Synephrine Extra Strength Nasal Spray	Phenylephrine HCl 1%	**Adults & Peds: ≥6 yrs:** Instill 2-3 sprays per nostril q4h.
Neo-Synephrine Mild Formula Nasal Spray	Phenylephrine HCl 0.25%	**Adults & Peds: ≥6 yrs:** Instill 2-3 sprays per nostril q4h.
Neo-Synephrine Regular Strength Nasal Decongestant Spray	Phenylephrine HCl 0.5%	**Adults & Peds: ≥12 yrs:** Instill 2-3 sprays per nostril q4h.
Nostrilla 12 Hour Nasal Decongestant	Oxymetazoline HCl 0.05%	**Adults & Peds: ≥6 yrs:** Instill 2-3 sprays per nostril q10-12h. **Max:** 2 doses q24h.
Vicks Sinex 12 Hour Ultra Fine Mist For Sinus Relief	Oxymetazoline HCl 0.05%	**Adults & Peds: ≥12 yrs:** Instill 2-3 sprays per nostril q10-12h.
Vicks Sinex Long Acting Nasal Spray For Sinus Relief	Oxymetazoline HCl 0.05%	**Adults & Peds: ≥12 yrs:** Instill 2-3 sprays per nostril q10-12h. **Max:** 2 doses q24h.
Vicks Sinex Nasal Spray For Sinus Relief	Phenylephrine HCl 0.5%	**Adults & Peds: ≥12 yrs:** Instill 2-3 sprays per nostril q4h.
Zicam Extreme Congestion Relief	Oxymetazoline HCl 0.05%	**Adults & Peds: ≥12 yrs:** Instill 2-3 sprays per nostril q10-12h. **Max:** 2 doses q24h.
Zicam Intense Sinus Relief	Oxymetazoline HCl 0.05%	**Adults & Peds: ≥12 yrs:** Instill 2-3 sprays per nostril q10-12h. **Max:** 2 doses q24h.
TOPICAL NASAL MOISTURIZERS		
4-Way Saline Moisturizing Mist	Water, Boric Acid, Glycerin, Sodium Chloride, Sodium Borate, Eucalyptol, Menthol, Polysorbate 80, Benzalkonium Chloride	**Adults & Peds: ≥2 yrs:** Instill 2-3 sprays per nostril prn.
Ayr Baby's Saline Nose Spray, Drops	Sodium Chloride 0.65%	**Peds:** Instill 2 to 6 drops in each nostril.
Ayr Saline Nasal Gel With Soothing Aloe	Water, Methyl Gluceth 10, Propylene Glycol, Glycerin, Glyceryl Polymethacrylate, Triethanolamine, Aloe Barbadensis Leaf Juice (Aloe Vera Gel), PEG/PPG 18/18 Dimethicone, Carbomer, Poloxamer 184, Sodium Chloride, Xanthan Gum, Diazolidinyl Urea, Methylparaben, Propylparaben, Glycine Soja Oil (Soybean), Geranium Maculatum Oil, Tocopheryl Acetate, Blue 1	**Adults & Peds:** Apply to nostril prn.
Ayr Saline Nasal Gel, No-Drip Sinus Spray	Water, Sodium Carbomethyl Starch, Propylene Glycol, Glycerin, Aloe Barbadensis Leaf Juice (Aloe Vera Gel), Sodium Chloride, Cetyl Pyridinium Chloride, Citric Acid, Disodium EDTA, Glycine Soja (Soybean Oil), Tocopheryl Acetate, Benzyl Alcohol, Benzalkonium Chloride, Geranium Maculatum Oil	**Adults & Peds: ≥12 yrs:** Instill 1 spray in each nostril as directed.
Ayr Saline Nasal Mist	Sodium Chloride 0.65%	**Adults & Peds: ≥12 yrs:** Instill 2 sprays per nostril prn.
ENTSOL Mist, Buffered Hypertonic Nasal Irrigation Mist	Purified Water, Sodium Chloride, Sodium Phosphate Dibasic Edetate Disodium, Potassium Phosphate Monobasic, Benzalkonium Chloride	**Adults & Peds:** Instill 1-2 sprays per nostril prn.
ENTSOL Single Use, Pre-Filled Nasal Wash Squeeze Bottle	Purified Water, Sodium Chloride, Sodium Phosphate Dibasic, Potassium Phosphate Monobasic	**Adults & Peds: ≥12 yrs:** Use as directed.
ENTSOL Spray, Buffered Hypertonic Saline Nasal Spray	Purified Water, Sodium Chloride Phosphate Dibasic, Potassium Phosphate Monobasic	**Adults & Peds: ≥12 yrs:** Instill 1 spray per nostril bid, 6 times daily

Table 20. NASAL DECONGESTANT/MOISTURIZING PRODUCTS (cont.)

BRAND NAME	INGREDIENT/STRENGTH	DOSE
ENTSOL Nasal Gel with Aloe and Vitamin E	Water (Purified), Propylene Glycol, Aloe, Glycerin, Dimethicone Copolyol, Poloxamer 184, Methyl Gluceth 10, Triethanolamine, Carbomer, Sodium Chloride, Vitamin E, Disodium EDTA, Xanthan Gum, Benzalkonium Chloride	**Adults & Peds:** Use prn.
Little Noses Saline Spray/Drops, Non-Medicated	Sodium Chloride 0.65%	**Peds:** 2-6 drops per nostril as directed.
Ocean Premium Saline Nasal Spray	Sodium Chloride 0.65%	**Adults & Peds: ≥6 yrs:** Instill 2 sprays per nostril prn.
Simply Saline Sterile Saline Nasal Mist	Sodium Chloride 0.9%	**Adults & Peds: ≥12 yrs:** Use prn as directed.
SinoFresh Moisturizing Nasal & Sinus Spray	Purified Water, Propylene Glycol, Monobasic Sodium Phosphate, Dibasic Sodium Phosphate, Sodium Chloride, Polysorbate 80, Sorbitol Solution, Essential Oil Blend (Wintergreen Oil, Spearmint Oil, Peppermint Oil, Eucalyptus Oil) Cetylpyridinium Chloride, Benzalkonium Chloride	**Adults & Peds: ≥12 yrs:** Instill 1-3 sprays per nostril bid.

Table 21. OPHTHALMIC DECONGESTANT/ANTIHISTAMINE PRODUCTS

BRAND NAME	INGREDIENT/STRENGTH	DOSE
KETOTIFEN		
Alaway	Ketotifen 0.025%	**Adults & Peds: >3 yrs:** 1 drop in affected eye bid. **Max:** 2 doses qd.
Zaditor	Ketotifen 0.025%	**Adults & Peds: >3 yrs:** Instill 1 drop in affected eye bid. **Max:** 2 doses qd.
NAPHAZOLINE		
Bausch & Lomb Advanced Eye Relief	Naphazoline HCl/Hypromellose 0.3%-0.5%	**Adults:** Instill 1-2 drops to affected eye qid.
Clear Eyes ACR Seasonal Relief	Naphazoline HCl/Glycerin/Zinc Sulfate 0.012%-0.2%-0.25%	**Adults:** Instill 1-2 drops to affected eye qid.
Clear Eyes Extra Relief Lubricant Eye Redness Reliever	Naphazoline HCl/Glycerine 0.012%-0.2%	**Adults:** Instill 1-2 drops to affected eye qid.
Opcon-A Allergy Relief Drops	Naphazoline HCl/Pheniramine Maleate 0.025%-0.3%	**Adults & Peds: >6 yrs:** Instill 1-2 drops to affected eye qid.
Rohto V Cool Redness Relief Drops	Naphazoline HCl/ Polysorbate 80 0.012%-0.2%	**Adults:** Instill 1-2 drops to affected eye qid.
Visine-A Allergy Relief Drops	Naphazoline HCl/ Pheniramine Maleate 0.025%-0.3%	**Adults & Peds: ≥6 yrs:** Instill 1-2 drops to affected eye qid.
OXYMETAZOLINE		
Visine L.R. Redness Reliever Drops	Oxymetazoline HCl 0.025%	**Adults & Peds: ≥6 yrs:** Instill 1-2 drops to affected eye prn.
PHENYLEPHRINE		
Allergan Relief Redness Reliever & Lubricant Eye Drops	Phenylephrine HCl/ Polyvinyl Alcohol 0.12%-1.4%	**Adults:** Instill 1-2 drops to affected eye qid.
TETRAHYDROZOLINE		
Murine Tears Plus Eye Drops	Tetrahydrozoline HCl/Polyvinyl Alcohol/ Povidone 0.05%-0.5%-0.6%	**Adults:** Instill 1-2 drops to affected eye qid.
Rohto Ice Eye Drops	Tetrahydrozoline HCl/Hypromellose/Zinc Sulfate 0.05%-0.2%-0.25%	**Adults:** Instill 1-2 drops to affected eye qid.
Visine Original Drops	Tetrahydrozoline HCl 0.05%	**Adults:** Instill 1-2 drops to affected eye qid.
Visine Advanced Redness Reliever Drops	Tetrahydrozoline HCl/Polyethylene Glycol 400/ Povidone/Dextran 70 0.05%-1%-1%-0.1%	**Adults:** Instill 1-2 drops to affected eye qid.
Visine A.C. Astringent Redness Reliever Drops	Tetrahydrozoline HCl/ Zinc Sulfate 0.05%-0.25%	**Adults:** Instill 1-2 drops to affected eye qid.

Table 22. PSORIASIS PRODUCTS

Brand Name	Ingredient/Strength	Dose
COAL TAR		
Denorex Therapeutic Protection 2-in-1 Shampoo	Coal Tar 2.5%	**Adults & Peds:** Use at least biw.
Denorex Therapeutic Protection Shampoo	Coal Tar 2.5%	**Adults & Peds:** Use at least biw.
DHS Tar Shampoo	Coal Tar 0.5%	**Adults & Peds:** Use at least biw.
Ionil-T Plus Shampoo	Coal Tar 2%	**Adults & Peds:** Use at least biw.
Ionil-T Shampoo	Coal Tar 1%	**Adults & Peds:** Use at least biw.
MG217 Ointment	Coal Tar 2%	**Adults & Peds:** Apply to affected area qd-qid.
MG217 Tar Shampoo	Coal Tar 3%	**Adults & Peds:** Use at least biw.
Neutrogena T/Gel Shampoo Extra Strength	Coal Tar 1%	**Adults & Peds:** Use at least biw.
Neutrogena T/Gel Shampoo Original Formula	Coal Tar 0.5%	**Adults & Peds:** Use at least biw.
Neutrogena T/Gel Stubborn Itch Shampoo	Coal Tar 0.5%	**Adults & Peds:** Use at least biw.
Polytar Shampoo	Coal Tar 0.5%	**Adults & Peds:** Use at least biw.
Polytar Soap	Coal Tar 0.5%	**Adults & Peds:** Apply to affected area prn.
Psoriasin Multi-Symptom Psoriasis Relief Gel	Coal Tar 1.25%	**Adults & Peds:** Apply to affected area qd-qid.
Psoriasin Multi-Symptom Psoriasis Relief Ointment	Coal Tar 2%	**Adults & Peds:** Apply to affected area qd-qid.
CORTICOSTEROIDS		
Aveeno Hydrocortisone 1% Anti-Itch Cream	Hydrocortisone 1%	**Adults & Peds:** ≥2 yrs: Apply to affected area tid-qid.
Cortaid Advanced 12-Hour Anti-Itch Cream	Hydrocortisone 1%	**Adults & Peds:** ≥2 yrs: Apply to affected area tid-qid.
Cortaid Intensive Therapy Cooling Spray	Hydrocortisone 1%	**Adults & Peds:** ≥2 yrs: Apply to affected area tid-qid.
Cortaid Intensive Therapy Moisturizing Cream	Hydrocortisone 1%	**Adults & Peds:** ≥2 yrs: Apply to affected area tid-qid.
Cortaid Maximum Strength Cream	Hydrocortisone 1%	**Adults & Peds:** ≥2 yrs: Apply to affected area tid-qid.
Cortaid Maximum Strength Ointment	Hydrocortisone 1%	**Adults & Peds:** ≥2 yrs: Apply to affected area tid-qid.
Cortizone-10 Cream	Hydrocortisone 1%	**Adults & Peds:** ≥2 yrs: Apply to affected area tid-qid.
Cortizone-10 Maximum Strength Anti-Itch Ointment	Hydrocortisone 1%	**Adults & Peds:** ≥2 yrs: Apply to affected area tid-qid.
Cortizone-10 Ointment	Hydrocortisone 1%	**Adults & Peds:** ≥2 yrs: Apply to affected area tid-qid.
Cortizone-10 Plus Intensive Healing Formula	Hydrocortisone 1%	**Adults & Peds:** ≥2 yrs: Apply to affected area tid-qid.
SALICYLIC ACID		
Dermarest Psoriasis Overnight Treatment	Salicylic Acid 3%	**Adults & Peds:** Apply to affected area qhs. **Max:** qid.
Dermarest Psoriasis Medicated Moisturizer	Salicylic Acid 2%	**Adults & Peds:** Apply to affected area qd-qid.
Dermarest Psoriasis Medicated Scalp Treatment	Salicylic Acid 3%	**Adults & Peds:** Apply to affected area qd-qid.
Dermarest Psoriasis Medicated Shampoo/Conditioner	Salicylic Acid 3%	**Adults & Peds:** Apply to affected area at least biw.
Dermarest Psoriasis Skin Treatment	Salicylic Acid 3%	**Adults & Peds:** Apply to affected area qd-qid.
Neutrogena T/Gel Conditioner	Salicylic Acid 2%	**Adults & Peds:** Use at least biw.
Psoriasin Therapeutic Shampoo and Body Wash	Salicylic Acid 3%	**Adults & Peds:** Use biw.
Psoriasin Therapeutic Shampoo With Panthenol	Salicylic Acid 3%	**Adults & Peds:** Use biw.

Table 23. SMOKING CESSATION PRODUCTS

Brand Name	Ingredient/Strength	Dose
Commit Stop Smoking 2mg Lozenges	Nicotine Polacrilex 2mg	**Adults:** If smoking first cigarettte >30 minutes after waking up use 2mg lozenge. **Weeks 1 to 6:** 1 lozenge q1-2h. **Weeks 7 to 9:** 1 lozenge q2-4h. **Weeks 10 to 12:** 1 lozenge q4-8h. **Max:** 5 lozenges/6 hours; 20 lozenges/day. Stop using at the end of 12 weeks.
Commit Stop Smoking 4mg Lozenges	Nicotine Polacrilex 4mg	**Adults:** If smoking first cigarettte within 30 minutes after waking up use 4mg lozenge. **Weeks 1 to 6:** 1 lozenge q1-2h. **Weeks 7 to 9:** 1 lozenge q2-4h. **Weeks 10 to 12:** 1 lozenge q4-8h. **Max:** 5 lozenges/6 hours; 20 lozenges/day. Stop using at the end of 12 weeks.
NicoDerm CQ Step 1 Clear Patch	Nicotine 21mg	**Adults:** If smoking >10 cigarettes/day. **Weeks 1 to 6:** Apply one 21mg patch/day. **Weeks 7 to 8:** Apply one 14mg patch/day. **Weeks 9 to 10:** Apply one 7mg patch/day.
NicoDerm CQ Step 2 Clear Patch	Nicotine 14mg	**Adults:** If smoking <10 cigarettes/day. **Weeks 1 to 6:** Apply one 14mg patch/day. **Weeks 7 to 8:** Apply one 7mg patch/day.
NicoDerm CQ Step 3 Clear Patch	Nicotine 7mg	**Adults:** Apply 1 patch qd Weeks 9 to 10 if smoking >10 cigarettes/day or Weeks 7 to 8 if smoking ≤10 cigarettes/day.
Nicorette 2mg, Original/Mint/Orange Gum	Nicotine Polacrilex 2mg	**Adults:** If smoking <25 cigarettes/day use 2mg gum. **Weeks 1 to 6:** 1 piece q1-2h. **Weeks 7 to 9:** 1 piece q2-4h. **Weeks 10 to 12:** 1 piece q4-8h. **Max:** 24 pieces/day.
Nicorette 4mg, Original/Mint/Orange Gum	Nicotine Polacrilex 4mg	**Adults:** If smoking ≥25 cigarettes/day use 4mg gum. **Weeks 1 to 6:** 1 piece q1-2h. **Weeks 7 to 9:** 1 piece q2-4h. **Weeks 10 to 12:** 1 piece q4-8h. **Max:** 24 pieces/day.
Habitrol Nicotine Transdermal System Patch Step 1	Nicotine 21mg/24hr	**Adults:** If smoking >10 cigarettes/day. **Weeks 1 to 4:** Apply one 21mg patch/day. **Weeks 5 to 6:** Apply one 14mg patch/day. **Weeks 7 to 8:** Apply one 7mg patch/day.
Habitrol Nicotine Transdermal System Patch Step 2	Nicotine 14mg/24hr	**Adults:** If smoking >10 cigarettes/day. **Weeks 1 to 4:** Apply one 21mg patch/day. **Weeks 5 to 6:** Apply one 14mg patch/day. **Weeks 7 to 8:** Apply one 7mg patch/day. If smoking <10 cigarettes/day. **Weeks 1 to 6:** Apply one 14 mg patch/day. **Weeks 7 to 8:** Apply one 7mg patch/day.
Habitrol Nicotine Transdermal System Patch Step 3	Nicotine 7mg/24hr	**Adults:** If smoking >10 cigarettes/day. **Weeks 1 to 4:** Apply one 21mg patch/day. **Weeks 5 to 6:** Apply one 14mg patch/day. **Weeks 7 to 8:** Apply one 7mg patch/day. If smoking <10 cigarettes/day. **Weeks 1 to 6:** Apply one 14mg patch/day. **Weeks 7 to 8:** Apply one 7mg patch/day.

Table 24. WEIGHT MANAGEMENT PRODUCTS

Brand Name	Ingredient/Strength	Dose
Alli Weight-Loss Aid	Orlistat 60 mg	**Adults:** 1 cap with each fat-containing meal. **Max:** 3 caps per day.
Applied Nutrition Green Tea Fat Burner	Chromium (From Chromium Picolinate), Green Tea Extract (Leaf, 50% EGCG, 2% Caffeine), Natural Caffeine, Xenedrol Blend [(Bitter Orange Extract) (Fruit, 6% Synephrine), Betaine HCl, Bladderwrack Powder, Cayenne Powder (Fruit), Eleuthero Powder (Root), Ginger Powder(Root), Gotu Kola Powder (Aerial), Licorice *(Glycyrrhiza glabra)* Powder (Root, rhizome), Maté (Yerba Maté) Powder (Leaf)]	**Adults:** Take 2 caps with meals bid.
Applied Nutrition Hoodia Diet Capsules	Green Tea Extract (Leaf, 20% Caffeine), *Hoodia gordonii* (Aerial, 20:1), Natural Caffeine, Garcinia Extract (Fruit, 50% Hydroxycitric Acid), Choline (as Choline Bitartrate), Inositol, L-Methionine	**Adults:** Take 2 caps with meals bid.
Applied Nutrition Natural Fat Burner Capsules	Vitamin C (as Ascorbic Acid), Vitamin E (as d-Alpha Tocopheryl Acetate), Niacin (as Niacinamide), Vitamin B6 (as Pyridoxine Hydrochloride), Folic Acid, Vitamin B12 (as Cyanocobalamin), Green Tea Extract (leaf, 50% EGCG), Natural Caffeine, Red Leaf Lettuce-powder, Cassia Extract (6:1 bark), Cranberry (*Vaccinium macrocarpon*) Extract (fruit), Grapefruit Extract, Noni Extract, Blueberry (*Vaccinium angustifolium*) Extract (fruit), Pomegranate Extract, Apple Cider Vinegar powder, Citrus (*Citrus spp.*) Bioflavonoids (fruit)	**Adults:** Take 2 caps with meals bid.
Applied Nutrition The New Grapefruit Diet Capsules	Vitamin B6 (as Pyridoxine HCl), Iodine, (Kelp), Chromemate (as Chromium Picolinate), Soy Lecithin, Grapefruit Powder Extract, Cider Vinegar Powder, Bioperine Black Pepper Extract (Fruit)	**Adults:** Take 1 or 2 caps qd-tid.
Aqua-Ban Maximum Strength Diuretic Tablets	Pamabrom 50mg	**Adults:** Take 1 tab qid. **Max:** 4 tabs q24h.
Atkins Essential Oils Vita-Nutrient Supplement Formula Softgels	Flaxseed Oil, Borage Seed Oil, Fish Oil, Oleic Acid, Linoleic Acid, Gamma Linolenic Acid, Eicosapentaenoic Acid (EPA), Docoshexaenoic Acid (DHA), Vitamin E (d-Alpha Tocopherol)	**Adults:** Take 1-2 caps daily with a meal.
BioMD Nutraceuticals Metabolism T3 Capsules	Calcium Phosphate, Gum Guggle Extract, L-Tyrosine, Garcinia cambogia, Dipotassium Phosphate, Sodium Phosphate, Disodium Phosphate, Phosphatidyl Choline	**Adults:** Take 2 caps with meal bid-tid. **Max:** 6 caps q24h.
Biotest Hot-Rox Capsules	A7-E Super-Thermogenic Gel Lauroyl Macrogol-32 Glycerides, P-Merthylcarboylethylphenol 3, 17-Dihydroxydelta 5-Etiocholane-7-One Diethyl-carbonate, Sclaremax (Proprietary Sclareolide), Yohimbine HCL, Piperine, Caffeine.	**Adults:** Take 1-2 caps bid. **Max:** 4 caps q24h.
Carb Cutter Original Formula Tablets	Vitamin C (as Ascorbic Acid), Chromium (as Chromium Dinicotinate Glycinate), Absorptive Vegetable Fiber, Banaba Leaf Extract (*Lagerstroemia speciosa*), Gymnema Sylvestre Leaf and Gymnema Sylvestre Leaf Extract (25% Gymnemic Acids), Fenugreek Seed Extract, Super Hydroxycitric Extract of *Garcinia cambogia* Fruit], Vanadium (as BMOV), Guarana Seed Extract (Supplying 60mg Caffeine), Korean Ginseng Root Extract (5% Ginsenosides), Eleuthero Root Extract (0.8% Eleutherosides), Green Tea Leaf Extract (36% Total Polyphenols)	**Adults:** Take 1-2 tabs with meals bid.

Table 24. WEIGHT MANAGEMENT PRODUCTS (cont.)

Brand Name	Ingredient/Strength	Dose
Carb Cutter Phase 2 Starch Neutralizer Tablets	*Gymnema Sylvestre* Leaf, Fenugreek Seed, *Garcina cambogia* Fruit Extract Hydroxycitric Acid, Vanadium (as Vanadyl Sulfate)	**Adults:** Take 1-2 tabs with meals bid.
Chroma Slim Apple Cider Vinegar Caplets	Buchu Extract (Leaf), Parsley (Leaf and Stem), Juniper (Berry), Uva-Usi (Leaf), Dandelion (Root)	**Adults:** Take 2 caps with meals qd or bid.
Dexatrim Max Caplets Evening Appetite Control	Proprietary Herbal Blend 450 mg (L-Theanine (From Green Tea Leaf); 5-HTP (Natural 5-Hydroxytryptophan From Griffonia Simplicifolia Seed); Chamomile Flower; English Lavender Flower; Lemon Balm Leaf and Orange Blossom]	**Adults:** Take 2 caps 30 minutes before evening meal. **Max:** 6 caps qd.
Dexatrim Max Maximum Weight, Effervescent Tablets	Thiamin (B1), Riboflavin (B2), Niacin (B3), Vitamin B6, Vitamin B12, Pantothenic Acid, Chromium, Potassium	**Adults:** Dissolve 2 tablets in 16 ounces of water.
Dexatrim Natural Extra Energy Formula Caplets	Calcium, Chromium, Green Tea Leaf Standardized Extract with Epigallocatechin Gallate (EGCG) and Caffeine, Asian (Panax), Ginseng Root	**Adults:** Take 1 cap with meals tid.
Dexatrim Natural Green Tea Formula Caplets	Calcium, Chromium, Green Tea Leaf Standardized Extract, Asian (Panax), Ginseng Root	**Adults:** Take 1 cap with meal tid.
Dexatrim Max Evening Appetite Control Caplets	L-Theanine (from Green Tea Leaf), 5-HTP (natural 5-hydroxytryptophan), Chamomile Flower, English Lavender Flower, Lemon Balm Leaf, Orange Blossom.	**Adults:** Take 2 caps 30 minutes before evening meal. **Max:** 6 caps q24h.
EAS CLA Capsules	Green Tea *(Camellia sinensis)* Leaf, Total Polyphenols, Catechins, Epigallocatechin Gallates (EGCG)	**Adults:** Take 2 caps with meals tid.
EAS Thermo DynamX Capsules	Cayenne Fruit (Capsicum annum) 500 mg, Scoville Heat Units 35,000, Polyphenols (from Green Tea, White Tea, [Camellia Sinensis] and Chocolate [Theobroma cacao L]) 360mg, Total Catechins (from Green Tea, Oolong Tea, White Tea [Camellia Sinensis]) 270mg, Eplgallocatechin Gallate (EGCG) (from Green Tea, White Tea [Camellia Sinensis]) 140mg, Total Methylxanthines (from Guarana [Paullinia Cupena], Green Tea, Oolong Tea [Camellia Sinensis] and Chocolate (Theobroma Cacao L]) 207mg, Gingerols (from Ginger [Zinglbe])	**Adults:** Take 2-3 caps bid before meals or exercise. **Max:** 5 days per week.
Estrin-D Capsules	Vitamin B6, Magnesium, Estrin-D Proprietary Blend (Yerbe Mate Leaf, Caffeine, Guarana Seed, Damiana Leaf and Stem, Green Tea, Ginger Root, Kola Nut, DHEA, Schisandra Fruit, Scutellaria Root, Coca Nut, Jujube Fruit, Thea Sinensis Complex Leaf)	**Adults:** Take 2 caps 30 minutes before meals. **Max:** 6 caps q24h.
Hydroxycut	Hydroxycitrate, Polynictinate, *Garcinia cambogia*, *Gymnema sylvestre* leaf extract, Soy Phospholipids, *Rhodiola rosea* extract, *Withania somnifera* extract, Hydroxytea, Green Tea Extract, White Tea Extract, Caffeine Anhydrous	**Adults:** Take 2 caps tid. **Max:** 6 caps q24h.
Hydroxycut Caffeine-Free Weight Loss Formula	Calcium, Chromium, Potassium, Hydroxagen Plus (Contains Garcinia cambogia extract, gymnema sylvestra leaf extract, soy phospholipids, rhodiola rosea extract, withania somnifera extract); HydroxyTea CF (Contains Caffeine-Free Green Tea Leaf Extract, Caffeine Free White Tea Extract, Caffeine Free Oolong Tea Extract	**Adults:** Take 2 caps with meals tid. **Max:** 6 caps q24h.

Table 24. WEIGHT MANAGEMENT PRODUCTS (cont.)

BRAND NAME	INGREDIENT/STRENGTH	DOSE
Isatori Lean System 7 Advanced Metabolic Support Formula	Yerba Maté, Guarana extract, *Citrus aurantium* Fruit Extract, *Forslean coleus forskohilli* extract, Dandelion Leaf and Root Powder, Green Tea Leaf Extract, Bioperine	**Adults:** Take 3 caps with meals bid. **Max:** 6 caps q24h.
Metab-O-Fx Extreme	Guarana Seed, Yerba Maté Leaf, Kola Nut Seed, Bitter Orange Extract, Green Tea Extract, Cocoa Nut, Black Tea Extract, Korean Ginseng Root, *Rhodiola rodsea* Extract	**Adults:** Take 1 tab with meal bid-tid. **Max:** 3 tabs q24h.
Metabolife Ultra Caplets	Thiamin (as Thiamin mononitrate), Riboflavin, Niacin (as Niacinamide), Vitamin B6 (as Pyridoxine HCl), Pantothenic Acid Calcium (as d-Calcium Pantothenate), (as Hydroxycitrate and Dicalcium Phosphate), Chromium (as Chromium Polymicotinate), Sodium, Potassium, Proprietary Blend of SuperCitrimax Garcinia Extract (Fruit; Standardized for Hydroxycitric Acid), Guarana Extract (Seed, Standardized for Caffeine).	**Adults:** Take 2 caps 1 hour before main meals with full glass of water. **Max:** 6 caps q24h.
Metabolife Ultra Caffeine Free Caplets	Thiamin (B1), Riboflavin (B2), Niacin (B3), Vitamin B6, Pantothenic acid, Calcium, Chromium, Potassium, Garcinia Extract (Fruit)	**Adults:** Take 2 tabs 30 minutes before meals bid-tid. **Max:** 6 tabs q24h.
Metabolife Ultra Weight Management Caplets	Proprietary Blend of Green Tea (Leaf) Extract, L-Tyrosine, Cayenne (Fruit), Caffeine	**Adults:** Take 2 tabs 30 minutes before meals bid-tid. **Max:** 6 tabs q24h.
MHP TakeOff, Hi-Energy Fat Burner Capsules	*Citrus aurantium* Extract, Guarana Seed Extract and Green Tea Leaf Extract, L-Tyrosine, Adrenal Support Blend, *Ginkgo biloba* Leaf Extract, Triple-Ginseng Concentrate (Contains: Panax Ginseng Root Extract, American Ginseng Root Extract and Siberian Ginseng Root Extract. Adrenal Support Blend: Licorice Root Extract, Astra-galus Root Extract and Schizandra Berry Extract.	**Adults:** Take 2 caps qd or bid.
Natrol Carb Intercept with Phase 2 Starch Neutralizer Capsules	White Kidney Bean Extract	**Adults:** Take 2 caps before carbohydrate-containing meals.
Natrol CitriMax Plus	Calcium (from (-) Hydoxycitric Acid), Chromium (as Chromium Polynicotinate), (10(-) HydroxyCitric Acid (HCA) (from Garcinia Cambogia (Fruit), Uva Ursi (Leaf), Cascara Sagrada (bark)	**Adults:** Take 1 cap ½ hr before meals tid.
Natrol Green Tea 500mg Capsules	Green Tea Extract, Polyphenols, Catechins, Caffeine	**Adults:** Take 1 cap with meals qd.
Natural Balance Fat Magnet Capsules	Chitosan, Psyllium Husk, Malic Acid, Vegetarian Lipase, Aloe Vera	**Adults:** Take 2 caps with meals bid.
Nature Made Chromium Picolinate, Extra Strength	Chromium 350mg	**Adults:** Take 1 tab qd.
Nature's Bounty Super Green Tea Diet Capsules	Green Tea *(Camellia sinensis)* (Leaf); Caffeine; Guarana *(Paullinia cupana)* (Seed); Ginger *(Zingiber officinale)* (Root); Bladderwrack Extract *(Fucus vesiculosus)* (Whole Plant); Uva Ursi *(Arctistaohylos uva-ursi)* (Leaf); Vitamin B-6 (as Pyridoxine Hydrochloride); Chromium (as Chromium Polynicotinate)	**Adults:** Take 1 cap bid.
Nature's Bounty Xtreme Lean Zn-3 Ephedra Free Capsules	Methylxanthines (Caffeine), Green Tea Extract (Camellia Sinensis) (Leaf) (Standardized for Epigallocatechin gallate, Caffeine, Polyphenols), Metabromine Cocoa Extract (Standardized for Theobromine, Caffeine), Bitter Orange Extract (Citrus Aurantium) (Fruit) (Standardized for Synepherine, N-Methyltyramine, Hordenine, Octopamine and Tyramine), Tyrosine Complex	**Adults:** Take 2 caps bid.

Table 24. WEIGHT MANAGEMENT PRODUCTS (cont.)

Brand Name	Ingredient/Strength	Dose
Nature's Bounty Xtreme Lean Zn-3 Ephedra Free Capsules *(continued)*	(L-Tyrosine and Acetyl L-Tyrosine), L-Methionine, Ginger Extract (Zingiber Officinale) (Root), Grape Seed Extract (seed), Flavone Complex (Proprietary Blend of 3, 3', 4', 5-7-Tetrahydroxyflavone), DMAE (Dimethyl-aminoethanol). Vitamin C as Ascorbic Acid; Vitamin B6 as Pyridoxine Hydrochloride, Pantothenic acid as d-Calcium Pantothenate, Magnesium as Magnesium Oxide	
Nunaturals LevelRight for Blood Sugar Management Capsules	*Gymenema sylvestre* Extract, Fenugreek Extract, Bitter Melon Extract, Siberian Ginseng Extract, Alpha Lipoic Acid, Cinnamon Bark Extract, Banaba Leaf Extract, Biotin, Chromium Polynicotinate, Chromium Picolinate, Vanadium	**Adults:** Take 1 cap with meals tid.
One-A-Day Weight Smart Dietary Supplement Tablets	Vitamin A (100% as Beta Carotene), Vitamin C, Vitamin D, Vitamin E, Vitamin K; Thiamin (B1); Riboflavin (B2); Niacin (B3); Vitamin B6, Vitamin B12; Folic Acid; Calcium; Iron; Magnesium; Zinc; Pantothenic Acid, Selenium; Manganese, Chromium, EGCG (from Green Tea Extract, Camilla Sinensis Leaf), Caffeine	**Adults:** Take 1 tab with meals qd.
PatentLean Effective and Trusted Fat and Weight Loss Supplement	3-Acetyl-7-Oxo-Dehydroepiandrosterone	**Adults:** Take 1 cap with meals bid. **Max:** 2 caps q24h.
Prolab Enhanced CLA	CLA (Conjugated Linoleic Acid), Flax Seed Oil, Alpha Linoleic Acid, Linoleic Acid, Sunflower or Safflower Oil	**Adults:** Take 3 caps with meals qd.
Stacker 2 Ephedra Free Capsules	Proprietary Blend: Green Tea Extract 60% (Leaves) [120mg Polyphenols] Grape Seed Extract [80% of Proanthocyanidins] Cactus Extract 12:1 Yerba Mate (Fruit) Guarana (Seeds) Caffeine Anhydrous 150mg.	**Adults:** Take 1 Capsule ½ hour to 1 hour before breakfast and lunch. Do not take prior to bedtime.
Tetrazene ES-50 Ultra High-Energy Weight Loss Catalyst Capsules	Vitamin B6 (as Pyridoxine HCl); Biotin; Tetrazene Proprietary Blend: KGM-90 (Super-Class) Pharmaceutical Grade Glucomannan), Glutamine, Olive Leaf Extract. ES-50 Thermogenic Complex: L-Tyrosine, *Camellia Sinensis* (Green Tea Leaf Extract, Standardized for EGCG and Caffeine), Pharmaceutical Grade Caffeine, Vinpocetine.	**Adults:** Take 2 caps with meals tid. **Max:** 6 caps q24h.
Tetrazene KGM-90 Rapid Weight Loss Catalyst Capsules	Vitamin B6; Biotin; Propietary Blend as Follows: KGM-90 (SuperClass Pharmaceutical Grade Glucomannan)	**Adults:** Take 2 caps with meals tid. **Max:** 6 caps q24h.
Thermogenics Plus Stimulant-Free Capsules	Niacin (Vitamin B3), Proprietary Blend (Phosphosterine): Calcium Phosphate, *Commiphora phytosterol* extract, *Garcinia cambogia*, L-Tyrosine, Dipotassium Phosphate, Sodium Phosphate, Disodium Phosphate, Phosphatidyl Choline, *Scutellaria* (Root), *Bupleurum* (Root), *Epimedium* (Herb)	**Adults:** Take 2 caps tid.
ThyroStart with Thydrazine, Thyroid Support Capsules	Vitamin A 6000IU, Vit C 20mg, Vit B2 10mg Vit B1 1.65mg, Vit B6 2mg, Vit B12 10mg, Biotin: 50mcg, Pantothenic Acid 10mg, Magnesium 20mg, Zinc 10mcg, Selenium: 10mcg, Copper 20mcg, Manganese 1mg, Molybdenum 10mcg, Proprietary Blend (Contains Kelp Meal, Niacinamide, L-Tyrosine, Horsetail Root, Nettles, Radish, Parathyroid Substance, Thymus Substance, Adrenal Substance, Pancrease Substance.	**Adults:** Take 2 caps with meals tid.
Twinlab GTF Chromium	Calicum from Dicalcium Phosphate Dehydrate; 200mcg tablets Chromium from Chromium Yeast; Brewers Yeast	**Adults:** Take 1 tab qd.

Table 24. WEIGHT MANAGEMENT PRODUCTS (cont.)

BRAND NAME	INGREDIENT/STRENGTH	DOSE
Twinlab Mega L-Carnitine	L-Carnitine 500mg	**Adults:** Take 1 tablet daily on an empty stomach.
Twinlab Metabolift, Ephedra Free Formula Capsules	Guarana Seed Extract, Citrus Aurantium Fruit Extract, Proprietary Thermogenic and Metabolic Blend, St. John's Wort Extract, L-Phenylalanine, Green Tea Leaf Extract, Quercetin Dihydrate, Citrus Bioflavonoid Complex, Ginger Root, Cayenne Fruit	**Adults:** Take 2 caps before each meal. **Max:** 6 caps q24h.
Ultra Diet Pep Tablets	Vitamin B12 (Cyanocobalamin), Vitamin B6 (as Pyridoxine HCl), Pantothenic Acid (as d-Calcium Pantothenate), DynaChrome Chromium (as Arginate/Chelidamate), Potassium (as Potassium Chloride), Green Tea Leaf Extract, Dandelion (Leaf); Ginger (Root), Passion Flower (Aerial Portion Extract)	**Adults:** Take 1 tab with meals bid.
Xenadrine EFX Capsules	Tyroplex (Proprietary Blend of L-Tyrosine and Acetyl-L-Tyrosine), Green Tea Extract (standardized for Epigallocatechin Gallate, Caffeine and Polyphenols), Seropo (Proprietary Cocoa Extract standardized for Tyramine and Theobromine), Yerba Maté (standardized for Caffeine and Methylxanthines), dl-Methionine, Guara Standardized for Theophylline), L-Theamine, Norabrolide Fermented Saliva Scalera Leaf Extract, Ginger Root (standardized for Gingerols), Isotherm (proprietary blend of 3, 3', 4', 5-7 Pentahydroxyflavone and 3, 3', 4', 7-Tetrahydroxyflavone), DMAE (2-Dimethylaminoethanol), Grape Seed Extract (standardized for Catechins), Long Pepper, Black Pepper, Red Cayenne Pepper (Standardized for 1% Capsaicin)	**Adults:** Take 2 caps bid, before breakfast and in mid-afternoon. **Max:** 4 caps q24h.
Xenadrine NRG 8 Hour Power Capsules	Proprietary Thermoxanthin Blend: Yerba Maté Leaf *(Ilex Paraguariensis)*, Guarana Seed *(Paullinia cupana)*, Cocoa Seed *(Theobroma cacao)*, Green Tea Leaf *(Camellia sinensis)*, Green Coffee Bean Extract *(Coffee arabica)*, Naturally Infused Caffeine	**Adults:** Take 2 caps qd.
XtremeLean Advanced Formula, Ephedra Free Capsules	Vitamin C (as Ascorbic Acid), Vitamin B-6 (as Pyridoxine Hydrochloride), Pantothenic Acid (as d-Calcium Pantothenate), Magnesium (as Magnesium Oxide), Proprietary XtremeLean, Thermo Complex (Yerba Maté Extract [Leaf])-(standardized for Methylxanthines [Caffeine])), Green Tea Extract *(Camellia sinensis)* (Leaf) (standardized for Epigallocatechin Gallate, Caffeine, Polyphenols), Metabromine Cocoa Extract (standardized for Theobromine, Caffeine), Bitter Orange Extract *(Citrus aurantium)* (Fruit) (standardized for Synepherine, N-Methyltyramine, Hordenine, Octopamine, Tyramine), Tyrosine Complex (L-Tyrosine, Acetyl L-Tyrosine), L-Methionine, Ginger Extract *(Zingiber officinale)* (Root), Grape Seed Extract (Seed); Flavone Complex (Proprietary Blend of: 3, 3', 4', 5-7- Pentahydroxyflavone, 3, 3', 4', 7 Tetrahydroxyflavone), DMAE (Dimethylaminoethanol)	**Adults:** Take 2 caps before meals bid.
Zantrex 3, Ephedrine Free	Rice Flour, Zantrex-3 Proprietary Blend Containing: Yerba Maté (Leaf), Caffeine, Guarana (Seed), Damiana (Leaf, Stem), Green Tea (Leaf), Kola Nut, *Schizonepeta* (Spica), *Piper nigrum* (Fruit), Tibetan Ginseng (Root), Panax Ginseng (Root), Maca Root, Cocoa Nut, Thea Sinensis Complex (Leaf).	**Adults:** Take 2 caps with meals qd. **Max:** 6 cap q24h.

Table 25. WOUND CARE PRODUCTS

Brand	Ingredient/Strength	Dose
NEOMYCIN/POLYMYXIN B/BACITRACIN COMBINATIONS		
Bacitracin Ointment	Bacitracin 500 U	**Adults & Peds:** Apply to affected area qd-tid.
Bactine Pain Relieving Protective Antibiotic	Neomycin/polymyxin B/bacitracin/pramoxine 3.5mg-10,000 U- 500 U- 1%	**Adults & Peds:** Apply to affected area qd-tid.
Neosporin Ointment	Neomycin/polymyxin B/bacitracin 3.5mg-5,000 U-400 U	**Adults & Peds:** Apply to affected area qd-tid.
Neosporin Plus Pain Relief Cream	Neomycin/polymyxin B/pramoxine 3.5mg-10,000 U-10mg	**Adults & Peds:** Apply to affected area qd-tid.
Neosporin Plus Pain Relief Ointment	Neomycin/polymyxin B/bacitracin/pramoxine 3.5mg-10,000 U-500 U-10mg	**Adults & Peds:** Apply to affected area qd-tid.
Neosporin To Go Ointment	Neomycin/polymyxin B/bacitracin 3.5mg-5,000 U-400 U	**Adults & Peds:** Apply to affected area qd-tid.
Polysporin Ointment	Polymyxin B/bacitracin 10,000 U-500 U	**Adults & Peds:** Apply to affected area qd-tid.
BENZALKONIUM CHLORIDE COMBINATIONS		
Bactine First Aid Liquid	Lidocaine HCl/benzalkonium chloride 2.5%-0.13%	**Adults & Peds:** ≥2 yrs: Apply to affected area qd-tid.
Bactine Pain Relieving Cleansing Spray	Lidocaine HCl/benzalkonium chloride 2.5%-0.13%	**Adults & Peds:** ≥2 yrs: Apply to affected area qd-tid.
BENZETHONIUM CHLORIDE COMBINATIONS		
Gold Bond First Aid Quick Spray	Menthol/benzethonium chloride 1%-0.13%	**Adults & Peds:** ≥2 yrs: Apply to affected area tid-qid.
Lanacane Maximum Strength Cream	Benzocaine/benzethonium chloride 20%-2%	**Adults & Peds:** ≥2 yrs: Apply to affected area tid-qid.
CHLORHEXIDINE GLUCONATE		
Hibiclens	Chlorhexidine gluconate 4%	**Adults & Peds:** Apply sparingly to affected area prn.
IODINE		
Betadine Skin Cleanser	Povidone-iodine 7.5%	**Adults & Peds:** Apply to affected area. Wash vigorously for 15 seconds and rinse.
Betadine Solution	Povidone-iodine 10%	**Adults & Peds:** Apply to affected area qd-tid.
MISCELLANEOUS		
Aquaphor Healing Ointment	Petrolatum, mineral oil, ceresin, lanolin	**Adults & Peds:** Apply to affected area prn.
Proxacol Hydrogen Peroxide	Hydrogen peroxide 3%	**Adults:** Apply to affected area qd-tid.
Wound Wash Sterile Saline Spray	Sterile sodium chloride solution 0.9%	**Adults & Peds:** Apply to affected area prn.